Nutrition for Professionals

Ultimate Nutrition Resource Textbook for Health and Fitness Professionals

Nutrition for Professionals

Copyright 1995, 2001, 2004, 2008
©Dr. Jane Pentz and Lifestyle Management Associates

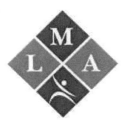

Printed in the United States

Required Textbook for

Nutrition Specialist®
Certification

Printed in the United States of America

ISBN 13: 978-1-892426-15-4
ISBN 10: 1-892426-15-3
Information Address:
LMA Publishing
111 Grove Street, Suite 1
West Roxbury, MA 02132
www.lifestylemanagement.com

Nutrition for Professionals

Reviewers of Nutrition for Professionals

Nicole Byrd, AS, BS
West Palm Beach, FL

Lindsay Cotter, BS Nutrition
Austin, TX

Erin Franklin, MS Nutrition, ASSA
Port Orange, FL

Pam Giese, BA, SCW
Port Orange, FL

Suzanne Moody
Wethersfield, CT

Tom Reynolds
Port Orange, FL

Greg Salgueiro, MS RD
Barrington, RI

QUESTIONS FOR PROFESSIONALS

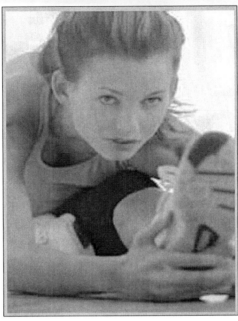

o Are your clients not able to lose weight even after exercising two to three hours a day?

o Are you confused about the role of supplements in fat utilization, muscle hypertrophy, and energy production?

o Are you unsure of what constitutes adequate protein intake necessary to build muscle?

o Are you frustrated because you can't seem to help your clients achieve their weight loss goals?

o Have you been told that nutrition education is beyond your scope of practice?

o Would you like to incorporate nutrition services into your program while still adhering to all state licensure laws and the ADA guidelines?

The Nutrition for Professionals Textbook has been specifically designed to provide answers to these and many other questions facing fitness and allied health professionals, as well as educators and athletic trainers. This book contains all the details needed to incorporate nutrition services safely and professionally while still adhering to all state licensure laws and the American Dietetic Association guidelines.

ACKNOWLEDGMENTS
From Dr. Jane Pentz

Upon receiving my degree, I entered the field of education for professionals because of a strong dedication and awareness of the tremendous need for an accurate and timely flow of information from the scientific community to the group directly teaching the general public—teachers and health and fitness professionals.

I began this undertaking by creating a company dedicated to providing the highest quality nutrition education to professionals. Lifestyle Management Associates is now a continuing education provider for: The National Athletic Trainers' Association, The National Academy of Sports Medicine, The National Strength and Conditioning Association, The American Council on Exercise, the American College of Sports Medicine, the Aerobics and Fitness Association of America, and the American Dietetic Association.

I initiated the task of designing a textbook that would include all relevant information pertaining to the topic of nutrition for professionals. The first version was simply an outline. The first text, in manual form, was published in 1995, culminating in this the eight edition of the textbook.

Thanks to the support of my faculty, students, friends, and family, our courses are now being taught on a national level. The steps taken to get here have been long and arduous, but the dream is now a reality.

My sincere gratitude and appreciation to my dedicated faculty who have so diligently worked with me—Greg Salgueiro, Sara Hauber, Ann Glora, Pam Giese, Nicole Byrd, Suzanne Moody and Tyler Aiken; many thanks for your dedication, inspiration and passion. Thanks for listening to my complaints and frustrations, and for continuously supporting me. I would also like to thank the class of October, 1996—Christine Lawson, Mattie Tiano, Karen Paolino, and other students—for their inspiration, enthusiasm, and motivation in convincing me to present my program to a national audience.

Thanks also to my beautiful children and my precious grandchildren. Their love underlies everything I do.

Finally, this endeavor would never have reached fruition without the emotional (and I must add financial) support of my best friend and "sweetie", my husband. Thanks Bob for loving me and having faith in me throughout all the years of schooling, and especially through the past several years while I was trying to decide what I wanted to be when I grew up. Thank God, I have finally decided.

FOREWORD

This manual is dedicated to all professionals involved in the pursuit of total fitness/wellness programming. Our nation is currently facing a major long-term public health crisis. In recent years, an unprecedented number of Americans of all ages are either overweight or obese. Obesity has accelerated and shows no signs of abating. If it is not reversed, the gains in life expectancy and quality of life resulting from medical advances will erode, and more health-related costs will burden our nation even further.

More than 90 million Americans are affected by chronic diseases and conditions that compromise their quality of life and well-being. Overweight and obesity are risk factors for premature death, diabetes, hypertension, dyslipidemia, cardiovascular disease, stroke, gall bladder disease, respiratory dysfunction, gout, osteoarthritis, and certain kinds of cancers. Poor diet and physical inactivity, resulting in an energy imbalance, are the most important factors contributing to the increase in overweight and obesity in this country. The total cost of obesity in the U.S. is up to $117 billion per year.

Our nation spends more on health care than any other country in the world. In 2001 the total health care cost was an astounding $1.4 trillion. This is an average of $5,035 for each American. If current policies and conditions hold true, by the year 2011, our nation will be spending over $2.8 trillion on health care. We just cannot afford this escalating cost.

Are there any solutions to this crisis? Former Secretary of Health and Human Services (HHS), Tommy Thompson, indicates that "our health care system is not equipped to meet the skyrocketing costs associated with chronic diseases due to obesity." The vision for prevention, says Mr. Thompson, "is to build a community-based public health infrastructure that embraces prevention as a priority." He calls on all health professionals to take an active role in reducing obesity rates at the community level.

In the past health and fitness professionals have been told that nutrition is beyond your scope of practice and that nutrition should be left to dietitians. This is no longer true. The problem is too huge and too out of control. I once heard a counselor tell me that the definition of mental health is living with reality. The reality is Americans are still getting fatter. Reality is they perceive you - the fitness professional - as the expert in exercise and nutrition. I experienced this reality when I worked in a large health club and members would go to the fitness staff for nutrition advice, even though I have a Ph.D. in nutritional biochemistry and I am a licensed dietitian in the state of MA.

After this experience, my mission changed from educating the public to educating you - the fitness professional. I am also not alone in believing that you are the ideal professional to reduce obesity rates. Margaret Moore, of Wellcoaches, witnessed a pilot program in Seattle, WA. The program was a doctor referred obesity clinic. Each patient was provided a physician, a psychologist, a dietitian, and a personal trainer. Guess which professional brought about the greatest lifestyle changes. You Got It: Personal trainers. According to Margaret, "fitness professionals" often have personalities better suited to coaching than other health professionals.

Do you need more convincing to become involved in disseminating nutrition education? Steps to a Healthier US (or simply STEPS), is an initiative that began in 2002 under a directive of the President and Health and Human Services (HHS). The HHS is advancing the president's initiative through this STEPS program. Important to note here is that The STEPS program is aimed at <u>prevention</u>. Rather than relying on our health care system, the STEPS program provides "action steps" for all professionals to disseminate the recommendations contained in the new dietary guidelines.

With this in mind, providing nutrition information **is** within your scope of practice. Defining a scope of practice is key to providing safe, effective programs that adhere to all state licensure laws and the ADA guidelines. A scope of practice by the American Academy of Sports Dietitian and Nutritionists is available at www.aasdn.org. With a professional scope of practice in place, you are now ready to disseminate lifesaving nutrition education in conjunction with your fitness programming.

This is our opportunity to take an active role! Together we can reduce obesity rates. As fitness/ wellness professionals, this is a perfect opportunity for us take up the cause "to help build this community-based public health infrastructure that embraces prevention as a priority". No longer are we compelled to sit back and hope that the medical community, or the dietetics community, will solve the problem.

Dr. Jane Pentz

INTRODUCTION

The goal of this textbook is to provide you with all the tools necessary to allow you to incorporate nutrition education into your wellness programming and serves as the text for the Nutrition Specialist certification.

PART 1 - The SCIENCE OF NUTRITION

- ☐ discussion of digestion, absorption, roles and utilization of essential nutrients
- ☐ discussion of energy nutrient utilization during rest, exercise, fasting, illness, and stress
- ☐ discussion of micronutrients
- ☐ discussion of nutrition and disease
- ☐ discussion of supplements
- ☐ discussion of the Dietary Supplement Health and Education Act and how this act altered the entire supplement industry
- ☐ discussion of integrity in science and development of skills to discern bias and unethical practices in the media and scientific journals

PART 2 - Incorporating Nutrition

- ☐ discussion of legal considerations, scope of practice and required skills to implement a nutrition program
- ☐ outline of client sessions; including discussion of the importance of body composition versus scale weight; calculation of body composition measures; total energy expenditure; analysis of food intakes through case studies; discussion of an appropriate scope of practice when incorporating nutrition while adhering to all state licensure laws and ADA guidelines
- ☐ discussion of the obstacles to success including the futility of diets, diet fads, etc.; deceptive labeling practices; deceptive definitions, etc.
- ☐ discussion of "The Business of Nutrition" including details of how to generate additional income by adding nutrition services
- ☐ discussion of nutritional needs of special populations

Nutrition for Professionals
8th Edition Outline

Part 1 – The Science of Nutrition

Part 2 - Incorporating Nutrition

Nutrition for Professionals

Part 1

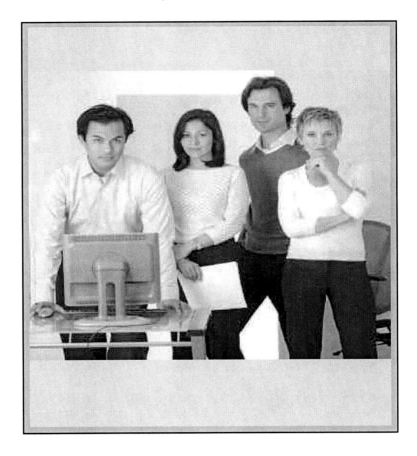

The Science of Nutrition

Chapter 1
The Basics

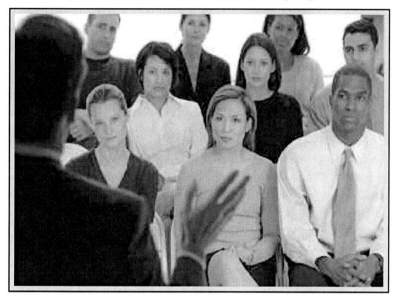

Before we can begin to understand how the body utilizes food or energy, we must first understand some basic principles of biology, physiology, etc.

Objectives:

There are a number of objectives this textbook will attempt to meet. After reading and studying this chapter, you should:

1. Be able to discuss the differences between plant and animal cells, and the differences among muscle cells, fat cells, nerve cells, and red blood cells.

2. Be able to define and recognize the organs involved in digestion and absorption.

3. Be able to recognize the major differences between macromolecules and micromolecules and identify the four basic micromolecules found in cells.

4. Be able to define and list the macronutrients and the energy they provide.

5. Be able to discuss Recommended Dietary Allowances in light of the new Dietary Reference Intakes.

6. Be able to discuss the 2005 Dietary Guidelines and the significance of the Guidelines.

7. Be able to define homeostasis and provide several examples.

INTRODUCTION

Any discussion concerning the basics of nutrition must start with the basic unit of life - the human cell. The body contains about 100 trillion cells. While these cells differ markedly from each other, all have basic characteristics that are alike. In all cells oxygen combines with carbohydrate, fat or protein to release the energy required for cell function. Each type of cell is adapted to perform one particular function. Cells organize into organs. Each organ in the body is an aggregate of many different types of cells held together in supporting structures.

PHYSIOLOGY

Cells consist of small membrane bounded compartments filled with concentrated aqueous solution (cytosol). Within the cell are smaller membrane bounded compartments known as organelles. Cells can be differentiated by whether or not they contain a nucleus. The nucleus holds most of the cell's genetic material or DNA. A cell without a nucleus is called a prokaryote and a cell with a nucleus is called a eukaryote. Bacteria are examples of prokaryotes, while plant cells and animal cells are examples of eukaryotes.[1]

Eukaryotic cells have a nucleus which contains most of the cell's DNA. The nucleus is enclosed by a double lipid layer membrane. The rest of the contents of the cell are suspended in what is known as the cytoplasm. The cytoplasm is a gel-like substance in which most of the cells' metabolic reactions occur.

Many of the differences between plants and animals in the areas of nutrition, digestion, growth, reproduction, and defense, can be traced to the differences in cell walls. *Plant cells have a rigid cell wall composed of tough fibrils of cellulose (fiber).* The plant cell wall is much thicker, stronger, and more rigid than animal cell walls. Rigid plant cell walls prevent the plant cell from movement.

Plant cells can only receive organic (carbon containing) nutrients through photosynthesis, which is the ability to absorb sunlight and to convert solar energy to chemical energy. The products of photosynthesis can be used directly by the cell for energy, or converted to a sugar that can be used by other tissues in the plant (roots). Plant cells also have large vesicles called vacuoles. As plant cells grow they accumulate water in these vacuoles.

Unlike plant cells, animal cells receive nutrients through the bloodstream and are bound together by a loose meshwork of large molecules called the extracellular matrix. *These animal cell membranes are composed of lipid bilayers.* These cell membranes have dynamic, fluid structures which allow the molecules to move about rapidly and freely in the plane of the membrane. These lipid layers also serve as impermeable barriers to the flow of most water-soluble molecules.

Mitochondria are a feature of many eukaryotic cells. Mitochondria are responsible for respiration (the energy released in the aerobic oxidation of food molecules); this process occurs nowhere else in the cell. In other words, mitochondria are the energy factories of the cell. Muscle cells contain many mitochondria while fat cells contain very few; i.e., muscle cells utilize many more calories than fat cells.

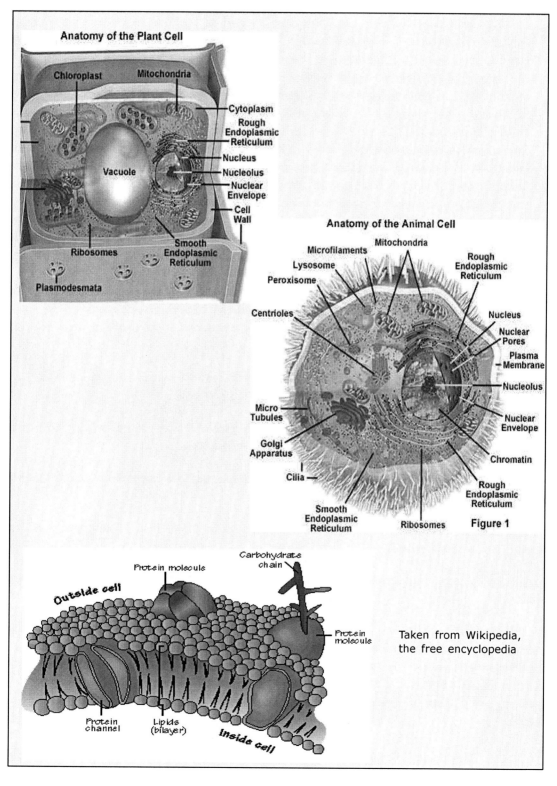

Taken from Wikipedia, the free encyclopedia

There are over 200 types of human cells. These cell types are assembled into a variety of different tissues such as: epithelia, connective, muscle, and nervous tissue.[2]

☐ Epithelia - Epithelial cells are cells on the surface of the skin and mucous membranes. Epithelial tissues serve as selective barriers between the body's interior and the environment (cornea, skin, respiratory and digestive tract lining).

☐ Connective - Connective tissue consists of extracellular structural and supportive elements of the body; i.e., tendons, ligaments, cartilage, and the organic matrix of bones.

☐ Muscle - Approximately 40 percent of the body is skeletal muscle, and almost another 10 percent is smooth and cardiac muscle. Smooth muscle is found in the eye, gut, bile ducts, uterus, and many blood vessels. Many of the same principles apply to skeletal muscle and smooth muscle; however, the internal physical arrangement of smooth muscle fiber is different. Smooth muscle fibers are composed of smaller fibers in contrast to the skeletal muscle fibers. Skeletal muscles are made of numerous fibers and each fiber in turn is made up of successively smaller subunits, myofibrils. Each myofibril contains about 1500 myosin filaments and 3000 actin filaments, which are large protein molecules that are responsible for muscle contraction. Cardiac muscle is similar to skeletal muscle, however special mechanisms in the heart maintain cardiac rhythmicity.

☐ Nerve - The nervous system is unique in the vast complexity of the control actions that it can perform. The nervous system, along with the endocrine system, provides most of the control functions for the body. This system controls the rapid activities of the body, and even the rates of secretion of some endocrine glands.

Four types of cells important in metabolism include the fat cell, the muscle cell, the nerve cell, and the red blood cell. Discussion will focus on these four types of cells.

A muscle cell has many mitochondria. It is important to remember that mitochondria are the energy producing factories of the body; they regulate caloric expenditure.

A fat cell has very few mitochondria; hormones are produced, but very few calories are expended by fat cells.

A nerve cell has no mitochondria and must obtain its energy from simple sugars (in the form of glucose) in the blood stream.

A red blood cell also has no mitochondria and must rely on glucose in the bloodstream for its energy supply.

The fact that certain cells have no mitochondria is very important in metabolism. These cells require a constant flow of glucose from the bloodstream. If there is too much glucose or too little glucose in the bloodstream, cells will become damaged and eventually die. Glucose concentrations in the bloodstream are controlled by hormones. If food is unavailable for long periods of time, the body must produce glucose for these cells. How the body makes glucose will be discussed in the next chapter.

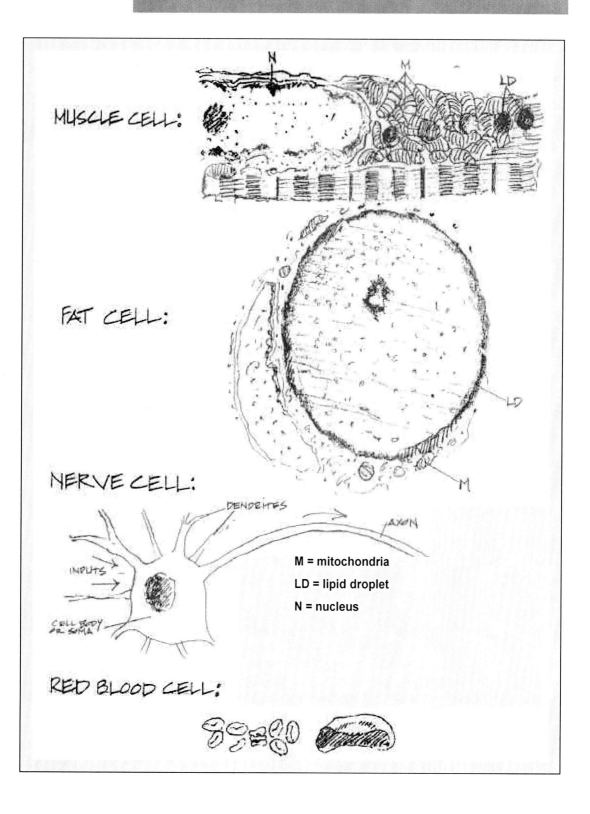

MUSCLE CELL:

FAT CELL:

NERVE CELL:

M = mitochondria
LD = lipid droplet
N = nucleus

RED BLOOD CELL:

DIGESTION

Digestion is the process by which ingested foods are broken down into smaller segments in preparation for absorption. Digestion occurs in the gastrointestinal tract (GI) which is a flexible muscular tube about 26 feet in length. Food enters the mouth, moves through the esophagus, stomach, small intestines, large intestine, and rectum to the anus. Only when a nutrient or other substance penetrates the GI tract wall does it enter the body. Many things pass through the GI tract without being absorbed. Endogenous refers to chemicals in the body (endo meaning within, gen meaning arising). Exogenous refers to chemicals from foods (exo meaning outside the body).

The breakdown of food into nutrients that are then absorbed requires secretions from five different organs: the salivary glands in the mouth, the stomach, the pancreas, the liver (via the gallbladder) and the small intestines.

The process of digestion involves the following:

Mouth: Chewing food begins the process of digestion. The food mixes with saliva which contains enzymes that begin the breakdown of foods. (Enzymes are proteins that facilitate chemical reactions). A semisolid mass called a bolus is formed.

Esophagus: At the top of the esophagus, a process known as peristalsis begins. Peristalsis is wavelike muscular contractions of the GI tract that push the contents down the tract. The entire GI tract is ringed with muscles that can squeeze it tightly. Outside these rings lie longitudinal muscles. Whenever the rings are relaxed and the long muscles are tight, the tube bulges. These actions push the contents down along the tract. A circular muscle at the entrance to the stomach, the cardiac sphincter, closes after the contents enter the stomach preventing these contents from returning to the esophagus.

Stomach: When the bolus reaches the stomach, acids, enzymes, and other fluids grind the food to a liquid mass called chyme. Chyme is the semiliquid mass of partly digested food expelled by the stomach into the duodenum (upper part of the small intestines).[3] Cells in the stomach secrete gastric juice, a mixture of water, enzymes, and hydrochloric acid. The acid is so strong that it registers below "2" on the pH scale - stronger than vinegar. The strong acidity prevents bacterial growth and kills most bacteria that enter the body with food. The cells of the stomach wall secrete mucus, a thick, slimy white substance which coats them and prevents their destruction from the acid. The only significant digestive event in the stomach is the partial breakdown of proteins. The stomach has the thickest walls and strongest muscles of the entire GI tract. It not only has circular and longitudinal muscles, but has a third layer of diagonal muscles that also alternately contract and relax. The contents of the stomach are churned and liquefied with the aid of juices released from the stomach wall. When the contents are liquefied they leave the stomach through another sphincter, the pyloric sphincter.

Small intestines: The food next reaches the small intestines through the pyloric sphincter. The small intestines is where most nutrients are broken down into small molecules and absorbed. There are three segments that make up the small intestines, the duodenum, the jejunum and the ileum; these three segments when stretched out are over 10 feet in length. The small intestines contain hundred of folds and each fold is contoured into thousands of fingerlike projections called villi. A single villus is composed of hundreds of cells each covered with its own microscopic hairs called microvilli. The villi are in constant motion and they can wave, squirm, and wriggle like the tentacles of sea anemone. Small nutrient molecules are trapped among the microvilli and are drawn into the intestinal cells. The pancreas and liver contribute additional juices through ducts leading into the upper level of the small intestines (duodenum). A process known as segmentation occurs. The contents are not only pushed, but periodically squeezed which forces the contents backwards allowing digestive juices to make better contact with the contents.

Liver: From cholesterol, the liver manufactures bile which is necessary for the absorption of fats. Bile is a compound made from cholesterol and is an emulsifier, i.e. can disperse and stabilize fat droplets in a watery solution. (See transport for more details).

Gallbladder: This organ stores bile for future use. Bile is necessary for the absorption of fat and fat soluble vitamins. Bile reaches the gall bladder from the bile duct which is connected to the liver.

Pancreas: The pancreas is connected to the small intestines by way of the pancreatic duct. The pancreas secretes enzymes and bicarbonate. The bicarbonate has a basic pH and neutralizes the acidic food coming from the stomach. The enzymes digest the food.

Large intestine: Undigested residues, such as some fibers are not absorbed. The unabsorbed nutrients flow to the large intestine where water and minerals are reabsorbed. Bacteria in the large intestine help to absorb digestible fiber as well.

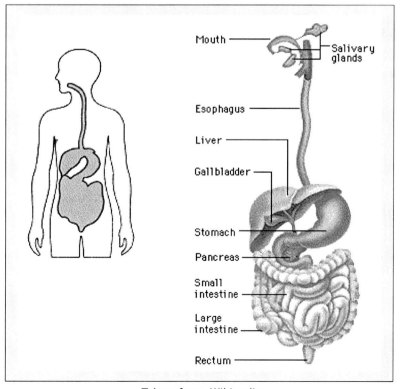

Taken from Wikipedia

ABSORPTION

Absorption is the process by which nutrients enter the intestinal cells in the small intestines and are absorbed into the body.[3] The intestines consist of the small intestines and the large intestine (colon). Most absorption takes place in the small intestines. The stomach has a poor absorptive area. Only a few highly fat-soluble substances, such as alcohol and some drugs, like aspirin, can be absorbed in small quantities in the stomach.

The small intestines are divided into three segments: the duodenum, the jejunum and the ileum. Visually, they look like a tube that has a one inch circumference. This tube extends about twenty feet and contains hundreds of folds. Because of these folds, the area of the intestines provides a surface comparable to a quarter of a football field. Each fold contains thousands of projections called villi. Villi are fingerlike projections from the folds of the small intestines. Nutrients are absorbed through blood and lymphatic vessels supplied to each villus. One villus is composed of hundreds of cells with their own microscopic hairs called microvilli. Microvilli are tiny, hairlike projections on each cell of every villus that can trap nutrient particles and transport them into the cells. The microvilli and their membranes contain hundreds of different kinds of pumps and enzymes producing tremendous specialization of absorption of nutrients. This fact combined with the large surface area allows for quick absorption of nutrients. Specialization also occurs in the segments of the small intestines. The nutrients that are ready for absorption early are absorbed near the top of the intestinal tract, those that take longer to be digested are absorbed further down the tract. Hence, the idea that people should not eat certain foods together because the digestive system cannot handle more than one task at a time is a myth. For example, if only fat is eaten, the protein and carbohydrate carriers for absorption would be idle, while the fat carriers would be working overtime. We will discuss absorption of individual nutrients in future chapters.

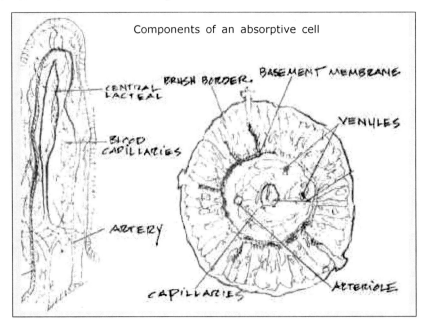

Components of an absorptive cell

TRANSPORT

Before discussion of what happens to nutrients once they are absorbed, it is essential to understand the body's circulatory systems - the vascular system and the lymphatic system.

The vascular system (blood circulatory system) is a closed system of vessels with continuous flow of blood. The heart serves as a pump, pumping blood to all cells through arteries. Arteries are vessels that carry blood away from the heart. Arteries branch into smaller vessels known as capillaries. As the blood circulates through arteries (then capillaries), it picks up and delivers materials to the cells of the body. All cells receive oxygen and nutrients from the blood and all cells deposit carbon dioxide and other wastes into the blood.

Blood entering the digestive system is carried by way of an artery just as with all organs. However, blood leaving the digestive system goes by way of a vein - the portal vein. The portal vein is unique in that it is a one-way system flowing directly to the liver. Once nutrients enter the intestinal cells they enter the bloodstream via the portal vein and are transported to the liver. The liver is placed in the circulation at this point so that it will have the first chance at the materials absorbed from the GI tract. The liver functions in preparing the absorbed nutrients for use by the body. The liver has many metabolic functions and is truly the body's major metabolic organ. The liver in many ways is an overworked and "heroic" organ. Functions of the liver include:
- make and store glycogen
- convert all sugars to glucose from amino acids (and glycerin)
- convert glucose to energy when needed
- build and break down triglycerides, phospholipids and cholesterol
- package extra fats into lipoproteins for transport
- manufacture bile and sends to the gallbladder
- make ketones (when needed)
- manufacture dispensable amino acids
- remove excess amino acids from the blood and "deaminates" them (removes the nitrogen)
- remove ammonia from the blood and converts it to urea (which is then sent to the kidneys)
- make DNA and RNA (genetic materials)
- make plasma proteins such as clotting factors
- detoxify alcohol, other drugs, wastes and poisons
- break up old blood cells and recycles the iron
- store some vitamins and minerals
- form lymph

The lymphatic system is also a one way-route. Lymphatic fluid (lymph) circulates between cells of the body and collects into tiny capillary-like vessels. Lymph is almost identical to blood except that it does not contain red blood cells or platelets. Molecules in the lymphatic system collect in the thoracic duct which terminates in a vein (subclavian vein). Contents are conducted towards the heart where they enter the circulation like other nutrients from the GI tract. One exception, however, are nutrients entering the blood stream from the lymphatic system which bypass the liver.

The fat products, once inside the intestinal cells, require packaging before they can be transported. They are anhydrous (water insoluble) and cannot be transported directly via the bloodstream. They are assembled into packaging systems called lipoproteins. Some of these lipoproteins - chylomircrons are too large to enter the bloodstream and enter the lymphatic system.

NUTRITION BASICS

The science of nutrition is the study of the nutrients in foods and how the body handles them (including ingestion, absorption, transport, metabolism, interaction, storage, and excretion). A chemical analysis of the body indicates that it is composed of materials similar to those found in foods.[3] The molecules found inside cells can be classified as micromolecules (small molecules) or macromolecules (large molecules). Do not confuse macronutrients (energy nutrients) with macro-molecules.[4]

Molecules

Micromolecules are organic (carbon) containing compounds; the word organic means carbon containing. Carbon is unique in the body, in that it alone has the ability to form four bonds with other atoms - hydrogen, nitrogen, oxygen, phosphorous, sulfur - or itself. Because of this unique feature, carbon is central to the biochemistry of life.

Nearly all of the solid matter in cells is organic and is present in four forms: proteins, polysaccharides, lipids, and nucleic acids. Proteins consist of amino acids; polysaccharides consist of simple sugars; lipids (fats) consist of fatty acids (and other components); DNA and RNA consists of nucleotides.

Anabolic reactions are reactions in which small molecules are put together to build larger ones and requires energy. Catabolic reactions are reactions in which large molecules are broken down to smaller ones releasing energy.

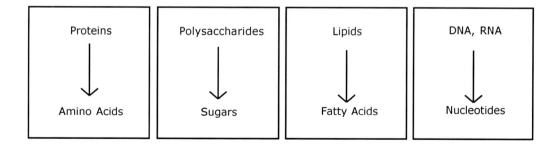

Essential Nutrients

The macronutrients—proteins, lipids, carbohydrates, along with vitamins, minerals, and water are the essential nutrients. Because the body can't make them, and they are necessary to sustain life, we must obtain these nutrients from foods. Eventually, cells will break down and become destroyed if these essential nutrients are not absorbed.

ESSENTIAL NUTRIENTS

	Nutrient	Calories per gram
Macronutrient:	Carbohydrates Fats Proteins	4 9 4
Micronutrient:	Vitamins Minerals	zero zero
Water	Neither a macronutrient nor a micronturient, but is an essential nutrient.	zero

The macronutrients - carbohydrates, fats, and proteins - provide the body with energy while the micronutrients, vitamins and minerals, do not yield energy.

Calories are the units by which energy released from foods is measured. A calorie is a unit by which energy is measured. Food energy is measured in kilocalories. One kilocalorie is the amount of heat necessary to raise the temperature of one kilogram of water one degree centigrade. While calories are listed on labels, the measurement is actually kilocalories.[3] One gram of carbohydrate equals 4 Kcal. One gram of protein also equals 4 Kcal. One gram of fat equals 9 Kcal. One gram of alcohol equals 7 Kcal. One ounce equals 28.35 grams (see page appendix for other conversion factors). One half cup of vegetables or juice weighs about 100 grams. One teaspoon of salt weighs about 5 grams. Another measure of food energy is the kilojoule (kJ). A joule is the amount of energy expended when one kilogram is moved one meter by a force of one newton. One gram of carbohydrate equals 17 KJ. One gram of protein also equals 17 KJ. One gram of fat equals 37 KJ. One gram of alcohol equals 29 KJ.[3] To convert from Kcal to KJ multiply by 4.2.

Carbohydrates are the number one energy source for the body. There are two categories of carbohydrates:

CARBOHYDRATES

Simple	Complex

One or two sugars linked together
Monosaccharide: glucose
    fructose
    galactose
Disaccharide: sucrose
    lactose
    maltose
	Many sugars linked together
	starch
	glycogen
	cellulose

Carbohydrate Foods

Fruits	Food Amount	Carbs (g)	TCalories
Apple	1 med	20	80
Orange	1 med	20	80
Banana	1 med	25	105
Raisins	$1/4$ cup	30	120
Vegetables			
Corn, canned	$1/2$ cup	18	80
Winter squash	$1/2$ cup	15	65
Peas	$1/2$ cup	10	60
Carrot	1 med	10	40
Green Beans	$1/2$ cup	7	30
Broccoli	1 stalk	5	30
Zucchini	$1/2$ cup	4	20
Bread			
Submarine roll	8" long	60	280
Branola wheat bread	2 slices	35	210
Lender's Bagel	1	30	160
Thomas's English	1	25	130
Pita pocket	$1/2$ of 8" round	22	120
Matzo	1 sheet	28	115
Saltines	6	15	90
Graham Crackers	2 squares	11	60
Grains, pasta, starches			
Baked potato	1 large	55	240
Baked beans	1 cup	50	330
Lentils, cooked	1 cup	40	215

Simple carbohydrates, or sugars, consist of one (mono) or two (di) sugar units. Glucose, fructose, and galactose are one unit sugars; while sucrose, lactose, and maltose are two sugar units. Simple carbohydrates are found in fruits, vegetables, table sugar, milk, and malt.

Complex carbohydrates are many sugar units linked together. Complex carbohydrates are found in pasta, potatoes, grains, rice, etc. Carbohydrates from plant foods are called starch. When the plant starches are stored in the body they are called glycogen. Certain parts of plant foods cannot be digested by enzymes in the body. These parts are known as fiber. We will discuss carbohydrates and fiber in detail in the next chapter.

Lipids, often referred to as fats, are divided into two broad categories, saturated and unsaturated. Unsaturated fatty acids are either monounsaturated or polyunsaturated.

Lipids	
Saturated Solid at Room Temperature	Unsaturated Liquid at Room Temperature
Animal Sources	Oils Exceptions include coconut oil, palm oil Unsaturated lipids consist of monounsaturated and polyunsaturated fatty acids. (see below)

Fat Content

	% Saturated	% Monounsaturated	% Polyunsaturated
Saturated			
Coconut oil	90	10	-
Palm oil	50	30	20
Butter	65	30	5
Beef fat	50	45	5
Chicken fat	30	50	20
Monounsaturated			
Olive oil	15	75	10
Canola oil	5	60	35
Combination			
Peanut oil	20	50	30
Soybean oil	23	62	15

*Margarine and other trans fatty acids are created when vegetable oils are hardened. Trans fatty acids have been associated with high rates of heart disease.

To make the picture more complicated, when unsaturated fats are turned into solids by hydrogenation, they become trans fatty acids. Trans fatty acids are similar to saturated fatty acids in that they are considered "unhealthy".

The major fats found in foods are: triglycerides, phospholipids, and cholesterol (sterol). Triglycerides are the storage form of fat, while phospholipids are part of all cell membranes and are involved in immune system function. It is, therefore, very important to have a certain portion of fat in the diet to provide stored energy for sustained activity, to maintain the integrity of cell membranes, for absorption of fat soluble vitamins and immune function. The third type of fat found in foods is cholesterol. We obtain cholesterol from our diets and the human body can also make cholesterol.

Proteins are a third energy source, in addition to carbohydrates and fats. Amino acids are the basic component of proteins (22 amino acids make up proteins).

Protein Foods

Item	Serving Size	Protein (g)
Meat, poultry, fish	3 oz. cooked	21
Milk	8 oz.	10
Yogurt	8 oz.	8
Cottage cheese	4 oz.	13
Eggs (whites)	1 large	4
Beans, dried peas, lentils	1/2 cup cooked	7

Amino acids contain the element, nitrogen. Nitrogen is anabolic (tissue building). The only way our bodies can obtain nitrogen is through amino acid intake. Traditionally amino acids have been distinguished by whether the body can make the amino acid (nonessential) or can not make the amino acid (essential). Metabolically, however, the distinctions are less clear because a number of essential amino acids can be formed by transamination - a chemical process of transforming one amino acid into another. Amino acid essentiality and protein quality will be discussed in detail in the Chapter 4 - Proteins.

In the traditional sense, protein sources that contain all of the essential amino acids (as well as the nonessential and conditional ones) include meats, milk and milk products, eggs, soybeans and wheat germ. Other legumes, grains, and vegetables contain some of the essential amino acids, but may be low or missing one or more of the essential amino acids; and for this reason, these foods are considered incomplete protein sources. Eating these foods in combination or with a complete protein source increases the protein value of the meal (see Chapter 4).

While proteins are a third energy source for the body, they are not a major or direct source of energy. Proteins must be broken down by the liver to produce glucose. Proteins have many varied roles in the body and the body uses them for energy only when other energy nutrients are not available.

The roles of proteins, as well as their digestion and absorption, will be discussed in Chapter 4.

The micronutrients include vitamins and minerals. Vitamins are a group of organic compounds other than protein, carbohydrates, and fats that cannot be manufactured by the body and are required in small amounts for specific functions of growth.[3] Minerals are inorganic elements essential to life that act as control agents in body reactions and cooperative factors in energy production, body building and maintenance of tissues. They retain their identity and cannot be destroyed by heat, air, acid, or mixing.[3]

Vitamins and minerals have many roles in the body. Certain vitamins help "derive" energy from the energy nutrients while not providing energy themselves. These vitamins attach to molecules involved in energy production. Some minerals are also involved in the energy cycle. Other vitamins and minerals have antioxidant properties whose role is to neutralize free radicals that can damage cells.

Vitamins

Water Soluble	Fat Soluble
B Vitamins Vitamin C	Vitamin A Vitamin D Vitamin E Vitamin K

Minerals

Major	Trace
Calcium, Phosphorus, Potassium, Sodium, Chloride, Magnesium	Iron, Zinc, Iodine, Copper, Manganese, Chromium, Selenium, Sulfur

These nutrients have many other roles that are pivotal to health and will be discussed in subsequent chapters.

Water

While discussion of water is not a major topic in this course, its importance in life and health cannot be minimized. A person can survive for long periods of time without food, but not without water. Water is inorganic and forms the major part of almost every body tissue. The amount of water that must be consumed is enormous relative to other nutrients: 6 to 8 cups or about 2 liters per day. Water provides the environment in which nearly all the body's activities occur. Water participates in almost all metabolic reactions and is the medium for transporting molecules in and out of cells. Water lubricates joints and acts as a shock absorber. Water is contained in the eye as well as in the spinal cord.

Water constitutes 55 to 60 percent of an adult's body weight.[3] Thirst acts to provide needed water; however, it lags behind the body's need. Therefore, responding to thirst will not remedy a water deficiency. Because of this, it is important to include large amounts of water each day. A general water requirement is difficult to establish since needs are so variable; water recommendations are expressed in proportion to the amount of energy expended under average environmental conditions.[4]

General water recommendations have been a topic of controversy. The actual research determining water needs does not appear to exist. Respected nutrition organizations differ on hydration needs. The following calculation, while not proven scientifically, is a good estimate of need. General recommendations under average environmental conditions is as follows: 1.0 to 1.5 ml water per calorie expended (1 ml = .03 ounces)[5]. For example, if a person expends 400 calories during exercise, that person should drink 400 to 600 ml, or 12 to 18 ounces. If a person expends 2000 calories per day, he or she should consume 60 to 90 ounces of water per day.

Water naturally suppresses the appetite and helps the body metabolize stored fat. Studies have shown that a decrease in water intake causes fat deposits to increase, while increasing water intake can actually reduce fat deposits. Also drinking water is the best treatment for fluid retention. Fluid retention shows up as excess weight. The best way to overcome the problem of water retention is to give the body adequate amounts of water. Overweight persons need more water since larger people have larger metabolic loads. An additional glass of water for every 25 pounds of excess weight is recommended. Water helps to maintain proper muscle tone by giving muscles their natural ability to contract and by preventing dehydration. It also helps sagging skin that usually follows weight loss. Shrinking cells are buoyed by water, which plumps the skin and leaves it clear, healthy and resilient.

Water can help relieve constipation. When the body doesn't get enough water, it siphons what it needs from internal sources. The colon is one primary source for water siphoning and the result is constipation.

HOMEOSTASIS

The human body is endowed with a vast network of feedback mechanisms that control the necessary balances for life. This high level of internal bodily control is called "homeostasis. In other words, homeostasis is the maintenance of constant internal conditions in body systems; i.e. balance.[2] A homeostatic system is constantly reacting to external forces so as to maintain limits set by the body's needs. Examples include glucose, calcium, alcohol, and cholesterol homeostasis (see individual topics for more information on each). The human body has a tremendous capacity to return to homeostasis. For example, without homeostasis, drinking carbonated beverages would produce large changes in the pH of the blood stream. Small changes in pH cause death. However, the body has a tremendous buffering system (chemical reactions) which does not allow the large changes to occur. In other words, homeostasis is the response of the body to maintain a constant pH by utilizing or producing other molecules that will return the internal conditions to "normal". In many instances, this is not simply one chemical reaction, but hundreds, even thousands of reactions. Hence, something so simple as drinking carbonated beverages causes the body to respond through chemical reactions to maintain constant internal conditions.

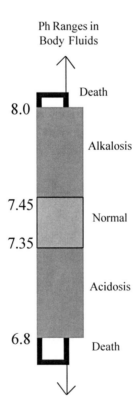

Ph Ranges in
Body Fluids

Death

8.0

Alkalosis

7.45

Normal

7.35

Acidosis

6.8

Death

CONTROLS OF METABOLISM

To view metabolism as what one eats is simplistic. Metabolism is defined as the complex set of physical and chemical processes occurring within a living cell or organism that are necessary for the maintenance of life; i.e., provide energy for maintaining life. There are many factors that control metabolism.[3] Some of these factors are enzymatic, others are hormonal, while still others are controlled at the cellular level through concentration and compartmentalization. The enzymatic controls of metabolism are beyond the realm of this textbook. However, we will examine several hormones as well as several controls at the cellular level - concentration and compartmentalization.

Hormonal control[3]

Hormones are chemical messengers secreted in trace amounts by one type of tissue. They are carried by the blood to a target tissue and they then stimulate activity in this target tissue.

Insulin: Every body cell depends on glucose for its fuel to some extent, and certain cells depend primarily on glucose for energy. Insulin moves glucose from the bloodstream into cells. When blood glucose levels rise, special cells of the pancreas secrete insulin into the blood. The circulating insulin binds to receptors on cell membranes which then allow the glucose to enter the cell. Most cells take up only the glucose they need (except muscle cells and liver cells which can store the glucose as glycogen). Thus, high serum glucose levels are returned to normal.

Glucagon: When blood glucose falls, cells of the pancreas secrete glucagon into the blood. Glucagon counteracts insulin and raises blood glucose by signaling the liver to release its glycogen stores.

Epinephrine: This hormone also elicits release of glucose from the liver cells. Under stress, epinephrine is released into the bloodstream. Like glucagon, epinephrine works to return glucose to the blood from liver glycogen. This hormone also elicits the breakdown of protein in muscle.

Thyroid hormones: The thyroid hormones control basal metabolic rate (calories expended at rest). Too much of these hormones will produce an increased basal metabolic rate, while low levels will produce a decreased metabolic rate.

Concentration[3]

Concentration of certain nutrients in certain parts of the cell also has an effect on metabolism. If too much of a product accumulates in a certain part of the cell, the increased amount of the product signals the cell to stop producing the product or transpose the product into another molecule. For example when too much glucose enters liver cells, the excess glucose signals the cells to store glycogen.

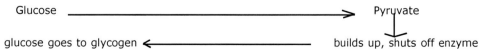

Glucose ————————————————→ Pyruvate

glucose goes to glycogen ←—————————— builds up, shuts off enzyme

Compartmentalization[3]

This occurs when certain nutrients in different parts of the cell build up and the increased amounts signal the cell to switch metabolism. For example, when fatty acids in the cytosol of the cell build up they become attached to a molecule called carnitine which carries these fatty acids into the mitochondria where they are oxidized for energy. If too many fatty acids build up in the mitochondria, the extra fatty acids are then turned into a chemical called citrate; the citrate leaves the mitochondria and goes back into the cytosol where the citrate can be turned back into fatty acids.

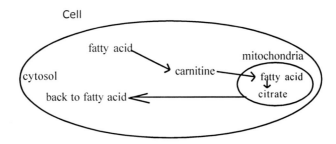

DIETARY REFERENCE INTAKES

The publication of the first edition of Recommended Dietary Allowances (RDAs) in 1941 was recognized as one of the most authoritative sources of information on recommendations for nutrient intakes for healthy people. Since publication of the last edition in 1989, rising awareness of the impact of nutrition on chronic disease has dictated an expanded review of uses and misuses of RDAs in the U.S. and Recommended Nutrient Intakes (RNIs) in Canada.

The new framework for this expanded approach developed by U.S. and Canadian scientists is now referred to as the Dietary Reference Intakes (DRIs). This new series of references greatly extends the scope and application of previous quantitative nutrient guidelines to include requirements based on how the nutrient may be related to chronic disease or developmental abnormalities. This new framework also identifies a new reference intake, the Tolerable Upper Intake Level (UL), which, if consumed consistently, may result in adverse effects. *Dietary Reference Intakes* represents a new paradigm for the nutrition community.

The following criteria have been used in establishing the new DRIs. They are an average daily dietary intake level sufficient to meet the nutrition requirement of nearly all (97 to 98 percent) healthy individuals in a particular life stage and gender group. They are intended to be used as a guide for daily intake by individuals. RDAs (US standards) depend on Estimated Average Requirements (EAR). If no EAR has been established, then no RDAs are set. If sufficient data is not available to calculate an EAR, then a reference intake - adequate intake (AI) is used instead of an RDA[7,8,9,10].

Less information is available on which to base allowances for certain nutrients (copper, manganese, chromium, molybdenum, and chloride). These nutrients are not included in the RDAs and figures are averages of Safe and Adequate Intakes as set by the National Academy of Sciences.[11]

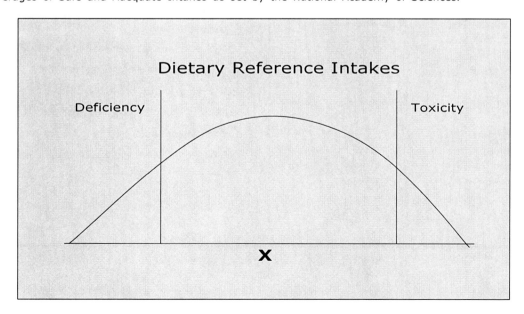

DAILY VALUES ON FOOD LABELS*

The Daily Values are standard values developed by the FDA for use on food labels. In establishing the Daily Values the FDA uses Reference Daily Intakes (RDI) when RDAs exist for the nutrient, and Daily Reference Values when RDAs do not exist for the nutrient. The Reference Daily Intakes are for vitamins and minerals and reflect allowances based on the RDA. Daily Reference Values are for fat, saturated fat, cholesterol, carbohydrate, fiber, sodium, potassium, and protein* which do not have established RDAs. Together they make up the Daily Values. The following are amounts used to determine Percent Daily Values of selected nutrients required on labels.[12]

Reference Daily Intakes		Daily Reference Values	
vitamin A	5,000 IU		
vitamin C	60 mg	fat	65 grams
calcium	1000 mg	saturated fatty acids	20 grams
iron	18 mg	cholesterol	300 mg
vitamin D	400 IU	total carbohydrate	300 grams
vitamin E	30 IU	fiber	25 grams
vitamin K	80 mcg	sodium	2,400 mg
thiamin	1.5 mg	potassium	3500 mg
riboflavin	1.7 mg		
niacin	20 mg		
vitamin B6	2.0 mg		
folate	400 mcg		
vitamin B12	6 mcg	* It is important to note that Daily Values	
biotin	300 mcg	reflect amounts as determined by the FDA	
pantothenic acid	10 mg	for the purposes of food labeling, and	
phosphorus	1000 mg	hence vary widely from the DRIs estab-	
Iodine	150 mcg	lished by The Food and Nutrition Board.	
magnesium	400 mg	Hence percentages listed on labels may	
zinc	15 mg	not be an accurate picture of actual needs.	
selenium	70 mcg		
copper	2.0 mg		
manganese	2.0 mg		
chromium	120 mcg		
molybdenum	75 mcg		
chloride	3,400 mg		

2005 DIETARY GUIDELINES

In January 2005, two federal agencies – The Department of Health and Human Services (the HHS) and the U. S. Department of Agriculture (the USDA) – released the new Dietary Guidelines for Americans. The sixth edition of Dietary Guidelines for Americans places stronger emphasis on reducing calorie consumption and increasing physical activity.

History of the guidelines[13]

Until 1977, no one really cared what Americans ate, as long as they ate enough to survive and didn't develop nutrient-deficiency diseases. But in 1977, Senator George McGovern, leader of the Senate Select Committee on Nutrition and Human Needs, issued a report stating that nutrition had a major impact on health, a concept that was considered "pioneering" at the time. The Committee on Nutrition and Human Needs recommended that Americans:

o Increase carbohydrate intake to 55 to 60 % of calories
o Decrease dietary fat intake to no more than 30% of calories, with a reduction in saturated fat, and approximately equivalent distribution of saturated, polyunsaturated, and monounsaturated fats.
o Decrease cholesterol intake to 300 mg per day
o Decrease sugar intake to 15% of calories
o Decrease salt intake to 3 grams per day

Even these simple guidelines met with a great deal of political debate and controversy from industry groups and the scientific community. The Senate Select Committee wanted to provide evidence of the science used to determine the recommendations.   Hence, the expertise of the U.S. Department of Agriculture and the Department of Health, Education, and Welfare were pulled together; and input from the scientific community throughout the country was collected.   The American Society for Clinical Nutrition formed a panel to study the relationship between dietary practices and health outcomes. The findings, presented in 1979, were reflected in the publication *Healthy People: The Surgeon General's Report on Health Promotion and Disease Prevention*.

In 1980, the first edition of the publication entitled *Nutrition and Your Health: Dietary Guidelines for Americans*, was issued jointly by the Department of Health and Human Services (HHS) and the U.S. Department of Agriculture (USDA). According to the publication, it was released in response to the public's desire for authoritative, consistent guidelines on diet and health. The guidelines were based on the most up-to-date information available at the time and were directed to healthy Americans. The guidelines also generated considerable discussion between nutrition scientists, consumer groups, and the food industry.

Also in 1980, under the Carter Administration, a U.S. Senate Committee on Appropriations report directed that a committee be established to review scientific evidence and recommend revisions to the *1980 Dietary Guidelines*. In 1983-1984, a Federal advisory committee of nine non-government nutrition scientists was convened to review and make recommendations to the HHS and USDA about the first edition of the *Dietary Guidelines for Americans*. The brochure centered on ways to build a healthful diet and lifestyle. The two departments were issued a directive to convene a Dietary Guidelines Advisory Committee.

In 1985 the HHS and USDA jointly issued a second edition of the *Dietary Guidelines for Americans*. This revised edition was nearly identical to the first. Some changes were made for clarity, while others reflected advances in scientific knowledge of the association between diet and a range of chronic diseases. The second edition received wide acceptance and was used as a framework for consumer education messages.

In 1990, The National Nutrition Monitoring and Related Research Act was passed, which requires publication of the *Dietary Guidelines for Americans* every 5 years. This legislation also required a review by the Secretaries of the USDA and HHS of all Federal publications containing dietary advice for the general public. In 2000, the fifth edition of the Dietary Guidelines was increased to 10 statements, with a new statement about physical activity, greater emphasis on fruits and vegetables, and a new guideline on safe food handling. In 1992 the first food pyramid was introduced. (See the file called "Development of the Dietary Guidelines – A chronology," on this course CD.)

As with the past guidelines, The 2005 Guidelines form the basis for federal food programs and nutrition education programs. However, the 2005 Dietary Guidelines for Americans affords remark- able new changes. The recommendations are based on the preponderance of scientific evidence for lowering risk of chronic disease and promoting health. The guidelines are now oriented toward policy makers, nutrition educators, nutritionists, and health care providers rather than the general public, as previous versions of the guidelines had been, and therefore they contain more technical informa- tion. They provide health education experts, such as doctors and nutritionists, with a compilation of the latest science-based recommendations.

So why did this big change occur? Our nation is currently facing a major long-term public health crisis. In recent years, an unprecedented number of Americans of all ages are either overweight or obese. Obesity has accelerated and shows no signs of abating. If it is not reversed, the gains in life expectancy and quality of life resulting from medical advances will erode, and more health-related costs will burden our nation even further.

More than 90 million Americans are affected by chronic diseases and conditions that compromise their quality of life and well-being. Overweight and obesity are risk factors for premature death, diabetes, hypertension, dyslipidemia, cardiovascular disease, stroke, gall bladder disease, respira- tory dysfunction, gout, osteoarthritis, and certain kinds of cancers. Poor diet and physical inactivity, resulting in an energy imbalance, are the most important factors contributing to the increase in overweight and obesity in this country. The total cost of obesity in the U.S. is up to $117 billion per year.

Our nation spends more on health care than any other country in the world. In 2001 the total health care cost was an astounding $1.4 trillion. This is an average of $5,035 for each American. If current policies and conditions hold true, by the year 2011, our nation will be spending over $2.8 trillion on health care, and we just cannot afford this escalating cost.

Why is health care for chronic disease so costly? Due to improvements in environment and social conditions, Americans are living longer than ever before. The average life expectancy in 1950 was 59 years; today it is nearly 77 years. The percentage of the population over age 65 has increased 11-fold since 1900. Health care expenditures for a 65-year old are now 4 times those of a 40-year old. By 2030, health care spending will rise by 25% simply because Americans will be older.

While chronic diseases are among the most common and costly of all health problems, they are also among the most preventable. People who are obese (BMI>30) have a 50% to 100% greater risk of premature death from all causes than people at a healthy weight. Thirty-three percent (33%) of all U.S. deaths can be attributed to smoking, lack of exercise, and poor eating habits.

Despite the evidence that prevention works, the focus of our health care system is on disease treatment. But clearly our health care system is not equipped to meet the needs of people with chronic diseases.

As stated in the introduction, *the vision of the Department of Health and Human Services is to build a community-based public health infrastructure that embraces prevention as a priority.* Hence, the HHS calls on all policy makers, health care providers, and all professionals and educators to work together on implementing the recommendations contained in the 2005 Dietary Guidelines for Americans.

Guidelines[14]

The guidelines were developed in a three-stage approach. In the first stage, a 13-member advisory committee prepared a report based on the best available science. The thirteen-member committee analyzed all the latest information and published their report in the Dietary Guidelines Advisory Committee Report. This report was the primary resource for development of the guidelines. The committee did not write the guidelines, they made suggestions and recommendations.

In the second stage, scientists and officials developed the guidelines after reviewing the committee's report and agency and public comments. The public included lay people, academic researchers, consumer and trade groups, and businesses. The advisory committee notes that they were continuously made aware of the food industry, the beverage industry, and the economic impact of their decisions. Committee members are confident that they remained above the influence of outside interests – especially the very strong food industry lobbying groups.

The final stage – the recommendations - rested with the politically appointed HHS and USDA secretaries, Tommy Thompson and Ann Veneman. Tommy Thompson refers to the relationship between the food industry and the government guidelines as a "partnership". This partnership introduced political aspects associated with the guidelines.

Political aspects - "partnership" with the food industry

The food industry spent over $48 million on lobbying politicians in 2004. The goal of every food-industry association is: to maintain the status quo; to delay; to fight; to lobby; and to obscure the facts so that manufacturers can reposition their products to compete for consumer demand". The quote is by Jeff Nadelman, a former lobbyist for the Grocery Manufactures of America at *www.menshealth.com*, April 20, 2005. The food industry was given a year to "reposition" their labels before the new guidelines took effect so consumers could glance at their food labels and believe they were eating foods that fit in with the new guidelines. And it's true that the food industry played a key role in the final dietary recommendations made by the government.

Because of this, quote, "partnership", as it is termed by the former HHS Secretary, Tommy Thompson, between the government agencies and the food industry, the guidelines were changed from the advisory committee's recommendations in several significant ways: trans-fats, and sugar, and sugar free.

The committee unanimously voted to reduce trans-fat intake to one percent or less of total calories, but that figure was removed from the final guidelines. Assigning a number would have resulted in a Daily Value Percentage being posted on the Nutrition Facts panel of every single packaged food. Consumers would have known that most pre-packaged foods would exceed daily recommended intake of trans-fat by 200 to 300%. Federally funded school lunch programs (worth $7.1 billion annually) would also be required to meet dietary guidelines. Manufacturers would have been required to modify their products just to remove all of the trans fats they include. So instead of taking the committee's recommendations, the guidelines instead read: "limit trans fats". Once again, the political aspects of the guidelines are making it even more challenging for the general public to safeguard our own health. What does "limit trans fats" mean? If we knew it meant 1% or less of total calories, and our food labels held a Daily Value Percentage, we could choose foods more wisely. But the vague guideline to limit trans fats still leaves health and fitness professionals with a lot of work to do.

As for sugars, the advisory committee recommended that added sugars make up less that 10% of daily calories. As with trans fats, however, politics prevailed and the guidelines now read: "limit sugars". The FDA requires that foods claiming "sugar-free" must indicate "Not For Weight Control" when they are not low-calorie foods. Low-calorie foods must be less than 40 calories per serving. A Snackwell's Sugar Free Fudge Brownie has 90 calories. It is NOT low-calorie.

For key recommendations of the 2005 Dietary Guidelines visit www.mypryamid.gov.

FOOD GUIDANCE SYSTEM

The Food Guidance System was established to improve the nutrition and well-being of Americans. MyPyramid.gov was developed to carry the messages of the 2005 Dietary Guidelines and to make Americans aware of the vital health benefits of simple and modest improvements in nutrition, physical activity and lifestyle behavior.

Imagine the monumental task of educating an entire population on lifestyle behaviors required to improve the health of our nation and reduce unmanageable health care costs. The Food Guidance System does a good job of tackling such an enormous task. There is a plethora of information available on how to make improvements in one's diet (and activity level) for individuals wishing to do so. For individuals not familiar with using the internet, there is also a book available, *A Healthier You*, reiterating the same information in an easy-to-understand format.

The limitations involved with disseminating the plethora of information contained in the Food Guidance System are multifaceted. One problem is that the topic is too complicated. Trying to simplify such a complicated topic provides problems of its own. "You can't learn algebra if you don't know how to add or subtract! You can't learn how to operate a computer and navigate the internet just by pressing your computer's "on" button". Could people learn to drive a car by simply reading the manual? The same holds true with the information contained in the Food Guidance System.

Whenever transforming a large amount of information into an "easier" format "loss of critical details" occurs. Thus, loss of detail is a serious outcome of generalization. And this holds true with the Food Guidance System. Loss of detail can be found in reference to the exercise recommendations as well. Cardiovascular exercise is "maximized", while resistance training is "minimized". As health professionals, we are well aware that maintaining/building muscle is just as important as cardiovascular fitness when it comes to health. Another limitation to the Food Guidance System is the emphasis on weight loss. See the chapter on diets for more details on why weight loss should not be a major emphasis.

Finally, one of the major limitations to using the Food Guidance System is "time". We have to ask: Will Americans visit www.mypyramid.com periodically and make the slow lifestyle changes necessary to improve their health? Will Americans read *A Healthier You* a little at a time and continuously make the needed changes. A year after the introduction of the 2005 Dietary Guidelines, when asked if the new food pyramid changed their eating habits, 68% of Americans said they had not made any dietary changes. Only 11% indicated that they changed the way they eat. Ten percent didn't even know what the food pyramid was; and 11% said they didn't understand the pyramid (December 14, 2005 poll of 3147 Americans).

SUMMARY

Eukaryotic cells have a nucleus which contains most of the cell's genetic material. The nucleus is enclosed by a double lipid layer membrane. The contents of the cell are suspended in what is known as the cytoplasm.

Plant cells have rigid cell walls composed of tough fibrils of cellulose. The plant cells wall is much thicker, stronger, and more rigid than animal cell walls. Rigid plant cell walls prevent the plant cell from moving. Animal cell membranes are composed of lipid bilayers. These cell membranes have dynamic, fluid structures which allow molecules to move about rapidly and freely in the plane of the membrane.

Mitochondria are responsible for respiration and this process occurs nowhere else in the cell. Muscle cells contain many mitochondria, while fat cells contain very few. Cells, such as nerve cells, red blood cells, brain cells, and other cells do not contain mitochondria and can not produce their own energy. These cells rely on glucose in the blood stream for energy.

Digestion is the process by which ingested foods are broken down into smaller segments in preparation for absorption. Absorption is the process by which nutrients enter the small intestinal cells and are absorbed into the body.

Nutrition is the science of how the body breaks down and utilizes the nutrients in foods. The essential nutrients include carbohydrates, fats, proteins, vitamins, minerals and water. The macronutrients - carbohydrates, fats, and proteins provide the body with energy. The micronutrients - vitamins and minerals - do not provide energy, but are just as critical in health. Water provides the environment in which nearly all the body's activities occur. Water participates in almost all metabolic reactions and is the medium for transporting molecules in and out of cells.

Homeostasis is the maintenance of relatively constant internal conditions in body systems by corrective responses to forces that, if left unopposed, would cause unacceptably large changes in those conditions. The human body has a tremendous capacity to return to homeostasis.

The Dietary Reference Intakes represent a new paradigm for nutrient recommendations. The new framework for this expanded approach developed by US and Canadian scientists identifies a new reference, the Tolerable Upper Intake Level, which, if consumed consistently, may result in adverse effects.

Daily Values are standard values developed by the FDA for use on food labels. In establishing the Daily Values the FDA uses Reference Daily Intakes when RDAs exist for the nutrient, and Daily Reference Values when RDAs do not exist for the nutrient. It is important to note that Daily Values reflect amounts as determined by the FDA for the purposes of food labeling, and hence vary widely from the DRIs established by the Food and Nutrition Board.

In January 2005, two federal agencies – The Department of Health and Human Services (the HHS) and the U. S. Department of Agriculture (the USDA) – released the new Dietary Guidelines for Americans. The sixth edition of Dietary Guidelines for Americans places stronger emphasis on reducing calorie consumption and increasing physical activity.

The guidelines were developed in a three-stage approach. In the first stage, a 13-member advisory committee prepared a report based on the best available science. The thirteen-member committee analyzed all the latest information and published their report in the Dietary Guidelines Advisory Committee Report. This report was the primary resource for development of the guidelines. The committee did not write the guidelines, they made suggestions and recommendations. In the second stage, scientists and officials developed the guidelines after reviewing the committee's report and agency and public comments. The public included lay people, academic researchers, consumer and trade groups, and businesses. The advisory committee notes that they were continuously made aware of the food industry, the beverage industry, and the economic impact of their decisions. Committee members are confident that they remained above the influence of outside interests – especially the very strong food industry lobbying groups.

The final stage – the recommendations - rested with the politically appointed HHS and USDA secretaries, Tommy Thompson and Ann Veneman. Tommy Thompson refers to the relationship between the food industry and the government guidelines as a "partnership". Because of this, quote, "partnership", as it is termed by the former HHS Secretary, Tommy Thompson, between the government agencies and the food industry, the guidelines were changed from the advisory committee's recommendations in several significant ways: trans-fats, and sugar, and sugar free. The committee unanimously voted to reduce trans-fat intake to one percent or less of total calories, but that figure was removed from the final guidelines. Assigning a number would have resulted in a Daily Value Percentage being posted on the Nutrition Facts panel of every single packaged food. Consumers would have known that most pre-packaged foods would exceed daily recommended intake of trans-fat by 200 to 300%. Federally funded school lunch programs (worth $7.1 billion annually) would also be required to meet dietary guidelines. Manufacturers would have been required to modify their products just to remove all of the trans fats they include. So instead of taking the committee's recommendations, the guidelines instead read: "limit trans fats". Once again, the political aspects of the guidelines are making it even more challenging for the general public to safeguard our own health. What does "limit trans fats" mean? If we knew it meant 1% or less of total calories, and our food labels held a Daily Value Percentage, we could choose foods more wisely. But the vague guideline to limit trans fats still leaves us with a lot of work to do. As for sugars, the advisory committee recommended that added sugars make up less that 10% of daily calories. As with trans-fats, however, politics prevailed and the guidelines now read: "limit sugars".

CHAPTER 1 - SAMPLE TEST

1. List the energy nutrients and how much energy is derived from each.

2. Explain what constitutes a complete protein (in the traditional sense), and list three sources of complete proteins.

3. What are two major differences between plant cells and animal cells?

4. What are the roles of vitamins and minerals in providing energy?

5. If a man expends 3000 calories per day, what would be his recommended water intake?

6. Define homeostasis and provide several examples.

7. What are the Dietary Reference Intakes? Discuss whether or not they are minimum standard requirements. Also discuss the differences between DRIs and Daily Values.

8. Discuss the 2005 Dietary Guidelines and provide details concerning the history of the guidelines; the scientific and political nature of the guidelines; and the challenges associated with the guidelines.

REFERENCES

1. Alberts, B, D Brag, J Lewis, M Raff, K Roberts, J Watson. *Molecular Biology of the Cell.* NY: Garland Publishing Co., 1983.

2. Guyton, A, *Textbook of Medical Physiology,* 10th ed. Phil: W.B. Saunders Co. 2005.

3. Whitney, E, S Rolfes. *Understanding Nutrition,* 8th ed. NY: West Publishing Co. 2005.

4. Lehninger, A. *Principles of Biochemistry,* NY: Worth Publishers, Inc, 2004.

5. Zar, J. *Biostatistical Analysis*, 2nd ed. NJ: Prentice-Hall Inc., 1984.

6. Shils, M, V Young. *Modern Nutrition in Health & Disease,* 10th ed. Philadelphia PA: Lea & Febiger, 2005.

7. Recommended Dietary Allowances, 10th ed. Subcommittee on the tenth edition of the RDAs, Food and Nutrition Board Commission on Life Sciences, National Research Council. Washington, DC: National Academy Press, 1989.

8. Institute of Medicine, Food and Nutrition Board. Dietary Reference Intakes for Vitamin C, Vitamin e, Selenium and Carotenoids. A report of the Panel on dietary Antioxidants and Related Compounds, Subcommittees on Upper Reference Levels of Nutrients and Interpretation and Uses of Dietary Reference Intakes, and the Standing Committee on the Scientific Evaluation of Dietary Reference Intakes. Washington, D.C, National Academy Press, 2000.

9. Institute of Medicine, Food and Nutrition Board. Dietary Reference Intakes for Thiamin, Riboflavin, Niacin, Vitamin B6, Folate, Vitamin B12, Pantothenic Acid, Biotin, and Choline. A Report of the Standing Committee on the Scientific Evaluation of Dietary Reference Intakes and its Panel on Folate, other B vitamins and Choline and Subcommittee on Upper Reference Levels of Nutrients. Washington, D.C, National Academy Press, 2000.

10. Institute of Medicine, Food and Nutrition Board. Dietary Reference Intakes Calcium Phosphorus, Magnesium, Vitamin D, and Fluoride. Standing Committee on the Scientific Evaluation of Dietary Reference Intakes. Washington, D.C, National Academy Press, 2000.

11. RDA, National Academy of Sciences, National Academy Press, Washington, D.C., 1989.

12. Office of the Federal Register, National Archives and Records Administration, Code of Federal Regulations.   U.S.   Government   Printing   Office.   www.access.gpo.gov/cgi-bin/ cfrassemble.cgi?title=200021

13. History of the 2005 Dietary Guidelines: http://www.health.gov/dietaryguidelines/history.htm

14. U.S. Department of Health and Human Services and U.S. Department of Agriculture. Dietary Guidelines for Americans, 2005. 6th Edition, Washington, DC: U.S. Government Printing Office, January 2005.

Chapter 2
Carbohydrates

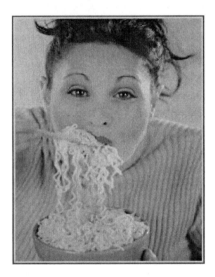

In the next three chapters we will take a more in-depth look at each of the energy nutrients. Carbohydrates, fats, and proteins provide the body with energy to perform all activities (moving, thinking, etc.) and life. For optimum health and fitness, these nutrients must be obtained in adequate amounts. In this chapter, we will examine carbohydrates in detail, including digestion, absorption, transport and importance in health.

Objectives

After reading and studying this chapter, you should:

1. Be able to describe digestion, absorption, transport and roles of carbohydrates.

2. Be able to discuss fiber and its role in health.

3. Be able to discuss the positive and negative effects of alcohol.

4. Discuss nonnutritive and nutritive sweeteners.

5. Discuss the controversy over high fructose corn syrup.

INTRODUCTION

The wild popularity of the Atkins, South Beach, and other low-carbohydrate diets has many Americans confused. These popular diets treat carbohydrates as evil, the root of all body fat and excess weight. That's a dangerous oversimplification, on a par with "fat is bad." There is a BIG difference between the natural, wholesome, 'good' carbs we are designed to eat and the unnatural, highly-processed, 'refined' carbs so many of us consume on a daily basis! See the section on diets for details on the futility of all diets.

This chapter will focus on the biochemistry of carbohydrates and discuss why and what types of carbohydrates are important in health. How much of our diet should contain carbohydrates will be discussed in a later chapter.

PHYSIOLOGY

Carbohydrates are found in a wide array of foods—bread, beans, milk, popcorn, potatoes, cookies, spaghetti, soft drinks, corn, and cherry pie. They also come in a variety of forms. The most common and abundant forms are sugars, fibers, and starches. The basic building block of every carbohydrate is a sugar molecule, a simple union of carbon, hydrogen, and oxygen. Starches and fibers are essentially chains of sugar molecules. Some chains are straight, others branch wildly.[1]

Carbohydrates were once grouped into two main categories. Simple carbohydrates included sugars such as fruit sugar (fructose), corn or grape sugar (dextrose or glucose), and table sugar (sucrose). Complex carbohydrates included everything made of three or more linked sugars. Complex carbohydrates were thought to be the healthiest to eat, while sugars weren't so great. It turns out that the picture is more complicated.

There are 3 classes of carbohydrates in foods. Monosaccharides consist of a one sugar molecule, oligosaccharides consist of a few sugar molecules (disaccharide-two sugars), and polysaccharides consist of many sugar molecules.[2]

The monosaccharides include glucose, fructose and galactose. Glucose is the simple sugar found in starch and glycogen. Fructose is the simple sugar found in fruit. Galactose is bound to glucose to form the disaccharide lactose found in milk. The disaccharides are the most common oligosaccharides and include sucrose (fructose and glucose), lactose (galactose and glucose), and maltose (glucose and glucose). Sucrose is a fructose and a glucose molecule that forms table sugar. Lactose is the disaccharide found in milk; and maltose occurs when starch is broken down.

The polysaccharides include starch, glycogen, and cellulose. Starch is a plant polysaccharide composed of glucose, digestible by human beings. Two forms of starch include amylose and amylopectin. Glycogen is the form of starch stored in the body. Glycogen is composed of glucose, manufactured and stored in the liver and muscle as a storage form of glucose. Starch and glycogen consist of many glucose molecules linked together as long branched chains. Glycogen, however, is more highly branched than starch.

MONOSACCHARIDE	OLIGOSACCHARIDE	POLYSACCHARIDE	
ONE	*FEW	MANY	
glucose fructose galactose	lactose maltose sucrose	HETEROGLYCAN (different) sugars linked together ↓ fibers ↓ pectin hemicellulose gums	HOMOGLYCAN (same) sugars linked together ↓ fructans glucans galactans

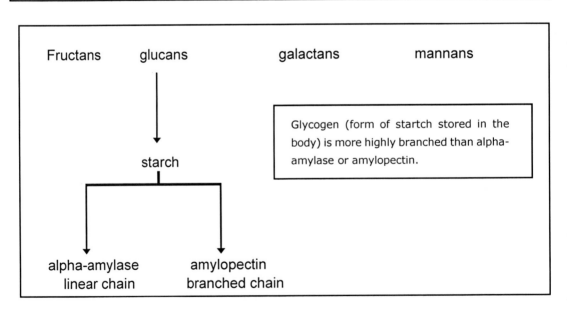

* Lactose consists of a galactose and a glucose molecule;
maltose consists of 2 glucose molecules; sucrose consists of a fructose and a glucose molecule.

DIGESTION

The goal of carbohydrate digestion is to degrade the carbohydrate into small compounds that the body can absorb.

> Mouth: Digestion of carbohydrates begins in the mouth. Glucose is unique in that small amounts can be absorbed through the lining of the mouth. But for the most part nutrient absorption takes place in the small intestines.
>
> An enzyme in saliva, known as salivary amylase hydrolyzes (breaks) starch to shorter polysaccharides. Because the food is soon swallowed, the job is incomplete.
>
> Stomach: The swallowed food mixes with the stomach's secretions. This halts starch digestion.
>
> Small Intestines: In the small intestines the major carbohydrate-digesting enzyme, pancreatic amylase, continues breaking down the polysaccharides to shorter glucose chains and disaccharides. This enzyme is secreted into the small intestines via the pancreatic duct. The final step takes place on the outer membranes of the intestinal cells where the disaccharides are broken down to monosaccharides. Only the indigestible fibers remain in the digestive tract and enter the large intestine. Here bacterial enzymes digest fiber. Fiber holds water, regulates bowel activity, and also binds cholesterol and some minerals, carrying them out of the body.[5]
>
> Large Intestines: Within one to four hours after a meal all the available carbohydrates are digested. Only the indigestible fibers remain in the large intestines.

ABSORPTION OF CARBOHYDRATES

Absorption of carbohydrates occurs when the monosaccharides or disaccharides enter small intestinal cells.

> Small intestines: The monosaccharides cross the small intestinal cells and are washed into the bloodstream by a rush of circulating blood which carries these monosaccharides to the liver.

TRANSPORT

Glucose is delivered through the blood stream to the Liver: The liver converts these different monosaccharides to glucose. There are five possible fates for glucose in the liver:[3]

> 1. Glucose can be converted into glycogen.
> 2. Glucose can be used for energy by liver cells.
> 3. Any amount beyond that which can be stored as carbohydrate will be turned into fatty acids which in turn can travel to the fat cells and be stored as fat.
> 4. The liver can add a phosphate group to glucose and store it as glucose-6-phosphate.
> 5. Glucose can also be made into nucleotides.

CARBOHYDRATE METABOLISM

In this section discussion will focus on the critical role of carbohydrates (glucose) in energy production. Carbohydrates are digested to simple sugars and absorbed as simple sugars (see absorption and digestion). Once absorbed, the liver converts all simple sugars to glucose. Glucose is the primary source of energy for the body.

Glucose is required by all cells for energy. Some cells can utilize glucose in conjunction with fat, while other cells must rely on glucose. In the absence of glucose some cells can switch to ketones (similar to glucose in structure) while other cells cannot.[2]

Glycogen

Glycogen is the storage form of glucose in the body. Glycogen can be stored in muscle cells and liver cells. Muscle and liver glycogen storage depots are independent of each other. The average 150 pound male can store approximately 1800 calories of carbohydrate (1400 calories in muscle in the form of glycogen, 320 calories in the liver in the form of glycogen, and approximately 80 calories of glucose in the blood).[2]

The glycogen stored in muscle tissue is energy for muscle cells only. A chemical reaction, called phosphorylation, takes place that "locks" the glucose in muscle cells. Phosphorylation is the process of adding a phosphate group to glucose. In muscle this process prevents glucose from the leaving the muscle cell. One might envision muscle cells as being "stingy" for not sharing their glucose. In fact, muscle cells cannot share stored glucose with the rest of the body because they do not contain the required enzyme for phosphorylation.

Many people are unaware of the fact that fat utilization in muscle cells can only occur when glucose is present. An old saying (still true) is: Fats burn in the flame of carbohydrates. In other words fat can not be used as an energy source by muscle cells if glycogen is depleted. See section on ketosis for exception under fasting circumstances. Muscle cells can utilize fat only in conjunction with glucose (or ketones in fasting), but not in isolation. If muscle cells are depleted of glycogen, energy ceases within seconds.[4]

Glucose Homeostasis

Glucose homeostasis is an example of one of the highest levels of homeostatic control in the human body. To reiterate, glucose is obtained from digestion and absorption of carbohydrate foods in the diet (see food sources in Chapter 1).

Two categories of cells are involved in maintaining glucose homeostasis - insulin-dependent and non-insulin-dependent cells. The body controls blood levels of glucose within a very narrow range - 80 to 120 mg/dl. If glucose levels in the blood stream are not maintained within this range, many types of cells become damaged and destroyed. The body maintains blood glucose levels through the use of hormones.[4]

Hormones are messenger molecules that carry instructions from the site of production, through the bloodstream, to other cells throughout the body. Each hormone affects one or more specific target tissues or organs and elicits specific responses to restore normal conditions. Insulin is secreted by groups of cells within the pancreas called islet cells. The pancreas is an organ that sits behind the stomach and has many functions in addition to insulin production.

Insulin is often called the "hyperglycemic" hormone because its role consists of removing excess glucose from the bloodstream after a meal. Sugars are absorbed from the intestines into the bloodstream after a meal. Insulin is then secreted by the pancreas in response to this detected increase in blood sugar. Many cells of the body have insulin receptors which bind the insulin. These types of cells are known as insulin-dependent cells.

When a cell has insulin attached to its surface, the cell activates other receptors designed to absorb glucose (sugar) from the blood stream into the inside of the cell. Hence, when glucose levels in the blood stream rise after a meal insulin helps remove the excess glucose from the bloodstream by allowing the glucose to be absorbed by insulin dependent cells. In this manner glucose levels are restored to normal.

The hormone responsible for controlling glucose levels in the blood stream when levels are low is glucagon, sometimes referred to as the "hypoglycemic hormone". Also, produced by the pancreas, it is released when glucose levels in the bloodstream are low allowing the liver to convert stored glycogen into glucose and releases it into the bloodstream. The action of glucagon is thus opposite to that of insulin.[4]

Epinephrine and norepinephrine produce a similar response as glucagon under stress conditions. During the fight-or-flight (stress) response, the adrenal gland releases epinephrine and norepinephrine into the blood stream, along with other hormones like cortisol signaling the liver to release its glycogen.

Most cells of the body are insulin-dependent cells with the exception of red blood cells, nerve cells, brain cells, and a variety of cells involved in vision. These cells, known as non-insulin-dependent cells, are quite different in that insulin has either little or no effect on glucose utilization or uptake. Also, these cells can only use glucose as an energy source. Therefore, it is essential that blood glucose levels be maintained within the homeostatic range.[3]

To reiterate, non-insulin-dependent cells do not have hormonal protection and are especially sensitive to fluctuating glucose levels in the blood stream.[3] The only role of insulin in this situation is to allow the glucose to flow from the bloodstream into insulin-dependent cells. This process returns blood glucose levels to normal thereby protecting non-insulin dependent cells from destruction (red blood cells, brain cells, nerve cells). When glucose levels are too low, glucagon is released from the pancreas. This event signals the liver to release glucose into the bloodstream, again protecting non-insulin dependent cells from destruction due to insufficient levels of glucose.

Glucose Time Curve

The body has a finite amount of glycogen that can be stored in the liver and muscle. As previously mentioned, the glycogen stored in muscle is not available to supply non-insulin dependent cells with glucose. Therefore these cells must rely on stored glucose from the liver when glucose is unavailable.[7]

The liver can store enough glycogen to supply brain cells, nerve cells, and other cells with glucose for about twelve to sixteen hours.[2] If liver glycogen stores are depleted and food is not eaten, the body must make glucose from other sources.

Consider the following example. An individual eats dinner consisting of complex and simple carbohydrates at 6 p.m. For the first four hours after this meal glucose is present in the bloodstream from the meal. At around 10 p.m. the individual goes to bed. Even while sleeping the body utilizes many calories for metabolic reactions (basal metabolic rate). Glycogen stored in the liver is released all night long providing the needed glucose for the glucose requiring reactions. When the individual gets up at 6 a.m. glycogen in the liver is nearly depleted and by 10 a.m. is guaranteed to be depleted. Since blood glucose levels must be maintained (homeostasis), if the individual does not eat, glucose will be formed through a process known as gluconeogenesis.

Glucose Time Curve

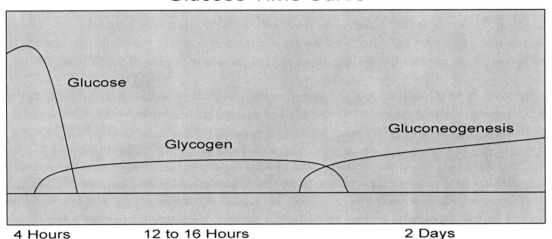

| 4 Hours | 12 to 16 Hours | 2 Days |

Gluconeogenesis

The only way the body can produce glucose after 12 to 16 hours of not eating is through gluconeogenesis, the making of glucose from non-carbohydrate sources. The only available source for glucose production in this stage is the breakdown of glucogenic amino acids (amino acids that can make glucose). The body cannot use fat for glucose production because fat cannot make glucose. (Glycerol, an alcohol can make small amounts of glucose, but the amount is inconsequential at this point.) To obtain these glucogenic (glucose-making) amino acids the body must break down whole proteins from skeletal muscle, and eventually other lean organ tissues. The process in which large molecules are broken down to smaller ones is known as catabolism.[7]

In the first few days of a fast, body proteins constitute over 90 percent of the needed glucose. Energy at this point is a homeostatic priority for the body and since energy from food is unavailable, the body must make it from glucogenic amino acids. As a reminder, fat cells utilize very few calories, while muscle cells can utilize 25% to 50% of daily caloric intake. This becomes an "expensive" way to obtain glucose since whole body proteins are broken down to provide amino acids for formation of glucose. Whole proteins are broken down to produce glucogenic and non-glucogenic amino acids (glucose forming and non-glucose forming amino acids). The nitrogen from glucogenic amino acids must be disposed of, along with nitrogen from the breakdown of non-glucogenic amino acids (this will be also discussed in detail in the section on proteins). This catabolic process becomes a huge sabotaging effect in weight management and health because fat burning machinery - muscle is lost. At this point the scale will go down, but is destined to go back up since over half the weight loss can be contributed to muscle loss (see also diets.)

Ketosis

Starvation begins to occur after two to three days of not eating. If the body were to use proteins at the same rate as in the first forty-eight hours, death would ensue within days. However, a process called ketosis begins to occur. Ketosis is a metabolic state that occurs when the liver converts fat into fatty acids and ketone bodies. These ketone bodies can then be used by certain cells for energy. Most medical resources regard ketosis as a physiological state associated with chronic starvation. Glucose is regarded as the preferred energy source for all cells in the body with ketosis being regarded as a crisis reaction of the body to a lack of carbohydrates in the diet.

Ketones can be thought of as "fake glucose". Biochemically ketones closely resemble glucose. Some cells (such as muscle cells) can switch to utilization of ketones for energy, while the non-insulin dependent cells previously discussed (brain cells, nerve cells, etc.) cannot. With the use of ketones by muscle cells and other cells, the body can survive weeks, and even months.[7] To reiterate, during the process of ketosis, the body must continuously catabolize muscle tissue to provide glucogenic amino acids for certain cells, such as brain cells, nerve cells, etc. So the process of ketosis - breakdown of fat into ketones - is always associated with breakdown of amino acids for energy. Death through starvation is the result of loss of muscle, acidosis and other contributing factors. At death there can still be substantial body fat with very little lean muscle remaining.

High levels of ketones in the bloodstream can produce serious health problems.[1] A process known as acidosis occurs (higher levels of acidity in the blood and body fluids). Acidosis can lead to coma and death. Excessive amounts of ketones in the bloodstream will slowly be broken down to acetone. Acetone is excreted in the breath and urine.

Ketosis should not be confused with ketoacidosis, which is severe ketosis causing the pH of the blood to drop below 7.2. Ketoacidosis is a medical condition usually caused by diabetes and accompanied by dehydration, hyperglycemia, ketonuria and increased levels of glucagon. Ketoacidosis is the accumulation of excessive keto acids (ketones) in the blood stream (specifically acetoacetate and beta-hydroxy bu-tyrate).

ABSORPTION RATE AND GLYCEMIC INDEX

After understanding the importance of carbohydrates in energy production, the next concept is understanding the types of carbohydrates that should make up a large part of a healthy eating plan.

Absorption Rate

Absorption rates of carbohydrates differ depending on several factors. Sugars are absorbed differently from complex carbohydrates. Absorption rates of simple sugars or complex carbohydrates are also different in the presence of other nutrients such as fiber, fat and protein. [7]

To reiterate larger than physiological levels of glucose (80 to 120 mg/dl) in the bloodstream are toxic to non-insulin dependent cells (red blood cells, nerve cells, etc.). The body protects these cells by removing the excess glucose rapidly from the blood stream. As long as individuals have adequate and effective insulin, the excess glucose is either shuttled into insulin-dependent cells, or transformed into triglycerides and stored as fat.

When large amounts of simple sugars are ingested in the absence of other nutrients, they enter the bloodstream very quickly. To prevent the damage described above, insulin shuttles the sugar (glucose) into insulin-dependent cells; i.e. muscle and fat cells. Exercise increases muscle sensitivity to insulin; hence, if the person is exercising, more of the glucose can be used for immediate energy, some will enter muscle cells, and excess will be transformed into triglycerides and stored in fat cells. If the person is not exercising very little will enter muscle cells and more of the glucose will be transformed into triglycerides and stored in fat cells.[7]

When complex carbohydrates (legumes, breads, etc.) or simple carbohydrates are absorbed in the presence of other nutrients such as fat, protein, or fiber, the absorption rate of the simple sugar is decreased (slowed). The sugars do not flood the bloodstream as quickly and the body does not have to shuttle the same large amount of glucose quickly as in the previous example; hence, less of the glucose (or none, depending on the total caloric intake) will be transformed into triglycerides.

To reiterate, calories from an 800 calorie soft drink are absorbed differently than 800 calories from fruit and cottage cheese. While 800 calories may or may not be too many calories (depending on the person and the activity level) much more of the calories from the soft drink will be transformed into triglycerides than the 800 calories from intake of fruit and cottage cheese.

Glycemic Index

Many people believe the glycemic index reflects absorption rate. However, the numbers do not add up. The glycemic index of various foods was initially developed for diabetics in the 1980's by Canadian researchers[28]. These researchers were investigating the possibility of using the index to determine healthier food choices for diabetics.

The glycemic index is theoretically based on how 50 grams of carbohydrates (not counting fiber) in a food will affect blood sugar levels. Glycemic index is determined by comparing an experimental food to a reference food. In some indexes the reference food is sugar, while in others the reference food is something other than sugar, such as white bread. In the Canadian research, white bread was the reference value (100) and sugar was compared to this value (glycemic index of 140).[7] *The New Glucose Revolution* by J. Brand-Miller uses glucose as the reference food and compares other foods to glucose.[8]

The theory is that the lower the glycemic index the healthier the food choice. But whole wheat bread has the same glycemic index as white bread. Carrots have a high glycemic index and people have eliminated them from their diets for

Canandian Research[7]	
Food	Index
potato	104
table sugar	83
couscous	93
Rice Krispies	117
All Bran	60
wh wheat br	100
white bread	100

Glucose Revolution[8]	
Food	Index
potato	93
table sugar	100
couscous	65
Frosted Flakes	55
All Bran	51
wh wheat br	70
white bread	70

this reason. But carrots are a wonderful, healthy food and a whole bag of carrots contains less than 50 calories. Sweet-tasting watermelon has a very high glycemic index. But a slice of watermelon has only a small amount of carbohydrate per serving (as the name suggests, watermelon is made up mostly of water). A Snickers bar has a glycemic index of 41, marking it as a low glycemic index food but it is certainly not a health food. To make the glycemic index even less meaningful, each of us has a differing daily glycemic response that can vary 43 percent on any given day.[7]

Part of the problem stems from the fact that starch comes in many different configurations. Some are easier to break into sugar molecules than others. The sugars in fiber are linked in ways that the body has trouble breaking down. The more fiber a food has, the less digestible carbohydrate, and so the less sugar, it can deliver. Ripe fruits and vegetables tend to have more sugar than unripe ones, and so tend to have a higher glycemic index. The more fat or acid a food or meal contains, the slower its carbohydrates are converted to sugar and absorbed into the bloodstream. Finely ground grain is more rapidly digested, and so has a higher glycemic index, than more coarsely ground grain.[10] Other factors include where the food was grown, ripeness, the amount eaten, fiber content, fat content, physical form, the way the food is prepared (mashed, baked, boiled), and if the food is eaten hot or cold.[9]

Too many factors influence a food's glycemic effect to be an effective tool in choosing healthy carbohydrates.

Glycemic Index and Athletes

An argument among athletes is that, unlike the general population that eat a combination of foods, they eat foods in isolation (a banana, a bagel). Should athletes use the glycemic index system to determine what to eat before, during and after exercise?[9]

According to Dr. Kathy Beals, athletes can disregard all the hype about the glycemic index and simply enjoy fruits, vegetables and whole grains without fretting about their glycemic effect. In theory low-glycemic-index foods (apples, yogurt, lentils, beans) provide a slow release of glucose into the blood stream. Could they help endurance athletes by providing sustained energy during long bouts of exercise? High-glycemic-index foods (sports drinks, jelly beans, bagel) quickly elevate blood sugar. The question becomes are they best to consume immediately after exercise to rapidly refuel the muscles and, thereby, enhance subsequent performance?[9]

According to Dr. Beals, well-trained muscles can readily take up carbohydrates from the blood stream. Hence, fit people need less insulin than unfit people. This means athletes have a lower blood glucose response to what would otherwise create a high blood glucose response in an unfit person. Exercise is very important to manage blood sugar — and help prevent Type II diabetes. All things considered, athletes should **not** have concern with a food's glycemic effect because they don't know their personal response to the food. Plus, research fails to clearly support the theories mentioned above. The research does indicate the best way to enhance endurance is to consume carbs before and during exercise — tried-and-true choices that taste good, settle well and digest easily. Hence, fit people need not choke down low-glycemic-index kidney beans thinking they will help you with sustained energy, when they actually might only create digestive distress![9]

Glycemic Index and Weight Gain

There is a popular myth that high-glycemic-index foods are fattening because they create a rapid rise in blood sugar, stimulate the body to secrete more insulin and thereby (supposedly) promote fat storage. This is wrong. Excess calories are fattening, not excess insulin. Dieters who lose weight because they stop eating high-glycemic-index foods lose weight because they eat fewer calories. A year-long study with dieters who ate high-glycemic or low-glycemic index meals indicates no difference in weight loss.[8]

Some people claim to be sugar sensitive; that is, after they eat sugar they report an energy "crash." If that sounds familiar, the trick is to combine carbs with protein or fat, such as bread and peanut butter, or apple and low-fat cheese. This changes the absorption rate of the carbohydrate.

Glycemic Load

Harvard researchers developed a related way to classify foods that takes into account both the amount of carbohydrate in the food and the impact of that carbohydrate on blood sugar levels. This measure is called the glycemic load.[14,15] A food's glycemic load is determined by multiplying its glycemic index by the amount of carbohydrate it contains. In general, a glycemic load of 20 or more is high, 11 to 19 is medium, and 10 or under is low.[9]

Food	Carb	x Index*	= Load
baked potato	34	1.04	35.4
sugar	4	.83	3.3
3/4 Rice Krispies	28	1.17	32.8
wh wheat bread	25	1.0	25
white bread	25	1.00	25
* changed to decimal			

Neither of these classification systems are ideal. When it comes to choosing healthy carbohydrates, the glycemic index is of no value. Instead, whenever possible, people should replace highly processed grains, cereals, and sugars with minimally processed whole-grain products.

INSULIN RESISTANCE

Insulin resistance is characterized by higher than normal insulin levels in the blood stream. Non-insulin-dependent diabetes (NIDDM) is characterized by insulin resistance (see section on Diabetes). These individuals have higher than normal levels of insulin (and body fat), because some of the insulin is "defective". The body makes more and more "defective" insulin while blood glucose levels continue to rise. The popular high protein diets put the horse before the cart. It's not that insulin makes people fat. It's the insulin resistance that is associated with obesity.[8] Ninety percent of adults with NIDDM are obese. As body fat increases, insulin resistance increases. Insulin resistance is a metabolic consequence of obesity. When obese individuals lose the fat, insulin once again becomes effective.

Syndrome X

Dr. Gerald Reaven, renowned and well respected professor of medicine at Stanford University, is the "insulin expert" quoted in all the bestselling anti-carbohydrate diet books - *The Zone, Dr. Atkins New diet Revolution, Protein Power.*[11,12] "They all misinterpret that work," says Dr. Reaven. He became so upset about the misinformation in these other books that he wrote his own book, *Syndrome X: Overcoming the Silent Killer That Can Give You a Heart Attack.*[13] Dr. Reaven coined the term Syndrome X in 1988 when referring to the unknown phenomenon of heart threatening abnormalities occurring in insulin-resistant people who did not get type II diabetes (now known as metabolic syndrome). In normal individuals insulin attaches to the insulin receptors on the cell surface and enables glucose to enter muscle and fat cells. But in Syndrome X the body is resistant to the insulin. To compensate, the pancreas secretes more and more insulin and the excess insulin manages to keep blood glucose levels within the normal range so diabetes does not occur. The high insulin levels lead to high triglyceride levels, low HDL levels, high blood pressure, smaller and denser LDL, and an increase in postprandial (after meals) accumulation of triglyceride rich lipoproteins in the blood. All these factors raise the risk of heart disease.[2,3,4]

When asked how many Americans have Syndrome X, Dr. Reaven explains that when his group measured insulin resistance in non-obese, nondiabetic individuals (without high blood pressure) about 25% to 30% were insulin resistant.

What are the causes of insulin resistance? The ability of insulin to do its job varies about ten fold in healthy populations - not counting diabetics.[13] According to Dr. Reaven, about half of that variability is genetic. The other half depends on how heavy you are and how fit you are. Dr. Reaven believes that obesity has been overplayed because most studies haven't taken into consideration that obese individuals are often sedentary. Hence about 25% of the risk of insulin resistance due to lifestyle depends on how heavy you are and another 25% depends on how fit you are. Smoking makes insulin resistance worse and two servings of alcohol a day makes it somewhat better (Note: two glasses or less for men and one glass or less for women). Greater amounts increase risk for prostate cancer in men, and breast cancer in women. See alcohol section for more information on benefits and risk.

How does someone know if they have Syndrome X? Dr. Reaven's team has identified 7 risk factors (see following table) that can be measured in any doctor's office. He cautions that these factors are not the only risk factors for a heart attack. Others include LDL over 130, smoking, having diabetes, age (over 45 for men; over 55 for women), and being male. Individuals can determine their risk of heart attack triggered by Syndrome X by answering the following questions (taken from Dr. Reaven's book):[13]

If Your	Give Yourself
1. Fasting glucose level is greater than 110, or your glucose at two hours into the Glucose Tolerance Test is greater than 140	3 points
2. Fasting triglyceride level is greater than 200	3 points
3. Fasting HDL cholesterol level is lower than 35	3 points
4. Blood pressure is greater than 145 over 90	3 points
5. Weight check reveals that you are more than 15 pounds overweight	1 point
6. Family has a history of heart disease, high blood pressure or diabetes	1 point
7. Lifestyle is characterized by physical inactivity in both work and leisure hours	1/2 point
Total Score_____	

If you scored	Your risk is
0-4 point ....Low	
5-8 points ....Moderate	
9-12 points ....High	
13 points or more ....Very High	

What do you do if you suspect that you have Syndrome X? Seek advice from a doctor who knows about Syndrome X and have the above tests done. The most powerful lifestyle changes, says Dr. Reaven, include how much you weigh and how fit you are. If you are insulin-resistant and overweight and you lose that weight you become less insulin-resistant and you stay that way as long as you keep the weight off. Whether or not you lose weight, exercise also makes you *less* insulin resistant. If you stop exercising, you lose the benefit.

Dr. Reaven also recommends a diet that is not high in carbohydrates since the body has to secrete more insulin to handle the carbs if you are insulin-resistant. He recommends around 45% carbohydrates. But unlike other high protein diets which recommend replacing carbs with protein and which do not differentiate between types of fats, Dr. Reaven recommends replacing the carbs with unsaturated fats -not proteins - like the high protein diets claim. Why? Protein stimulates insulin secretion for one reason, and also because protein is often accompanied by saturated fat and cholesterol, for another reason, states Dr. Reaven.

It must also be reiterated that while Dr. Reaven's recommendations may be scientifically sound, it has not been proven to be easily incorporated or effective in reducing the effects of insulin resistance. If individuals mistakenly add saturated fatty acids instead of the unsaturated, essential fatty acids, serum lipid levels will increase, and heart disease risk will increase.

Metabolic Syndrome

Described and defined in 1988 by G.M. Reaven, Syndrome X became known as the metabolic syndrome. The metabolic syndrome is characterized by a group of metabolic risk factors in one person.[14] They include:

- Abdominal obesity (excessive fat tissue in and around the abdomen)
- Atherogenic dyslipidemia (blood fat disorders — high triglycerides, low HDL cholesterol and high LDL - cholesterol — that foster plaque buildups in artery walls)
- Elevated blood pressure
- Insulin resistance or glucose intolerance (the body can't properly use insulin or blood sugar)
- Prothrombotic state (e.g., high fibrinogen or plasminogen activator inhibitor–1 in the blood)
- Proinflammatory state (e.g., elevated C-reactive protein in the blood)

People with metabolic syndrome are at increased risk of coronary heart disease and other diseases related to plaque buildups in artery walls (e.g., stroke and peripheral vascular disease) and type 2 diabetes. The metabolic syndrome has become increasingly common in the United States. It's estimated that over 50 million Americans have it. The dominant underlying risk factors for this syndrome appear to be abdominal obesity and insulin resistance. Insulin resistance is a generalized metabolic disorder, in which the body can't use insulin efficiently. This is why the metabolic syndrome is also called the insulin resistance syndrome. Other conditions associated with the syndrome include physical inactivity, aging, hormonal imbalance and genetic predisposition.

Some people are genetically predisposed to insulin resistance. Acquired factors, such as excess body fat and physical inactivity, can elicit insulin resistance and the metabolic syndrome in these people. Most people with insulin resistance have abdominal obesity. The biologic mechanisms at the molecular level between insulin resistance and metabolic risk factors aren't fully understood and appear to be complex.

Metabolic Syndrome Diagnosed

The criteria proposed by the National Cholesterol Education Program (NCEP) Adult Treatment Panel III (ATP III), with minor modifications, are currently recommended and widely used.[15]

The American Heart Association and the National Heart, Lung, and Blood Institute recommend that the metabolic syndrome be identified as the presence of three or more of these components:

> Elevated waist circumference:
> Men — Equal to or greater than 40 inches (102 cm)
> Women — Equal to or greater than 35 inches (88 cm)
>
> Elevated triglycerides:
> Equal to or greater than 150 mg/dL
>
> Reduced HDL ("good") cholesterol:
> Men — Less than 40 mg/dL

Women — Less than 50 mg/dL

Elevated blood pressure:
Equal to or greater than 130/85 mm Hg

Elevated fasting glucose:
Equal to or greater than 100 mg/dL

The primary goal of clinical management of the metabolic syndrome is to reduce the risk for cardiovascular disease and type 2 diabetes. Hence, the first-line therapy is to reduce the major risk factors for cardiovascular disease: stop smoking and reduce LDL cholesterol, blood pressure and glucose levels to the recommended levels.

For managing both long- and short-term risk, lifestyle therapies are the first-line interventions to reduce the metabolic risk factors. These lifestyle interventions include:
- Weight loss to achieve a desirable weight (BMI less than 25 kg/m^2)
- Increased physical activity, with a goal of at least 30 minutes of moderate intensity activity on most days of the week
- Healthy eating habits that include reduced intake of saturated fat, trans fat and cholesterol

FIBER

Fibers are the structural part of plants. Most are complex carbohydrates, but this does not include starch. Fiber looks like starch biochemically; however, the simple sugars are linked differently. Our bodies do not have the enzymes necessary to break these links; hence fibers are not absorbed in the small intestines. The indigestible fibers enter the large intestine where bacterial enzymes can digest some of them.

Crude fiber is defined as the residue remaining after treatment with harsh chemicals. Dietary fiber is the residue remaining after breakdown of the carbohydrate by digestive enzymes.[2]

Different types of fiber include cellulose, hemicellulose, pectin, gums, and lignin. Cellulose is the primary constituent of plant cell walls and therefore occurs in all vegetables, fruits and legumes. Hemicellulose is the main constituent of cereal fibers. Gums are found in oatmeal, dried beans, and other legumes. Lignin is a non-carbohydrate fiber found in the cell wall portion of plants, i.e. cobs, hulls. Because of its toughness, few of the foods people eat contain much lignin.

Fibers can be also be classified according to their solubility in water.[7] The insoluble fibers include cellulose, some hemicelluloses, and lignin; the soluble fibers include gums, pectin, and some hemicelluloses. In general, water soluble fibers dissolve in hot water and occur in high concentrations in fruits, whole grains, oats, barley, legumes, some vegetables; and water insoluble fibers are found in higher concentrations in vegetables, wheat, and cereals.

Benefits of Fiber

Water soluble fibers delay the stomach's emptying and the transit of chyme through the intestines; they have also been shown to lower blood cholesterol levels. Water insoluble fibers accelerate the transit time of chyme and increase fecal weight. In the body both types of fiber slow starch breakdown and delay glucose absorption into the blood.

The benefits of including adequate amounts of fiber in the diet are many. A large Harvard Study involving 69,000 female nurses, and other smaller studies, confirm that fiber appears to lower the risk of heart disease (23% reduction in women, and a 36% reduction in men).[16] It is estimated that about 1/5 of the benefit comes from fiber's ability to lower cholesterol levels.[17] The cholesterol benefit comes from soluble fibers. The theory is that these fibers work by inactivating digestive acids that are made from cholesterol, forcing the liver to pull cholesterol out of the blood to make more acids. It is estimated that adding about 5 grams of soluble fiber a day can lower total cholesterol levels by about 8 points.[17]

Other benefits of fiber include its ability to slow the conversion of carbohydrates into sugar in the blood. Refined products, such as white rice, white bread, etc. have much of the fiber removed. Digestion of these foods resembles the digestion and absorption of simple sugars.

Research suggests that an extra 14 grams of total fiber per day can lower both systolic and diastolic blood pressure by about 2 points in normotensive individuals, and even more in hypertensive individuals.[17] Such a decline lowers heart attack risk by 5 percent, and stroke risk by 8 percent.

Other Benefits of Fiber

Fiber can also help in weight loss. Soluble fiber mixes with liquids in the stomach to form a gelatinous mass, reducing appetite by making a meal feel larger and more satiating. In several studies, an addition of fiber resulted in an average of 4 extra pounds of weight loss over a two to three month period.

While not conclusive, research seems to suggest that soluble fiber in the gut may indirectly inhibit the formation of blood clots. Individuals that eat lots of fiber have lower levels of clot-promoting compounds. The evidence concerning fiber and colon and breast cancer is conflicting. Insoluble fiber (abundant in whole grain, beans, most vegetables and fruits) might reduce the risk of colon cancer by speeding potentially cancer causing waste through the colon, enlarging the stool, thus diluting their concentration. Also the fermentation of insoluble fibers in whole grains appears to create cancer fighting chemicals. No positive benefits were seen in the Harvard nurses study; however, even the women who ate the most fiber overall got little of it from whole grains. As for the benefits of fiber in breast cancer reduction, the evidence is hopeful, but inconclusive.

Fiber can help prevent diverticulosis (pouches forming in the wall of the colon).[14] Researchers used to think that fiber caused diverticulosis, but not so. It's the opposite. Fiber can actually help prevent diverticulosis by warding off constipation. Constipation results in an increase in colonic pressure that contributes to pouch formation.

It is better to rely on foods for fiber than supplements. Fiber rich foods, such as fruits, vegetables, and whole grains also reduce the risk of heart disease due to other factors (antioxidants, no saturated fat, etc.).

Recommended Intake

The recommended daily minimum intake of fiber is 12 grams, while the maximum intake recommended is 40 grams per day.[18] Amounts larger than 40 grams may interfere with absorption of minerals. A compound not classified as fiber but often found with fiber is phytic acid. Most of this compound is found in foods from seeds such as cereal grains. Minerals can become bound to phytic acid and be excreted (especially calcium, iron, and zinc). Another negative side of excessive amounts of fiber is abdominal discomfort. Increasing fiber in the diet should be done slowly to allow adaptation of the absorptive cells and to minimize abdominal discomfort.

Recommended intake of fiber:		
	Men	Women
Adults under 50	38 grams	25 grams
Adults over 50	30 grams	21 grams

Individuals can easily increase fiber intake by:[18]

   1. Switching to whole grain breads. Most breads called wheat or multigrain are made from refined flour. To make sure the product is whole grain look on the label for: whole wheat or 100 percent whole grain; whole wheat flour listed as the first ingredient; or at least 2 grams of fiber

per slice.

2. Switch from white flour to whole grain flour in baking

3. Choose brown rice over white rice

4. Substitute whole, unpeeled fruits for fruit juices

5. Add beans, barley, and other whole grains to soups

6. Eat cold salads that combine cooked whole grains, or beans with chopped raw vegetables

7. Begin to make meatless meals with beans, vegetables, and meat substitutes, such as soy

Fiber Content of Foods

Cereals	Serving Size	grams Total Fiber	grams Soluble Fiber	grams Insoluble Fiber
All Bran Bran Buds	1/3 cup	13.0	4.0	9.0
All Bran Extra Fiber	1/2 cup	13.0	1.0	12.0
Fiber One	1/2 cup	13.0	1.0	12.0
Quaker Oat Bran	1/2 cup	6.0	3.0	3.0
Raisin Bran	1/2 cup	4.0	0.5	3.5
Cheerios	1 cup	3.0	1.0	2.0
Shredded Wheat	1 1/4 cup	2.9	0.2	2.7
Oatmeal	1/2 cup	2.0	1.2	0.8
Corn Flakes	1 cup	1.0	0.0	1.0
Legumes (cooked)				
Lentils	1/2 cup	9.2	1.5	7.7
Red Kidney Beans	1/2 cup	8.2	3.4	4.9
Split Peas	1/2 cup	8.1	2.5	5.6
Pinto Beans	1/2 cup	7.4	2.7	4.6
Great Northern Beans	1/2 cup	6.2	1.1	5.1
Navy Beans	1/2 cup	5.8	1.7	4.1
Lima Beans	1/2 cup	4.9	1.2	3.8
Breads/Grains/Pasta				
Barley	1/2 cup	6.8	1.4	5.4
Whoe Wheat Spaghetti	1/2 cup	3.2	0.4	2.7
Whole Wheat Bread	1 slice	2.2	0.5	1.7
Brown Rice	1/2 cup	1.8	0.2	1.6
Wheat Bread	1 slice	1.6	0.2	1.4
Bagel	1/2 medium	1.3	0.5	0.8
Spaghetti	1/2 cup	1.1	0.5	0.6
White Bread	1 slice	0.6	0.3	0.3
White Rice	1/2 cup	0.6	0.1	0.4
Nuts and Seeds				
Almonds	1/4 cup	3.9	0.4	3.5
Peanut Butter	2 tbsp	2.1	0.6	1.5
Walnuts	1/4 cup	1.4	0.5	0.9

Fiber Content of Foods (continued)

Fruits (fresh)	Serving Size	grams Total Fiber	grams Soluble Fiber	grams Insoluble Fiber
Apple with skin	1 large	4.2	1.6	2.6
Pear with skin	1 medium	4.0	0.8	3.2
Blackberries	1/2 cup	3.8	0.9	2.9
Orange	1	3.6	2.1	1.5
Dried Prunes	4	3.1	1.3	1.8
Banana	1	2.8	0.9	1.9
Peach with skin	1	2.1	0.8	1.3
Grapefruit	1/2 large	1.8	1.3	0.5
Strawberries	1/2 cup	1.7	0.6	1.1

Vegetables (cooked)				
Corn	1/2 cup	4.7	0.2	4.4
Green Peas	1/2 cup	4.4	0.6	3.8
Avocado	1/2 cup	3.8	1.5	2.2
Brussels sprouts	1/2 cup	3.6	1.7	1.9
Sweet Potato(no skin)	1 medium	3.4	1.7	1.7
Potato (no skin)	1 large	2.8	0.7	2.1
Broccoli	1/2 cup	2.3	1.0	1.3
Carrot Slices	1/2 cup	2.3	1.0	1.3
Spinach	1/2 cup	2.1	0.6	1.4
Green Beans	1/2 cup	2.0	0.8	1.2
Cauliflower	1/2 cup	1.5	0.2	1.3

Vegetables (raw)				
Tomato	1 medium	1.3	0.3	1.0
Celery	1/2 cup	0.9	0.2	0.7
Green Pepper	1/2 cup	0.9	0.3	0.6
Romain Lettuce	1 cup	0.7	0.3	0.4

Information taken from ESHA Research, Salem, Oregon and manufacturers data
as reprinted in Consumer Reports, August, 1999.

ALCOHOL

Alcohols are a class of organic compounds, and they arise naturally from carbohydrates when certain microorganisms metabolize them in the absence of oxygen (fermentation).[1]

Most alcohols are toxic. They have the ability to dissolve the lipids out of cell membranes allowing the alcohol to penetrate rapidly into cells, destroying cell structures and killing cells. Ethanol, the type of alcohol we drink, is less toxic, and when sufficiently diluted, produces euphoria with low enough risk to be tolerated by the body.

Alcohol is a DRUG (a substance that can modify one or more of the body's functions). From the moment alcohol enters the body the tiny molecules need no digestion and are quickly absorbed. About 20 percent of the alcohol molecules are absorbed right through the walls of an empty stomach and can reach the brain within a minute. The stomach produces a small amount of an enzyme that breaks down alcohol (alcohol dehydrogenase) and can thus reduce the amount entering the blood. The amount of this enzyme is genetically determined. Men have more of this enzyme then women. When the stomach is full of food, the molecules have less chance of being absorbed as quickly and the influence on the brain is slightly delayed.

The alcohol that leaves the stomach is then absorbed in the intestines and circulates through the blood stream to the liver. Liver and stomach cells are the only cells that can produce alcohol dehydrogenase. The amount of alcohol that the liver can break down is limited to about 1/2 ounce of alcohol per hour; the maximum amount determined by the amount of alcohol dehydrogenase. The extra alcohol travels to all parts of the body, circulating until the liver can finally process it.[7]

Alcohol metabolism disrupts the liver. The liver can package excess fatty acids into triglycerides and ship them out to other tissues. When metabolizing alcohol, liver cells are forced to metabolize the alcohol and fatty acids accumulate. The presence of alcohol in the liver can also alter protein metabolism in the liver. Synthesis of some proteins important in the immune system slows down, weakening the body's defenses against infection. With excessive alcohol consumption, protein deficiency can develop.

Alcohol calories are not utilized as carbohydrate calories. A molecule involved in energy production, known as NADH, is required for the metabolism of alcohol and is thus not available to produce energy from glucose. The energy cycle is blocked, fatty acids accumulate and hydrogen ions change the pH in the body.

Alcohol is non-nutritive, contains 7 calories per gram, displaces nutrients from the diet, and can affect every tissue's metabolism of nutrients. Stomach cells begin to oversecrete acid and histamine. These changes make the stomach and esophagus linings vulnerable to ulcer formation. Intestinal cells fail to absorb B vitamins (thiamin, folate, and vitamin B12. Most dramatic is the effect of alcohol on folate. When alcohol is present, folate is removed from all its sites of action and storage. The liver secretes folate into the blood and as the blood concentration rises the kidneys excrete the folate. Liver cells lose efficiency in activating vitamin D and alter their production and excretion of bile.

Alcohol is also dehydrating.   The water loss includes loss of important minerals such as magnesium, potassium, calcium, and zinc.

The original studies examining possible cardiovascular benefits of alcohol were based on men.[19] Possible benefits include increased HDL levels. When similar studies were reproduced in women, a direct relationship between alcohol consumption and increased risk of breast cancer was observed.[16,17] It is now known that higher intake of alcohol is directly associated with increased risk of prostate cancer in men, as well as increased risk of certain other types of cancer in both men and women. When weighing the benefits and risks of alcohol consumption a host of other important risk factors, including high blood pressure, cigarette smoking, diabetes, body weight, physical activity, and lipid abnormalities must also be considered.

Summary of the latest evidence concerning possible benefits of alcohol is that light to moderate consumption confers the greatest benefits without increased risk for the above mentioned types of cancer. In middle-aged men this benefit is seen at less than two drinks per day.[19] Other study results revealed similar benefits in women, but at a consumption of less than one drink per day.[20]

Contrary to popular belief, alcohol should not be generally recommended to reduce risk of heart disease and stroke. Possible benefits begin only when a person reaches the age when the risk of these diseases increases - after the age of 40 for men and after menopause for women. As aging continues (after the age of 70) and caloric intake decreases, any possible benefits are far outweighed by the negatives of possible nutrient deficiencies.

Alcohol content

	total cal.	carb cal.	alcohol cal.
12 oz. beer	150	50	100
12 oz. lite beer	100	24	76
Apr. brandy (3-4 oz.)	65	-	65
80 pr. whiskey (1.5 oz.)	95	-	95
90 pr. whiskey (1.5 oz.)	110	-	110
7 oz. red wine	150	20	130
7 oz. white wine	160	30	130
7 oz. dry vermouth	210	10	200

One drink is the amount that delivers 1/2 ounce of pure ethanol (3 to 4 ounces wine, 10 ounces wine cooler, 12 ounces beer, 1 ounce hard liquor).

NUTRITIVE SWEETENERS

Sugar and sugar alcohols are each considered nutritive sweeteners because they provide calories when consumed. In the United States, sweeteners fall under the Generally Recognized as Safe (GRAS) list or as food additives under the 1958 Food Additives Amendment to the Federal Food, Drug, and Cosmetic Act.[21]

For a GRAS substance, generally available data and information about the use of the substance are known and accepted widely by qualified experts, and there is a basis to conclude that there is consensus among qualified experts that those data and information establish that the substance is safe under the conditions of its intended use.[21]

For a food additive, privately held data and information about the use of the substance are sent by the sponsor to FDA and FDA evaluates those data and information to determine whether the substance is safe under the conditions of its use.[21]

Sugar alcohols, or polyols, contain fewer calories than sugar. Sugar provides 4 kcal/gram and sugar alcohols provide an average of 2 kcal/gram (range from 1.5 kcal/gram to 3 kcal/gram). The reason that sugar alcohols provide fewer calories than sugar is because they are not completed absorbed.[21]

Sugar alcohols include sorbitol, mannitol, xylitol, erythritol, isomalt, lactitol, and malitol.[7] Contrary to their name, sugar alcohols are neither sugars nor alcohols. They are carbohydrates with structures that only resemble sugar and alcohol. They naturally occur in many fruits and vegetables but are most widely consumed in sugar-free and reduced-sugar foods. The sweetness of sugar alcohols varies from 25% to 100% as sweet as table sugar (sucrose). The amount and kind being used will be dependant on the food.

Sorbitol and mannitol are found in hard and soft candies, chewing gum, flavored jam and jelly spreads, frozen food and baked goods. Xylitol is found in chewing gum, hard candies and pharmaceutical products. Erythritol is found in chewing gum and some beverages. Isomalt is found in hard and soft candies, ice cream, toffee, fudge, lollipops, wafers and chewing gum. Lactitol is found in chocolate, cookies, cakes, hard and soft candies and frozen dairy desserts. Maltitol is found in sugar-free chocolate, hard candies, chewing gum, baked goods and ice cream.[21]

Because sugar alcohols are not completely absorbed, high intakes of foods containing them can lead to abdominal gas and diarrhea. Any foods that contain sorbitol or mannitol must include a warning on their label that "excess consumption may have a laxative effect." The American Dietetic Association advises that intakes greater than 50 grams/day of sorbitol or greater than 20 grams/day of mannitol may cause diarrhea.

The presence of sugar alcohols in foods does not mean that you can eat unlimited quantities. Sugar alcohols are lower in calories, gram for gram, than sugar but they are not calorie-free, and if eaten in large enough quantities, the calories can be comparable to sugar-containing foods. It's important to read the food labels for the calorie and carbohydrate content regardless of the claim of being sugar-free, low-sugar, or low-carb.

NONNUTRITIVE SWEETENERS

The five FDA-approved nonnutritive sweeteners are saccharin, aspartame, acesulfame potassium, sucralose, and neotame. Each of these is regulated as a food additive. These sweeteners are evaluated based on their safety, sensory qualities (for example, clean sweet taste, no bitterness, odorless), and stability in various food environments. They are often combined with other nutritive and/or nonnutritive sweeteners to provide volume that they lack on their own and a desired flavor. An Acceptable Daily Intake (ADI) for each additive has been established. The ADI is the amount of food additive that can be consumed daily over a lifetime without appreciable health risk to a person on the basis of all the known facts at the time of the evaluation.[21]

Saccharin[21]

Saccharin has been around for over 100 years and claims to be the best researched sweetener. Saccharin is also known as Sweet and Low, Sweet Twin, Sweet'N Low, and Necta Sweet. It does not contain calories, does not raise blood sugar levels and is 200 to 700 times sweeter than sucrose (table sugar).

There was a great deal of controversy surrounding the safety of saccharin back in the 1970s. In 1977, research showed bladder tumors in male rats with the ingestion of saccharin. The FDA proposed a ban on saccharin based on the Delaney Clause of the Federal Food, Drug, and Cosmetic Act, enacted in 1958. This clause prohibits the addition to the human food supply of any chemical that had caused cancer in humans or animals. Congress intervened after public opposition to the ban and allowed saccharin to remain in the food supply as long as the label carried this warning: "Use of this product may be hazardous to your health. This product contains saccharin which has been determined to cause cancer in laboratory animals." Further research was required to confirm the tumor findings. Since then, more than 30 human studies have been completed and found that the results found in rats did not translate to humans, making saccharin safe for human consumption. The original study published in 1977 has since been criticized for the very high dosages, that were hundreds of times higher than "normal" ingestion for humans, that were given to the rats. In 2000, the National Toxicology Program (NTP) of the National Institutes of Health concluded that saccharin should be removed from the list of potential carcinogens. The warning has now been removed from saccharin-containing products.

The FDA's guidelines on the use of saccharin for beverages are not to exceed 12 mg/fluid ounce, and in processed food, the amount is not to exceed 30 mg per serving. The Acceptable Daily Intake (ADI) for saccharin is 5 mg/kg of body weight. To determine your ADI, divide your weight in pounds by 2.2 and then multiply it by 5. For example, if you weighed 180 lbs., your weight in kg would be 82 (180 divided by 2.2) and your ADI for saccharin would be 410 mg (5 x 82). Saccharin is used in tabletop sweeteners, baked goods, jams, chewing gum, canned fruit, candy, dessert toppings, and salad dressings. It is also used in cosmetic products, vitamins, and pharmaceuticals.

The safety concerns of consuming products with saccharin remain even with the removal of the warning. According to a report written in 1997 written by the Center for the Science in Public Interest (CSPI) in response to the National Toxicology Program (NTP) removing saccharin from the list of potential carcinogens:

"It would be highly imprudent for the NTP to delist saccharin. Doing so would give the public a false sense of security, remove any incentive for further testing, and result in greater exposure to this probable carcinogen in tens of millions of people, including children (indeed, fetuses). If saccharin is even a weak carcinogen, this unnecessary additive would pose an intolerable risk to the public. Thus, we urge the NTP on the basis of currently available data to conclude that saccharin is "reasonably anticipated to be a human carcinogen," because there is "sufficient" evidence of carcinogenicity in animals (multiple sites in rats and mice) and "limited" or "sufficient" evidence of carcinogenicity in humans (bladder cancer) and not to delist saccharin, at least until a great deal of further research is conducted."

Another claim made against saccharin is the possibility of allergic reactions. The reaction would be in response to it belonging to a class of compounds known as sulfonamides which can cause allergic reactions in individuals who cannot tolerate sulfa drugs. Reactions can include headaches, breathing difficulties, skin eruptions, and diarrhea. It's also believed that the saccharin found in some infant formulas can cause irritability and muscle dysfunction. For these reasons, many people still believe that the use of saccharin should be limited in infants, children, and pregnant women. Without research to support these claims, the FDA has not imposed any limitations.

Aspartame[21]

Aspartame was discovered in 1965 and approved by the FDA in 1981 for dry uses in tabletop sweeteners, chewing gum, cold breakfast cereals, gelatins, and puddings. It was able to be included in carbonated beverages in 1983. In 1996, the FDA approved its use as a "general purpose sweetener," and it can now be found in more than 6,000 foods.

Aspartame is also known as Nutrasweet, Equal, and Sugar Twin. It does provide calories, and because it is 160 to 220 times sweeter than sucrose, very small amounts are needed for sweetening. The FDA has set the Acceptable Daily Intake (ADI) for aspartame at 50 mg/kg of body weight. To determine your ADI, divide your weight in pounds by 2.2 and then multiply it by 50. For example, if you weighed 200 lbs., your weight in kg would be 91 (200 divided by 2.2) and your ADI for aspartame would be 4550 mg (50 x 91). The amount of aspartame in some common foods is:

> 12 oz. diet soda—up to 225 mg of aspartame
> 8 oz. drink from powder—100 mg of aspartame
> 8 oz. yogurt—80 mg of aspartame
> 4 oz. gelatin dessert—80 mg of aspartame
> ¾ cup of sweetened cereal—32 mg of aspartame
> 1 packet of Equal—22 mg of aspartame
> 1 tablet of Equal—19 mg of aspartame

Aspartame has been approved for use in over 100 countries. An editorial in the British Medical Journal states that the "evidence does not support links between aspartame and cancer, hair loss, depression, dementia, behavioral disturbances, or any of the other conditions appearing in Web sites. Agencies such as the Food Standards Agency, European Food Standards Authority, and the Food and Drug Administration have a duty to monitor relations between foodstuffs and health and to commission research when reasonable doubt emerges. It concluded from biochemical, clinical, and behavioral research that the acceptable daily intake of 40 mg/kg/day of aspartame remained entirely safe—except for people with phenylketonuria."

Aspartame is one of the most controversial nonnutritive sweeteners. There are numerous Web sites, books, and articles stating various reasons why aspartame should not be consumed. Some cite studies to support their theories while others base their claims on industry-related conspiracies. Conflicts of interest in the studies performed on aspartame and the way in which its approval was obtained is an ongoing controversy.

H.J. Roberts, MD, coined the term "aspartame disease" in a book filled with over 1,000 pages of information about the negative health consequences of ingesting aspartame. He surveyed the studies of aspartame in the peer-reviewed medical literature. He states that "of the 166 studies felt to have relevance for questions of human safety, 74 had Nutrasweet industry related funding and 92 were independently funded. One hundred percent of the industry-funded research attested to aspartame's safety, whereas 92% of the independently funded research identified a problem." Other reports of federal employees working for the companies responsible for the testing and distribution of aspartame are cited on all of the sites and books opposing the use of aspartame.

Dr. Roberts reports that by 1998, aspartame products were the cause of 80% of complaints to the FDA about food additives. Some of these symptoms include headache, dizziness, change in mood, vomiting or nausea, abdominal pain and cramps, change in vision, diarrhea, seizures/convulsions, memory loss, and fatigue. Along with these symptoms, links to aspartame are made for fibromyalgia symptoms, spasms, shooting pains, numbness in your legs, cramps, tinnitus, joint pain, unexplainable depression, anxiety attacks, slurred speech, blurred vision, multiple sclerosis, systemic lupus, and various cancers. While the FDA has assured us that the research does not show any adverse health complications from aspartame, there has been some evidence to suggest that some of these symptoms can be related to aspartame:

One study confirmed that individuals with self-reported headaches after the ingestion of aspartame were indeed susceptible to headaches due to aspartame. Three randomized double-blind, placebo-controlled studies with more than 200 adult migraine sufferers showed that headaches were more frequent and more severe in the aspartame-treated group. In a study of the effect of aspartame on 40 patients with depression, the study was cut short due to the severity of reactions within the first 13 patients tested. The outcome showed that individuals with mood disorders were particularly sensitive to aspartame and recommended that it be avoided by them. In an initial study, 12 rats out of 320 developed malignant brain tumors after receiving aspartame in an FDA trial. There have been other studies to both support and contradict this finding. A recent study, conducted by Italian and French researchers indicates there is no association between low-calorie sweeteners and cancer. The researchers evaluated a variety of studies between the years of 1991 and 2004. These studies assessed the relationship between low-calorie sweeteners and many cancers, including oral and pharynx, esophagus, colon, rectum, larynx, breast, ovary, prostate and renal cell carcinomas. The researchers examined the eating habits of more than 7,000 men and women in their middle ages (mainly 55 years and over). Based on the data evaluated, there was no evidence that saccharin or other sweeteners (mainly aspartame) increase the risk of cancer at several common sites in humans. The debate continues while more research is conducted.

A study done with 14 dieters comparing the effects of aspartame-sweetened and sucrose-sweetened soft drinks on food intake and appetite ratings found that substituting diet drinks for sucrose-sweetened ones did not reduce total calorie intake and may even have resulted in a higher intake on subsequent days. In another study of 42 males given aspartame in diet lemonade versus sucrose-sweetened lemonade, there was no increase in hunger ratings or food intake with the diet group. Weight loss results from consuming fewer calories than your body needs. When you replace a caloric beverage with a noncaloric beverage, you will be saving calories and could lose weight if it is enough calories to put you in a negative balance. For aspartame to increase weight, there would have to be something else going on. There is not enough research to determine if something does exist so the jury is still out on this one.

Sucralose[21]

Sucralose is the newest nonnutritive sweetener on the market. It is well known for its claim to be made from sugar. Sucralose is made from sugar but cannot be digested because humans do not possess the enzymes to break the bonds between the sugars. It is sold as Splenda and is 600 times sweeter than sucrose. Maltodextrin, a starchy powder is added so it will measure like sugar. It provides essentially no calories and is not fully absorbed. Sucralose was approved in 1998 after 110 studies in animals and human over a period of over 20 years. ADI has been set at 5 mg/kg/body weight/day. No effects were observed at 500 mg/kg/bodyweight/day. To determine your ADI, divide your weight in pound by 2.2 and then multiply it by 50. For example, if you weighted 200 lbs., your weight in kg would be 91 (200 divided by 2.2) and your ADI for sucralose would be 455 mg (91 x 5).

Controversy surrounding sucralose stems from the fact that it was discovered while trying to create a new insecticide. The claim that it is made from sugar is a misconception about the final product. According to the book *Sweet Deception*, sucralose is made when sugar is treated with trityl chloride, acetic anhydride, hydrogen chlorine, thionyl chloride, and methanol in the presence of dimethylformamide, 4-methylmorpholine, toluene, methyl isobutyl ketone, acetic acid, benzyltriethlyammonium chloride, and sodium methoxide, making it unlike anything found in nature. The Splenda Web site even states that "although sucralose has a structure like sugar and a sugar-like taste, it is not natural." The product Splenda is also not actually calorie-free. Sucralose does have calories, but because it is 600 times sweeter than sugar, very small amounts are needed to achieve the desired sweetness. The first two ingredients in Splenda are dextrose and maltodextrin, which are used to increase bulk and are carbohydrates that are not free of calories. One cup of Splenda contains 96 calories and 32 grams of carbohydrates, which is substantial for people with diabetes but unnoticed due to the label claiming that it's a no calorie sweetener.

The name sucralose is another misleading factor. The suffix -ose is used to name sugars, not additives. Sucralose sounds very close to sucrose, table sugar, and can be confusing for consumers. A more accurate name for the structure of sucralose was proposed. The name would have been trichlorogalactosucrose, but the FDA did not believe that it was necessary to use this so sucralose was allowed. The presence of chlorine is thought to be the most dangerous component of sucralose. Chlorine is considered a carcinogen and has been used in poisonous gas, disinfectants, pesticides, and plastics. The digestion and absorption of sucralose is not clear due to a lack of long-term studies on humans. The majority of studies were done on animals for short lengths of time. The alleged symptoms associated with sucralose are gastrointestinal problems (bloating, gas, diarrhea, nausea), skin irritations (rash, hives, redness, itching, swelling), wheezing, cough, runny nose, chest pains, palpitations, anxiety, anger, moods swings, depression, and itchy eyes. The only way to be sure of the safety of sucralose is to have long-term studies on humans done.

Acesulfame K[21]

Acesulfame K has been an approved sweetener since 1988, and yet most people are not even aware that this is a nonnutritive sweetener being used in their food and beverages. It is listed in the ingredients on the food label as acesulfame K, acesulfame potassium, Ace-K, or Sunett. It is 200 times sweeter than sucrose (table sugar) and is often used as a flavor-enhancer or to preserve the sweetness of sweet foods. The FDA has set an Acceptable Daily Intake (ADI) of up to 15 mg/kg of body weight/day. The problems surrounding acesulfame K are based on the improper testing and lack of long-term studies. Acesulfame K does contain the carcinogen methylene chloride. Long-term exposure to methylene chloride can cause headaches, depression, nausea, mental confusion, liver effects, kidney effects, visual disturbances, and cancer in humans. There has been a great deal of opposition to the use of acesulfame K without further testing, but at this time, the FDA has not required that these tests be done.

Neotame[21]

In 2002, the FDA approved a new version of aspartame called Neotame. Neotame is chemically related to aspartame without the phenylalanine dangers for individuals with PKU. It is much sweeter than aspartame with a potency of approximately 7,000 to 13,000 times sweeter than sucrose (table sugar). The FDA has set an Acceptable Daily Intake (ADI) at 18 mg/kg of body weight/day. Neotame entered the market much more discreetly than the other nonnutritive sweeteners. While the Web site for neotame claims that there are over 100 scientific studies to support its safety, they are not readily available to the public. Opponents of neotame claim that the studies that have been done do not address the long-term health implications of using this sweetener. Without scientifically sound studies, done by independent labs, the opponents of neotame will continue to refute its use.

When To Use Artificial Sweeteners

Nonnutritive sweeteners were developed in hopes of reducing sugar intake in the U.S. These sweeteners allow diabetics the benefit of having "sweet tasting" foods. But consumers must be careful not to exceed Acceptable Daily Intakes.

Stevia

Stevia is a genus of about 150 species of herbs and shrubs in the sunflower family (Asteraceae), native to subtropical and tropical South America and Central America. The species *Stevia rebaudiana* Bertoni, commonly known as sweetleaf, sweet leaf, sugarleaf, or simply stevia, is widely grown for its sweet leaves. As a sugar substitute, stevia's taste has a slower onset and longer duration than that of sugar, although some of its extracts may have a bitter or liquorice-like aftertaste at high concentrations.[22] With its extracts having up to 300 times the sweetness of sugar, stevia has attracted attention with the rise in demand for low-carbohydrate, low-sugar food alternatives. Health and political controversies have limited stevia's availability in many countries. Stevia has not been approved as a sugar substitute in the U.S., Canada, or Europe because it is a known carcinogen in larger amounts.

Stevia is widely used as a sweetener in Japan, and it is now available in the US and Canada as a dietary supplement, although not as a food additive. Rebiana is the trade name for a stevia-derived sweetener being developed jointly by The Coca-Cola Company and Cargill with the intent of marketing in several countries and gaining regulatory approval in the US and EU. The United States banned it in the early 1990s unless labeled as a supplement.[34]

HIGH FRUCTOSE CORN SYRUP

High-fructose corn syrup (HFCS) is any of a group of corn syrups which have undergone enzymatic processing in order to increase their fructose content and are then mixed with pure corn syrup (100% glucose) to reach their final form. The typical types of HFCS are: HFCS 90 (used almost exclusively in the production of HFCS 55) which is approximately 90% fructose and 10% glucose; HFCS 55 (most commonly used in soft drinks) which is approximately 55% fructose and 45% glucose; and HFCS 42 (used in a variety of other foods, including baked goods) which is approximately 42% fructose and 58% glucose.[23]

The process by which HFCS is produced was first developed by Richard O. Marshall and Earl R. Kooi in 1957[23] and refined by Japanese researchers in the 1970s. HFCS was rapidly introduced in many processed foods and soft drinks in the US over the period of about 1975–1985.[23] In terms of sweetness, HFCS 55 is comparable to table sugar (sucrose), which is a disaccharide of fructose and glucose.[23] This makes it useful to manufacturers as a possible substitute for sucrose in soft drinks and other processed foods. HFCS 90 is sweeter than sucrose, while HFCS 42 is not as sweet as sucrose.[23]

Since its introduction, HFCS has begun to replace sugar in various processed foods in the USA.[24] The main reasons for this switch are: HFCS is somewhat cheaper due to the relative abundance of corn and the relative lack of sugar beets, as well as farm subsidies and sugar import tariffs in the United States; HFCS is easier to blend and transport because it is a liquid and usage leads to products with much longer shelf life.[23]

Cane sugar and Beet sugar are both relatively pure sucrose. While the glucose and fructose which are the two components of HFCS are monosaccharides, sucrose is a disaccharide *composed* of glucose and fructose linked together with a relatively weak glycosidic bond. A molecule of sucrose (with a chemical formula of $C_{12}H_{22}O_{11}$) can be broken down into a molecule of glucose ($C_6H_{12}O_6$) plus a molecule of fructose (also $C_6H_{12}O_6$ — an isomer of glucose) in a weakly acidic environment. Sucrose is broken down during digestion into fructose and glucose through hydrolysis by the enzyme sucrase, by which the body regulates the rate of sucrose breakdown. Without this regulation mechanism, the body has less control over the rate of sugar absorption into the bloodstream.[23]

The fact that sucrose is composed of glucose and fructose units chemically bound complicates the comparison between cane sugar and HFCS. The accuracy of saying that sucrose is "composed of 50% glucose and 50% fructose" depends on the context and point of view. Sucrose, glucose and fructose are unique, distinct molecules. Sucrose is broken down into its constituent monosaccharides - namely fructose and glucose - in weakly acidic environments by a process called inversion. This same process occurs in the stomach and in the small intestine during the digestion of sucrose into fructose and glucose.[23] Both HFCS and sucrose have approximately 4 kcal per gram of solid if the HFCS is dried; HFCS has approximately 3 kcal per gram in its liquid form.[25]

Some controversy has arisen over the use of HFCS as a food additive as manufacturers now use HFCS in an increasing variety of foods, such as breads, cereals, soft drinks, and condiments. The preference for high-fructose corn syrup over cane sugar among the vast majority of American food and beverage manufacturers is largely due to U.S. import quotas and tariffs on sugar. These tariffs significantly increase the domestic U.S. price for sugar, forcing Americans to pay more than twice the world price for sugar, thus making high-fructose corn syrup an attractive substitute in U.S. markets. For instance, soft drink makers like Coca-Cola use sugar in other nations, but use high-fructose corn syrup in their U.S. products.

The above-referenced studies have addressed fructose specifically, not sweeteners such as HFCS or sucrose which contain fructose in combination with other sugars. Thus, although they indicate that high fructose intake should be avoided, they don't necessarily indicate that HFCS is worse than sucrose intake, except insofar as HFCS contains 10% more fructose. Studies which have compared HFCS to sucrose (as opposed to pure fructose) find that they have essentially identical physiological effects. For instance, Melanson, et. al. (2006) studied the effects of HFCS and sucrose sweetened drinks on blood glucose, insulin, leptin, and ghrelin levels. They found no significant differences in any of these parameters.

Perrigue et. al. (2006) compared the effects of isocaloric servings of colas sweetened HFCS 45, HFCS 55, sucrose, and aspartame on satiety and subsequent energy intake. They found that all of the drinks with caloric sweeteners produced similar satiety responses, and had the same effects on subsequent energy intake. Taken together with Melanson et al (2006), this study suggests that there is little or no evidence for the hypothesis that HFCS is different from sucrose in its effects on appetite or on metabolic processes involved in fat storage. Both the Perrigue, et. al. study and the Melanson, et. al. study were funded by "the American Beverage Institute and the Corn Refiners Association."[30,31]

One much-publicized 2004 study found an association between obesity and high HFCS consumption, especially from soft drinks.[32] However, this study did not provide any evidence that this association is causal. In fact, one of the study coauthors, Dr. Barry M. Popkin, is quoted in the New York Times as saying, "I don't think there should be a perception that high-fructose corn syrup has caused obesity until we know more." In the same article, Walter Willett, chair of the Nutrition Department of the Harvard School of Public Health, is quoted as saying, "There's no substantial evidence to support the idea that high-fructose corn syrup is somehow responsible for obesity.[32]

In May 2006, the Center for Science in the Public Interest (CSPI) threatened to file a lawsuit against Cadbury Schweppes for labeling 7 Up as "All Natural" or "100% Natural", despite containing high-fructose corn syrup. While the U.S. FDA has no definition of "natural", CSPI claims that HFCS is not a "natural" ingredient due to the high level of processing and the use of at least one genetically modified (GMO) enzyme required to produce it.[32] On January 12, 2007, Cadbury Schweppes agreed to stop calling 7 Up "All Natural." They now call it "100% Natural Flavors."[33]

Experts Weigh in on HFCS

Many experts have given their views on the possible side effects of high fructose corn syrup. Here are some of their comments.

"There's no substantial evidence to support the idea that high-fructose corn syrup is somehow responsible for obesity. If there was no high-fructose corn syrup, I don't think we would see a change in anything important. I think there's this overreaction." (Dr. Walter Willett, Chairman of the Nutrition Department, Harvard School of Public Health; as quoted in The New York Times article, "Does This Goo Make You Groan?" [print]/"A Sweetener with a Bad Rap" [online]; by Melanie Warner; 07/02/06).[32]

"It's basically no different from table sugar. Table sugar is glucose and fructose stuck together. Corn sweeteners are glucose and fructose separated. The body really can't tell them apart ..." (Dr. Marion Nestle, Paulette Goddard Professor of Nutrition, Food Studies, and Public Health, New York University, author of "What to Eat" and "Food Politics").[32]

"The authors of this paper misunderstand chemistry, draw erroneous conclusions and have done a disservice to the public in generating this controversy." (Dr. Michael Jacobsen, Executive Director, Center for Science in Public Interest comparing HFCS to table sugar at the TIME/ABC News Summit on Obesity; 06/03/04).[32]

"HFCS is the chemical and nutritional equivalent of table sugar (sucrose). The two substances have the same calories, the same chemical composition and are metabolized identically. The increase in the prevalence of obesity in the U.S. coincides with the increased use of HFCS and it is tempting for some of the experts to pose the obvious question: Does HFCS cause obesity? We know, of course, that the simultaneous occurrence of two events does not necessarily mean that one caused the other and, in the case of HFCS, it is fair to say that there is no causal relationship between the two. The prevalence of obesity and diabetes is increasing even more rapidly in parts of the world where HFCS is not used in any significant amounts." (Dr. Arthur Frank, M.D., Medical Director, George Washington University Weight Management Program; in the commentary "Carbs and calories, confusion and chaos", published in *The Washington Times*; 12/06/06).[32]

"It was a theory meant to spur science, but it's quite possible that it may be found out not to be true. I don't think there should be a perception that high-fructose corn syrup has caused obesity until we know more." (Dr. Barry M. Popkin, Professor, Department of Nutrition, University of North Carolina at Chapel Hill; as quoted in *The New York Times* article, "Does This Goo Make You Groan?" [print]/"A Sweetener with a Bad Rap" [online]; by Melanie Warner; 07/02/06).[32]

"I don't think it is likely that things would be very different if people consumed increased amounts of either sucrose or high-fructose corn syrup. Over consumption of either sweetener, along with dietary fat and decreased physical activity, could contribute to weight gain." (Dr. Peter J. Havel, Associate Researcher, Department of Nutrition, University of California, Davis; as quoted in *The New York Times* article.)[32]

"Like all nutritive sweeteners, it contains calories. But critics who attack a single ingredient as the sole cause of obesity are wrong and counterproductive. A quixotic search for an easy answer means true solutions to the obesity problem are not being found. (Dr. John S. White, Caloric Sweetener Expert and President of White Technical Research Group; in a letter to the editor published in *The New York Times*; 07/09/06).[32]

SUMMARY

Carbohydrates contain 4 calories per gram and are the number one energy nutrient for the body. Every cell in the body requires carbohydrates in the form of glucose. Carbohydrates can be stored in muscle and liver in the form of glycogen. Glycogen storage in muscle is energy for muscle cells only. Glycogen in the liver can be released into the bloodstream and provide glucose for cells that can not produce their own energy. The amount of glucose in the bloodstream must be controlled within a very narrow range since these cells are susceptible to damage from excess or insufficient glucose. Homeostasis is the term to describe this fine tuning of the body's glucose environment. If glucose is unavailable, the body must produce it (gluconeogenesis) and in the first few days of a fast over 90% of glucose production comes from the breakdown of muscle (gluconeogenic amino acids). To prevent the body from running out of glucose, carbohydrate stores need to be continuously replenished. Absorption rates differ widely depending on the form of the carbohydrate. Large amounts of simple sugars, in the absence of other nutrients known to decrease absorption rate, will force the body to store these rapidly absorbed sugars as fatty acids. Insulin resistance occurs in approximately 25% to 30% of the population. Insulin-resistant individuals need to moderate their carbohydrate intake, not eliminate it.

Fiber is critical for maintaining the health of the gastrointestinal tract. Dangers of low carbohydrate diets which limit fiber include increased risk for GI disorders, and micronutrient deficiencies.

While some studies indicate that small amounts of alcohol may provide health benefits, chronic alcohol consumption can take a serious toll on health.

Sugar and sugar alcohols are each considered nutritive sweeteners because they provide calories when consumed. In the United States, sweeteners fall under the Generally Recognized as Safe (GRAS) list or as food additives under the 1958 Food Additives Amendment to the Federal Food, Drug, and Cosmetic Act.

The five FDA-approved nonnutritive sweeteners are saccharin, aspartame, acesulfame potassium, sucralose, and neotame. Each of these is regulated as a food additive. These sweeteners are evaluated based on their safety, sensory qualities (for example, clean sweet taste, no bitterness, odorless), and stability in various food environments. They are often combined with other nutritive and/or nonnutritive sweeteners to provide volume that they lack on their own and a desired flavor. An Acceptable Daily Intake (ADI) for each additive has been established. The ADI is the amount of food additive that can be consumed daily over a lifetime without appreciable health risk to a person on the basis of all the known facts at the time of the evaluation.

Some controversy has arisen over the use of HFCS as a food additive as manufacturers now use HFCS in an increasing variety of foods, such as breads, cereals, soft drinks, and condiments. Many experts have given their views on the possible side effects of high fructose corn syrup. Many of these experts believe that HFCS is no more harmful that other sugars.

CHAPTER 2 - SAMPLE TEST

1. List three different food sources of carbohydrates.

2. Discuss the role of carbohydrates in energy.

3. Which cells require glucose for energy?

4. Discuss the value of the glycemic index.

5. Define insulin resistance and the metabolic syndrome.

6. Discuss the types of fiber and importance of fiber in the diet.

7. Discuss nutritive and nonnutritive sweeteners.

8. Discuss the controversy surrounding high fructose corn syrup.

REFERENCES

1. http://www.hsph.harvard.edu/nutritionsource/carbohydrates.html

2. Shils, M, V Young. *Modern Nutrition in Health & Disease*, 10th ed. Philadelphia PA: Lea & Febiger, 2005.

3. Guyton, A. *Textbook of Medical Physiology*, 10th ed. Phil: W.B. Saunders Co. 2005.

4. Lehninger, A. *Principles of Biochemistry,* NY: Worth Publishers, Inc, 2004.

5. Slavin, J.L. Dietary fiber: classification, chemical analyses, and food sources, *J of the Amer Dietetic Assoc*, 8:1164-1171, 1987.

6. http://www.diabetes.org/about-diabetes.jsp.

7. Whitney, E, S Rolfes. *Understanding Nutrition,* 8th ed. NY: West Publishing Co. 2005.

8. Brand-Miller, J. *The New Glucose Revolution*. 2003.

9. http://www.active.com/story.cfm?story_id=14047&category=Nutrition.

10. http://www.hsph.harvard.edu/nutritionsource/carbohydrates.html.

11. Sears, B. *Enter the Zone*, NY: HarperCollins Publishers, 1995.

12. Atkins, R. *Dr. Atkins' New Diet Revolution*, NY: National Book Network, 1997.

13. Reaven, G. *Syndrome X,* NY: Simon and Schuster, 2000.

14. http://jama.ama-assn.org/cgi/content/full/295/7/850.

15. Johnson LW, Weinstock RS. The metabolic syndrome: concepts and controversy. Mayo Clinic Proceedings. 2006; 81:1615-20.

16. Harvard Nurses Study, *New England Journal of Medicine*, Jan 1999.

17. Bell, P. Cholesterol-lowering effects of soluble-fiber cereals as part of a prudent diet for patients with mild to moderate hypercholesterolemia, *American Journal of Clinical Nutrition* 52: 1020-1026, 1990.

18. http://www.dietbites.com/Diet-Articles-3/dietary-fiber.html.

19. Berger, K. Et al. Light-tomoderate alcohol consumption and risk of stroke among US male physicians. *New Eng J of Medicine,* 341(2),1557-64, 1999.

20. Smith-Warner, SA et al. Alcohol and breast cancer in women; a polled analysis of cohort studies. *J of the Amer Medical Assoc*, 279(7)535-40, 1998.

21. http://www.medicinenet.com/artificial_sweeteners/article.htm.

22. http://en.wikipedia.org/wiki/Stevia.

23. http://en.wikipedia.org/wiki/High_fructose_corn_syrup.

24. Bray, 2004 & U.S. Department of Agriculture, Economic Research Service, Sugar and Sweetener Yearbook series, Tables 50–52).

25. Nutrition information for HFCS at *The Calorie Counter. http://www.thecaloriecounter.com/Foods/1900/19351/Food.aspx.*

26. http://sugar.lin.go.jp/japan/data/j_html/j_1_01.htm.

27. Archer Daniels Midland: A Case Study in Corporate Welfare. cato.org. Retrieved on July 12, 2007.

28. Diabetes fears over corn syrup in soda. New Scientist (04 September 2007). Retrieved on 2007-11-17.

29. Bantle, John P.; Susan K. Raatz, William Thomas and Angeliki Georgopoulos (November 2000). "Effects of dietary fructose on plasma lipids in healthy subjects". *American Journal of Clinical Nutrition* 72 (5): 1128-1134.

30. http://www.eb2006-online.com/LBApdfs/600540.PDF.

31. http://www.foodproductdesign.com/hotnews/64h1411309.html.

32. Warner, Melanie (July 2, 2006). A Sweetener With a Bad Rap. The New York Times.

33. 7UP, Now 100% Natural Flavors. Dr Pepper/Seven Up (2007). Retrieved on 2007-09-24.

34. http://www.cspinet.org/nah/4_00/stevia.html

Chapter 3
Fats

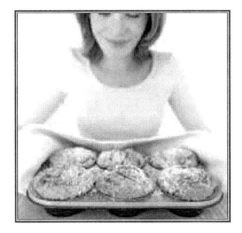

In this chapter we will take a more in-depth look at the biochemistry of fats.   We will examine fats in detail, including digestion, absorption, transport and biochemical roles.

Objectives

After reading and studying this chapter, you should:

1. Be able to describe digestion, absorption, transport and roles of fats, as well as the Recommended Daily Values.

2. Be able to discuss the types of fats and fatty acids.

3. Be able to discuss essential fatty acids and their importance in health.

INTRODUCTION

Fats consist of a wide group of compounds that are generally soluble in organic solvents and largely insoluble in water. Fats are the only essential nutrients that are anhydrous (do not mix with water) and, therefore, cannot be absorbed directly. To be absorbed, they must be emulsified by molecules that can mix with water. Once absorbed, fats must then be packaged to be transported throughout the body. They are packaged in what are known as lipoproteins.

Fats may be either solid or liquid at normal room temperature, depending on their structure and composition. Although the words "oils", "fats" and "lipids" are all used to refer to fats, "oils" is usually used to refer to fats that are liquids at normal room temperature, while "fats" is usually used to refer to fats that are solids at normal room temperature. "Lipids" is used to refer to both liquid and solid fats. The word "oil" is used for any substance that does not mix with water and has a greasy feel, such as petroleum (or crude oil) and heating oil, regardless of its chemical structure.[1]

PHYSIOLOGY

The major fats found in the foods we eat are triglyceride, phospholipid, and cholesterol (a sterol found only in animal products).

Approximately 90% to 95% of the fat in animal products is in the form of triglycerides.[2] The major role of triglycerides is energy. Triglycerides consist of a glycerol molecule and three fatty acids.

Another 5% to 9% of the fat in animal fats is phospholipid. Phospholipids consist of a glycerol molecule, two fatty acids and a phosphate head group. The major roles of phospholipids include membrane structure and immune system function. As a reminder, plant cell membranes are composed of fiber, while animal cell membranes are composed of phospholipids. Because animal cell membranes are composed of lipids, they have the ability to move and communicate with each other.

About 1% of the fat in animal products is cholesterol. Cholesterol is a circular molecule that does not contain fatty acids or glycerol. (Physiological roles of cholesterol will be discussed in the next section.)

Unlike animal products, plant products contain larger amounts of phospholipids, smaller amounts of triglycerides, and no cholesterol.

Triglyceride

Phospholipid

Cholesterol

TRIGLYCERIDES

As already mentioned, triglycerides make up 90 to 95% of the fat in animal products.[2] A glycerol molecule is the backbone of triglycerides and three fatty acids are attached. In nature, the two outside fatty acids prefer to hold a saturated fatty acid, whereas the middle position prefers an essential fatty acid (if available). Beef contains mostly saturated and very little monounsaturated fatty acids in all positions (there are almost no essential fatty acids). Completely hydrogenated fats carry almost 100% saturated fatty acids in all positions. Flax oil and safflower oil must carry essential fatty acids in outside positions because both of these oils contain more than 70% essential fatty acids.[2]

The major role of triglycerides is stored energy. Triglycerides form a layer around the body under the skin for insulation and surrounds organs to protect against shock and injury. Most of the stored fat in the body is triglyceride. One tablespoon of butter has approximately 15 grams of fat, most of which is triglyceride with almost no essential fatty acids present. One tablespoon of flax oil or safflower oil, also approximately 12 to 15 grams of fat (most of which is phospholipid), contains 60% to 75% essential fatty acids (see section on phospholipids).[3]

In addition to obtaining triglycerides from the diet, the body can make triglycerides from excess sugars, hence providing a safety mechanism since high blood levels of sugar can be toxic. The body begins by reducing the sugar to a 2-carbon fragment called acetate. The body makes saturated fatty acids out of these excess acetate fragments by hooking them end to end. Glycerol is then added and the resulting triglyceride is stored as body fat. The body can also make triglycerides from alcohol, fats and proteins.

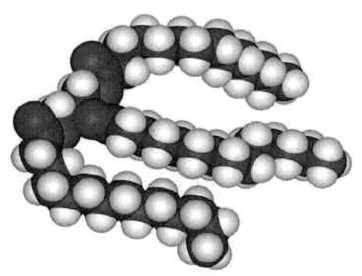

Triglyceride - Taken from Wikipedia

PHOSPHOLIPIDS

Phospholipids (also known as phosphatides) are the second type of fat found in foods. A phospho-lipid also has a glycerol molecule, but has only two fatty acids. The third fatty acid is replaced by a phosphate group.

The phosphate group mixes with water while the fatty acid portion mixes with fat.[2] The phosphate group attached to phospholip-ids is polar and water-soluble, while its fatty acids are oil-soluble. The phospholipids spread out in a thin layer over surfaces of water, and form double-layered membranes that surround every living cell of all living organisms. They also form membranes around subcellular organs (mitochondria, nucleus, lysosomes, etc.). Because of this property, phospholipids are <u>not</u> used as an energy source, but are part of all cell mem-branes. These phospholipid membranes form a barrier. They keep certain molecules out and certain molecules in cells. Also em-bedded within the phospholipid structure are proteins, cholesterol, and vitamin E. Fat-

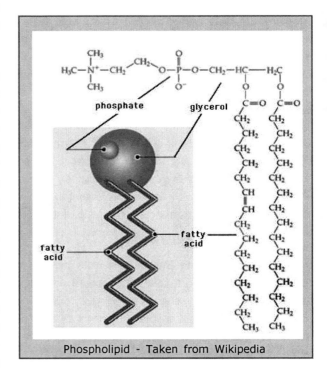

Phospholipid - Taken from Wikipedia

soluble toxic substances such as alcohol, barbiturates, drugs, and carcinogens can dissolve in these membranes and can exert their toxic effects.

Membranes can contain between 20 and 80% phospholipids, depending on the type of cell or or-ganelle.[4] RBC's contain about 45% phospholipids and 55% proteins in their membranes; nerve cell membranes (myelin sheath) contain 80% phospholipids and only 20% proteins, Mitochondrial mem-branes contain 25% phospholipids, while liver cell membranes contain about 50% phospholipids. Membranes account for 1 to 3% of the cell's total weight.[4]

Phospholipids "fluidize" cell membranes. The middle fatty acid of phospholipids is usually an essen-tial fatty acid which, being highly unsaturated, is bent and does not pack tightly. It takes up more space than a straight saturated fatty acid and keeps membranes from hardening. These phospho-lipids also supply the cell with essential fatty acids which are required to make eicosanoids, regula-tors of cell activities (see section on essential fatty acids).[4]

The phosphate groups attached to the phospholipid can have other chemical groups attached, such as choline, inositol, serine ethanolamine.[4] Phosphatidyl choline, or lecithin is the best known phospholipid. Lecithin, (a major constituent of cell membranes) is used by food manufacturers to combine ingredients such as water and oil. Lecithin advocates claim that it is necessary to purchase bottles of lecithin in order to receive the daily dose. This is false. The digestive enzyme lecithinase in the intestine hydrolyzes most of the lecithin before it enters the body. Also, all the lecithin a person needs for building cell membranes is made from scratch in the liver. Therefore, lecithin is not an essential nutrient.[4]

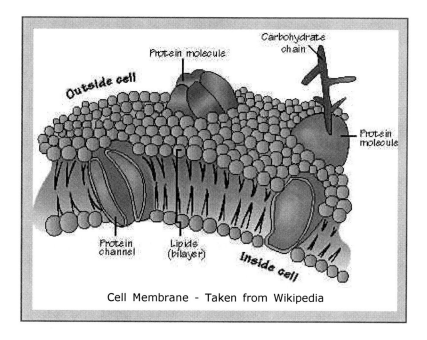

Cell Membrane - Taken from Wikipedia

CHOLESTEROL

Cholesterol is the third type of fat found in animal products. Cholesterol is a sterol. Sterols contain a multiple-ring structure and look different than triglycerides and phospholipids. Sterols do not contain fatty acids; they are circular molecules made from fatty acids. Cholesterol is a hard, waxy substance that melts at 149 degrees centigrade. It is made by the body, and is therefore not an essential nutrient. It is manufactured from simple 2-carbon acetate groups which are derived from the breakdown of sugars, fats, and in rare circumstances proteins. The 2-carbon fragments are hooked end to end until 30 of them are chained together. Each step involves enzymes, the chain is cyclized, and 3 carbons are removed to produce the 27 carbon cholesterol molecule.

Cholesterol is important in biochemistry. It forms part of cell membranes and is the precursor molecule to testosterone, estrogen, bile, and over 30 other steroid hormones. Cholesterol, along with sunlight, provides us with vitamin D. The average human body contains about 150 grams of cholesterol (150,000 mg). Most of this cholesterol is in membranes with about 7 grams in the bloodstream.[4] If a membrane has too little cholesterol it becomes too fluid and falls apart. If there is too much cholesterol, the membrane becomes stiff and breaks. The content of fatty acids in the diet varies hence the fatty acids used to build the basic structure of membranes varies. The more highly unsaturated fatty acids make membranes more fluid, and the more saturated ones make it more "stiff". Cholesterol has the function of compensating for the changes in membrane fluidity, keeping it within narrow limits that assure optimal membrane function. This function is so important that nature has equipped each cell with the ability to synthesize its own membrane cholesterol.[4]

The cells in the body can make varying amounts of cholesterol depending on homeostatic requirements. For example, when someone drinks alcohol, the alcohol dissolves in the membranes, making them more fluid. In response, the cells will manufacture cholesterol, build it into the membrane, and thereby bring the membrane back to its proper (less fluid) state. As the alcohol wears off and the membrane becomes stiffer, no more cholesterol is made and some of the cholesterol in the membrane is removed, again establishing the normal membrane fluidity. The extra cholesterol is then shipped off to the liver to be changed into bile acids (provided the vitamins and minerals necessary for this change are present). The bile acids are transported into the intestine where they aid in digestion of fats and are then removed from the body.[4]

Besides the cells' production of cholesterol, the liver, intestine, adrenal glands, and sex glands all make cholesterol for the other varied functions such as male and female steroid hormones. Testosterone, estrogen, and progesterone are the best known steroid hormones (there are over 30 other steroid hormones made from cholesterol). The adrenal corticosteroid hormones which regulate the body's water balance (through the kidneys) are derived from cholesterol. Cortisone promotes the synthesis of glucose in the flight or fight response to stress; it also suppresses inflammation reactions.

Cholesterol is one of the substances secreted by the glands in the skin and covers/protects the skin against dehydration, cracking, and the wear and tear of the sun, wind, and water.

The more sugars and non essential fatty acids present in the diet, the more pressure there is for the body to produce acetate groups, hence more pressure to make triglycerides and cholesterol.

FATTY ACIDS

Fatty acids can contain between 4 and 28 carbons. The fatty acid component can be saturated or unsaturated.

saturated fatty acid: c-c-c-c-c-c-c-c

monounsaturated fatty acid: c-c=c-c-c

polyunsaturated fatty acid: c-c=c-c-c=

The single lines between the c's (carbon atom) represent a saturated carbon atom (saturated with hydrogen). A saturated fatty acid has all single lines (bonds). The double lines (double bond) between the carbons represent an unsaturated carbon atom—not totally saturated with hydrogen. If there is one double bond the fatty acid is a monounsaturated fatty acid; if there are two or more double bonds the fatty acid is a polyunsaturated fatty acid. Fat that occurs naturally in living matter such as animals and plants is used as food for human consumption and contains varying proportions of saturated and unsaturated fatty acids.

Saturated Fatty Acids

Saturated fatty acids are the simplest of the fatty acids. Saturated fatty acids have no double bonds between the carbon atoms of the fatty acid chain; hence, they are fully saturated with hydrogen atoms. The saturated molecule is straight, has no kinks in it, contains no double bonds, and is slow to react with other chemicals. Saturated fats are popular with manufacturers of processed foods because they are less vulnerable to rancidity and are generally more solid at room temperature than *unsaturated* fats.

There are several kinds of naturally occurring saturated fatty acids, their only difference being the number of carbon atoms - from 1 to 24. Some common examples of saturated fatty acids are butyric acid with 4 carbon atoms (contained in butter), lauric acid with 12 carbon atoms (contained in breast milk, coconut oil, palm oil), myristic acid with 14 carbon atoms (contained in cow milk and dairy products), palmitic acid with 16 carbon atoms (contained in palm oil, hence the name, and meat), and stearic acid with 18 carbon atoms (also contained in meat and cocoa butter).

Foods that contain a high proportion of saturated fat are butter, suet, tallow, lard, coconut oil, cotton-seed oil, and palm kernel oil, dairy products (especially cream and cheese), meat, chocolate, and some prepared foods.[5]

While nutrition labels usually lump them together, the saturated fatty acids appear in different proportions among food groups. Lauric and myristic acids are most commonly found in "tropical" oils (e.g. palm kernel, coconut) and dairy products. The saturated fat in meat, eggs, chocolate and nuts is primarily palmitic and stearic acid.

The body uses saturated fatty acids up to 14 carbons in length for the production of energy. Longer chain saturated fatty acids (14 or more carbons) have melting points higher than body temperatures, are insoluble in water and tend to aggregate or stick together to form droplets or, if hard, plaques.

When intake of these saturated fatty acids is high, they tend to stick together and deposit within cells, within organs, and within the arteries.[6,]

Unsaturated Fatty Acids

An unsaturated fat is a fat or fatty acid in which there are one or more double bonds in the fatty acid chain. A fat molecule is monounsaturated if it contains one double bond, and polyunsaturated if it contains more than one double bond. Where double bonds are formed, hydrogen atoms are eliminated.

Long chain unsaturated fatty acids are used to build cell membranes as part of phospholipids. Their tendency to disperse balances the tendency of saturated fatty acids to aggregate. Both kinds of fatty acids are found in membranes. Unsaturated chains have a lower melting point hence increase the fluidity of cell membranes.

Double bonds in unsaturated fatty acids may be in either a *cis* or *trans* isomer, depending on the geometry of the double bond. In the *cis* conformation hydrogens are on the same side of the double bond, whereas in the *trans* conformation they are on opposite sides (see trans fats).

Natural sources of fatty acids are rich in the cis isomer. In this configuration, the hydrogen atoms on

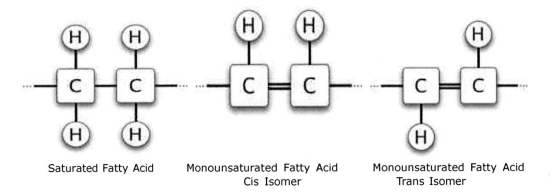

| Saturated Fatty Acid | Monounsaturated Fatty Acid Cis Isomer | Monounsaturated Fatty Acid Trans Isomer |

the carbons involved in the double bond are on the same side of the molecule. The hydrogen atoms repel each other and the fatty acid kinks. The kink changes the shape and the properties of the molecule.

The cis shape determines the way in which the molecule will function in the body. The kinks make it difficult for the fatty acid chains to fit together, hence they do not aggregate. This property of unsaturated fatty acids provides the fluidity needed in membranes. It allows molecules within the membrane the freedom to move, to fulfill their important chemical and transport functions. Unsaturated fatty acids are more <u>unstable</u>, chemically more active and can react with light, air, and other chemical groups. They melt at lower temperatures than saturated fatty acids identical except for the double bond. This makes these fatty acids vulnerable to destruction. Light or air can destroy the double bonds.

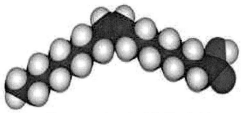
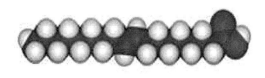

Monounsaturated Fatty Acid   Monounsaturated Fatty Acid
        Cis Isomer   Trans Isomer

Taken from Wikipedia

The body can also add double bonds into the saturated fatty acid chain by removing two hydrogen atoms causing the cis double bond configuration.

Trans Fatty Acids

Trans fat is the common name for a type of unsaturated fat with fatty acids in the "trans" configuration. Trans fats may be monounsaturated or polyunsaturated.

Most trans fats consumed today are industrially created by partially hydrogenating plant oils — a process developed in the early 1900s and first commercialized as Crisco in 1911. The goal of partial hydrogenation is to add hydrogen atoms to unsaturated fats, making them more saturated. These more saturated fats have a higher melting point making them attractive for baking, and extending their shelf-life. Another particular class of trans fats, vaccenic acid occurs naturally in trace amounts in meat and dairy products from ruminants.

Chemically, trans fats are made of the same building blocks as non-trans fats, but have a different arrangement. In trans fatty acid molecules, the hydrogen atoms bonded to pair(s) of doubly bonded carbon atoms (characteristic of all unsaturated fats) are in the *trans* rather than the *cis* arrangement.

In the trans configuration, hydrogen atoms on the carbons involved in the double bonds are on opposite sides of the molecule resulting in a non-kinked configuration. The molecule now has the same straight configuration of saturated fatty acids, and hence produces many of the same arterial damaging effects as saturated fatty acids. The trans configuration is more stable, it cannot be changed back to a cis configuration, and cannot complete the functions of the cis form. Hence, trans fatty acids are useful only as energy, and not in cell membrane structure or immune functions. If trans fatty acids are the only fatty acids available they can become embedded into cell membranes. This reaction changes the fluidity of the cell membrane. Recent research hypothesizes that this change in fluidity may lead to insulin resistance.

Trans fatty acids are formed when hydrogen is added to unsaturated fats. In the process of hydrogenation, an oil which contains unsaturated fatty acids in their natural cis state are reacted at high temperatures with hydrogen gas in the presence of a metal catalyst for 6 to 8 hours. If the process is brought to completion (completely hydrogenated), all of the hydrogen bonds in the oil are saturated with hydrogen. The fatty acids that result contain no double bonds, and have no essential fatty acid activity. This fat does not spoil, (is dead) and has a long shelf life. The completely hydrogenated fat can be used for frying, baking and cooking without being further chemically altered; however, these fats still add to increased risk of heart disease.

When the process of hydrogenation is not brought to completion partial hydrogenation occurs (the process is stopped when a desired consistency is achieved). The product can contain dozens of intermediate substances. Double bonds may turn from cis to trans, double bonds may shift, and fragments may be produced. Since the hydrogenation occurs at random, it is impossible to predict the outcome. Partial hydrogenation is the process by which margarines, shortenings, and shortening oils are made.

Unlike other dietary fats, trans fats are neither required nor beneficial for health[7] and in fact, the consumption of trans fats increases one's risk of coronary heart disease[8] by raising levels of "bad" LDL cholesterol and lowering levels of "good" HDL cholesterol.[9] Health authorities worldwide recommend that consumption of trans fat be reduced to trace amounts. Trans fats from partially hydrogenated oils are generally considered to be more of a health risk than naturally occurring oils.[10]

Trans fatty acids have been shown to increase blood cholesterol levels by as much as 15% and triglycerides levels by as much as 47%. Recent research indicates that trans fatty acids are eaten in much larger amounts than saturated fats, and is now a greater risk factor for heart disease than saturated fats.

ESSENTIAL FATTY ACIDS

Two unsaturated fatty acids are essential; i.e. the body cannot make them; hence they must be obtained from food for life to be sustained. These two unsaturated fatty acids, linoleic and linolenic acid, contain 18 carbons. Linoleic acid has two double bonds and is an omega 6 fatty acid; while linolenic has three double bonds and is an omega 3 fatty acid. Because of the double bonds, both essential fatty acids are easily destroyed. Linolenic acid is even more sensitive to destruction than linoleic acid because it contains three double bonds.   Linoleic acid is involved in the production of hemoglobin. Both essential fatty acids have a function in holding oxygen in cell membranes, where they acts as a barrier to foreign organisms. These foreign organisms will not thrive in the presence of oxygen. Both essential fatty acids form a structural part of all cell membranes. They hold proteins in the membrane by the attractive force of their double bonds; hence, they are involved in the traffic of substances in and out of cells. They are also structural parts of subcellular organelle membranes within the cell.[6]

Essential fatty acids are precursors to hormone-like substances called eicosanoids. Eicosanoids exert important effects on the immune system, cardiovascular system, reproductive and central nervous system. All cells can form eicosanoids, but tissues differ in enzyme profile and hence in the prod-

Recommended Intake of Essential Fatty Acids		
	Men	Women
Linoleic Acid	17 grams	12 grams
Linolenic Acid	1.6 grams	1.1 grams

ucts they form.[6] Eicosanoids are not stored and are synthesized in response to immediate cellular need. The production of eicosanoids is complex and further discussion is beyond the scope of this course. It is important to note, however, that fatty acid deficiency can lead to immune system dysfunction, as well as reproductive and central nervous system dysfunction.[2]   Individuals deficient in essential fatty acids (it takes a long time to become deficient) will have red rashy skin, compromised immune system (lots of colds and flu), and eventually liver damage.

Controversy remains concerning daily requirements of essential fatty acids for optimum health. The amount needed varies, depending on physical activity, stress, nutritional state, and hormonal differences. Optimum levels are estimated to be in the range of 3 to 10% of daily caloric intake, or 9 to 30 grams per day.

The best sources of essential fatty acids are oils of certain seeds and nuts. The richest food sources containing both essential fatty acids are flax seed and flax oil. Rich sources of linoleic acid include canola oil, safflower oil, sesame seed and oil, sunflower seed and oil, soybean and oil, and walnuts. The best food sources of linoleic acid are flax seed and flax oil; smaller amounts are found in canola oil, soybean and soybean oil.

It is important to note that because essential fatty acids are easily destroyed, the oils must be reasonably fresh. If fresh oils are not available, the seeds are the most nutritionally complete way to obtain the essential fatty acids. Flax oil spoils when exposed to light, oxygen, or heat, and care needs to be taken in pressing, filling, storing, and shipping of this oil. The oil must be less than 30 days old, stored in a dark, unopened bottle, and once opened, must be discarded after 30 days. Fish, while not containing essential fatty acids directly, contain important molecules made from fatty acids. Eicosapentaenoic acid (EPA) is a 20 carbon omega 3 fatty acid with 5 double bonds, and docasahexaenoic acid (DHA) is a 22 carbon omega 3 fatty acid with 6 double bonds. Both can be manufactured by the body from linolenic acid. EPA and DHA being highly unsaturated, have a strong urge to disperse, have extremely low melting points and help to disperse aggregation of the saturated fatty acids in cell membranes. EPA also produces a family of eicosanoids known as prostaglandins--the PG3 series--which have potent anti-clotting properties.[4] Fatty fish such as salmon, sardines, mackerel, trout, and eel are excellent sources of EPA and DHA.

Healthy Fat

Some fats produce health benefits while others do not. To understand which types of fats are heart healthy one must understand the role of prostaglandins. A prostaglandin is any member of a group of lipid compounds that are derived enzymatically from fatty acids and have important functions in the human body. Every prostaglandin contains 20 carbon atoms, including a 5-carbon ring. They are mediators and have a variety of strong physiological effects.[11]

A major effect of prostaglandins is control of platelet aggregation. Platelets, along with red cells and plasma, form a major portion of both human and animal blood. Platelets are actually fragments of the cells in bone marrow, called megakaryocytes. Under hormonal control, platelets break off the megakaryocytes and enter the blood stream, where they circulate for about 10 days before ending their short lives in the spleen. Specifically, platelets provide the necessary hormones and proteins for coagulation.[11]

Collagen is released when the lining of a blood vessel is damaged. The platelet recognizes collagen and begins to work on coagulating the blood by forming a kind of stopper, so further damage to the blood vessel is prevented. However, too much clotting of the blood can lead to formation of blood clots that can cause stroke.[11]

Three major types of prostaglandins found in platelets are: Series 1 prostaglandins; Series 2 prostaglandins; and Series 3 prostaglandins. Series 1 prostaglandins are formed from plant products such as flax, safflower, sunflower, sesame, soybean, and walnut. These prostaglandins are less inflammatory and anti-aggregating. In other words these prostaglandins reduce clotting. Series 2 prostaglandins are formed from animal products. Series 2 prostaglandins are more inflammatory and aggregating. These prostaglandins increase clotting. And finally, Series 3 prostaglandins are formed from plant products and fish. These prostaglandins are the least aggregating and inflammatory. Hence Series 3 prostaglandins produce the least amount of clotting and are the "heart healthiest".

When choosing essential fats for optimum health, one should choose plant products and fish.

ESSENTIAL FATTY ACIDS

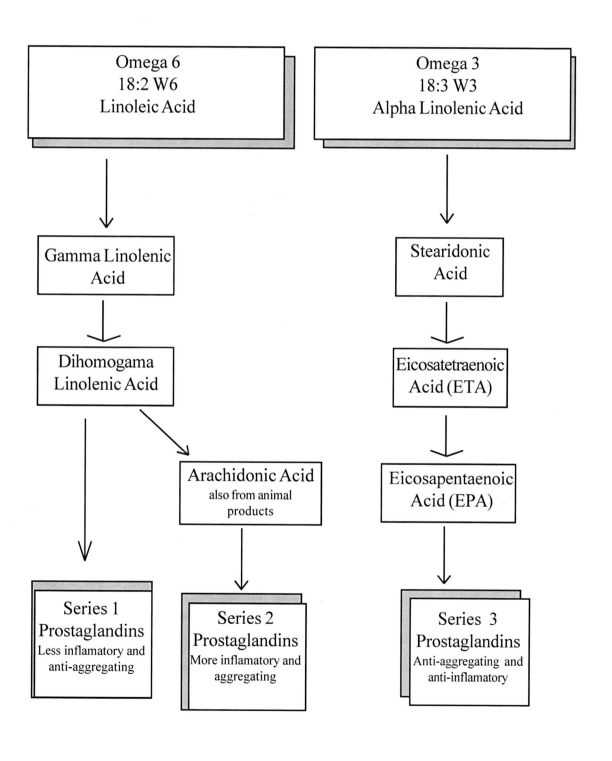

Heating Fats

Free radicals are formed when vegetable oils are heated. Trans fats are also formed, but the process becomes significant only when the oil is heated at very high temperatures and for prolonged periods (which occurs in some restaurants where the oil is reused). Reheating the oil is especially damaging. Various mutagens occur in the food being fried which can damage human DNA and increase cancer risk. When exposed to extreme heating, the highly polyunsaturated oils produce the highest levels of trans fats and free radicals. Olive oil and canola oil are less susceptible to oxidation and are healthier choices when cooking. It is true that partially hydrogenated oils and highly saturated fats (butter, coconut oil) are damaged less by heating, but they are already heart damaging before heating and are unhealthy choices.[12]

Mercury in Fish

Fish and shellfish are an important part of a healthy diet. They also contain high-quality protein, are low in saturated fat, and contain omega-3 fatty acids. A well-balanced diet that includes a variety of fish and shellfish can contribute to heart health. So everyone should include fish or shellfish in their diets due to the many nutritional benefits.[13]

However, nearly all fish and shellfish contain traces of mercury. For most people, the risk from mercury by eating fish and shellfish is not a health concern. Yet, some fish and shellfish contain higher levels of mercury that may harm an unborn baby or young child's developing nervous system. The risks from mercury in fish and shellfish depend on the amount of fish and shellfish eaten and the levels of mercury in the fish and shellfish. Therefore, the Food and Drug Administration (FDA) and the Environmental Protection Agency (EPA) are advising women who may become pregnant, pregnant women, nursing mothers, and young children to avoid some types of fish and eat fish and shellfish that are lower in mercury.[13]

By following these 3 recommendations for selecting and eating fish or shellfish, women and young children will receive the benefits of eating fish and shellfish and be confident that they have reduced their exposure to the harmful effects of mercury.[13]

- Do not eat Shark, Swordfish, King Mackerel, or Tilefish because they contain high levels of mercury.
- Eat up to 12 ounces (2 average meals) a week of a variety of fish and shellfish that are lower in mercury.
- Five of the most commonly eaten fish that are low in mercury are shrimp, canned light tuna, salmon, pollock, and catfish.
- Another commonly eaten fish, albacore ("white") tuna has more mercury than canned light tuna.

So, when choosing your two meals of fish and shellfish, you may eat up to 6 ounces (one average meal) of albacore tuna per week.

Check local advisories about the safety of fish caught by family and friends in your local lakes, rivers, and coastal areas. If no advice is available, eat up to 6 ounces (one average meal) per week of fish you catch from local waters, but don't consume any other fish during that week.

Follow these same recommendations when feeding fish and shellfish to your young child, but serve smaller portions. You can approximate your intake of mercury by using the mercury calculator at: http://www.nrdc.org/health/effects/mercury/index.asp?gclid=CK3L86eNgJECFSG8GgodIzGjGg.

PCB's in Fish

Headlining the good news has been salmon, one of several species high in omega-3 fatty acids. It seems that salmon may decrease the risk of coronary artery disease and help lower blood pressure.[14] A three-ounce serving of salmon provides half of the weekly dietary allowance of omega-3 oils. Two servings of fish every week, each about the size of a deck of cards, offer protection to those at risk of heart disease, according to the American Heart Association.[14] But salmon has been shown to have high levels of PCB's. As consumers eat more and more salmon, the fishing industry has struggled to keep up with demand. One of the solutions has been the advent of farmed fish. Initially, farming fish, particularly the high-profile salmon, seemed the answer to providing sufficient quantities of fish for health-conscious Americans. More fish could be produced at lower prices on a local level. Farmed fish would be healthier for consumers, as polluted oceans and waterways threatened the quality of the fish.[14] But salmon and other fish produced may not be as healthful as was once hoped. News reports and scientific studies vary widely in opinions of the safety of eating farmed salmon vs wild. On one side are the proponents of farmed salmon and on the other are the environmentalist groups.[14]

The PCB's, it appears, are introduced through farming practices and via the feed used to grow the salmon in captivity. Farm raised fish are fed pellets rich in fish oils. Because PCBs are stored in fat, the oil-rich feed pellets harbor concentrated amounts of PCBs. A controlled diet and an environment that restricts natural movement mean that farmed salmon usually are fattier than those caught in the wild. More fat means more potential for elevated levels of PCBs.[14]

How much PCB is allowable? The current Federal Drug Administration limits for PCBs in fish are 2 ppm (parts per million.) These standards, however, have not been updated since 1984. The stricter, 1999 Environmental Protection Agency recommendations are that no more than 8 ounces a month of fish with PCB levels of between .024 and .048 ppm should be eaten. The average level of PCBs in salmon is .027 ppm.[14]

Three years ago, the Environmental Working Group reported that farmed salmon sold in the United States contained 16 times the amount of PCBs found in wild caught salmon. In 2004, Science Journal reported 10 times the amounts of toxins in farmed salmon as that of wild caught salmon.[14] Toxins in wild salmon can vary based on where it is caught. Wild salmon caught in the vicinity of fish farms have shown increased levels of mercury in their flesh, according to an April 2006 article from the American Chemical Society.[14] Further confusing the issue, salmon marketed as "organic" has shown up in supermarket fish cases across the country, even though organic standards for the seafood industry have not yet been set by the United States Department of Agriculture.[14]

Should fish be eliminated from the diet? According to Nancy Crevier, PCBs occur in many other foods that are part of the daily diet. Meat, milk, and other dairy products can contain far higher percentages of contaminants than farmed or wild caught fish. And because most Americans eat larger portions of these foods more frequently, toxins in the diet are more likely to come from these than from the consumption of fish.[14] Totally eliminating fish from the diet because of perceived dangers could lead to health consequences that outweigh the alternatives. The facts remain that all salmon is lower in saturated fats than red meat. All salmon are an excellent source of omega-3 fatty acids. As with so many other choices in the modern world, a moderate approach to fish consumption is key to reaping the benefits.[14]

According to experts at Tufts University, Center for Science in the Public Interest and University of California Berkeley to reduce your exposure to PCBs, trim fat from fish before cooking. Also, choose broiling, baking, or grilling over frying, as these cooking methods allow the PCB-laden fat to cook off the fish. When possible, choose wild and canned Alaskan salmon instead of farmed, and eat farmed salmon no more than once a month.

Fresh versus Frozen

The term 'fresh' in the seafood industry implies that the fish has never been frozen, from catch to market to consumer. It has been kept in a chilled state until it ends up with the final consumer, you. In reality, the term fresh should equate with Quality. Certainly a fish just caught and consumed that same day would be very high in quality if caught from the right waters. However, consumers should be asking, "When and Where was the fish caught? The California Sea Grant program, a cooperative extension of the University of California offers consumer tips for purchasing high quality seafood. Consumers should base their seafood purchases on quality. Frozen seafood can be superior in quality to fresh products. Many fish and shellfish are "flash frozen" within hours of harvest. It might take several days for the same seafood to make it to your local seafood dealer as "fresh". With recent technological advances, fishing fleets are able to clean and flash-freeze fish virtually moments after they are caught. Flash-freezing freezes fish instantly, in as little as 3 seconds. The process freezes the water inside fish tissues, thus preserving juices and maximizing flavor and texture when cooked. Modern fishing trawlers have become virtual fishing factories at sea. The seafood they harvest is cleaned, processed and flash frozen (minimum temperature of -40°F) aboard ship within 2 hours of catch. Quality and freshness are maintained because the seafood is packed and shipped frozen, held in sub-zero freezers, and never thawed. The seafood is kept in optimum condition during its trip to distributors. There is never a need to ask the questions you would ask about "fresh" seafood: how long it traveled to distributors, whether it was kept cold enough in route to maintain its flavor and safety, or how long it has been on ice.[16,17,18,19] Roger Fitzgerald, editor of Seafood Leader, states: "A fish that's good - unspoiled - is one that looks, tastes and smells like it just came out of the water. The issue isn't whether a fish is frozen or fresh, but whether it's spoiled or unspoiled."

To determine if a fish has been properly frozen, as with fresh fish, check its appearance. It should be somewhat shiny and have no white freezer-burn spots. It should be hard as a rock, showing no evidence of previous defrosting. And always remember food safety. Check fresh fish carefully before buying (bruised or brown spots indicate decomposition, which may mean that bacteria are present), or buy fish that was frozen immediately after it was caught and stored frozen before it came to the market. Cook fish and shellfish thoroughly. Handle raw fish as you would handle other raw meat products. Take care not to contaminate cooked food or vegetables with the utensils used to cook raw fish, and wash utensils and hands thoroughly in between handling.

DIGESTION OF FATS

Digestion of fat begins in the stomach, very little breakdown occurs in the mouth.[2]

Mouth: No digestion of fats occurs in the mouth.

Stomach: In the stomach, fat floats as a layer above the other components of swallowed food. As a result, little digestion takes place. Mixing does occur; and enzymes that can split fats into their components are present, but the enzymes are inactive in stomach acids.

Small Intestines: In the small intestines a hormone, cholecystokinin, signals the gall bladder to release bile which emulsifies the fat. The liver manufactures bile acids from cholesterol, and the gallbladder stores the bile until called for by cholecystokinin. The churning action of the intestines mixes the fat with bile. The fat is emulsified; i.e. broken down to tiny droplets.

ABSORPTION OF FATS

Fats, not the bile acid, are absorbed into the cells of the small intestine. The melting point of triglycerides and phospholipids is important for intestinal absorption. During digestion the fatty acids are separated from the glycerol component by enzymes. Typically the fatty acids are removed and absorbed individually. However, often the middle fatty acid is not removed and the glycerol is absorbed with this fatty acid.   The fatty acid on the middle position of the triglyceride (mono and polyunsaturated fatty acids with lower melting points) is easily absorbed after digestion as monoglycerides even if normally poorly absorbed when present as free fatty acid. This mechanism assures greater absorption of the essential fatty acids which are preferentially attached to the number two position. Attached molecules are removed from cholesterol, and then the cholesterol is absorbed.[2]

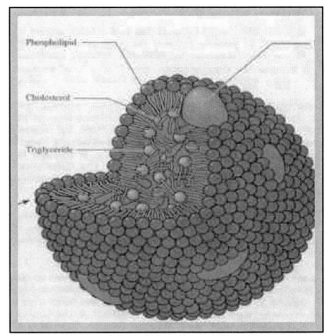

Lipoprotein - Taken from Wikipedia

Absorption of fats requires bile acids which surround the fats and makes them water soluble. Once absorbed, the fats must be reassembled to be transported throughout the body.

TRANSPORT OF FATTY ACIDS AND CHOLESTEROL

Once in the intestinal cell, the fatty acids and glycerol are then reassembled.   As previously stated, fats do not mix with water and must be made water soluble to be transported.   The packaging systems that transport fats are known as lipoproteins.   Lipoproteins are not a type of fat, but are packaging systems that transport fats.[3]

The handling of lipoproteins in the body is referred to as lipoprotein metabolism. It is divided into two pathways, exogenous and endogenous, depending in large part on whether the lipoproteins in question are composed chiefly of dietary (exogenous) lipids or whether they originated in the liver (endogenous).[15]

Exogenous pathway[15]

Epithelial cells lining the small intestines readily absorb lipids from the diet. These lipids, including fatty acids and cholesterol, are assembled into chylomicrons. These chylomicrons are secreted from the intestinal epithelial cells into the lymphatic circulation because they are too large to enter the bloodstream.   As they circulate through the lymphatic vessels, they bypass the liver circulation and are drained elsewhere into the bloodstream.

In the bloodstream, HDL particles donate proteins to the chylomicron; the chylomicron is now considered mature. An enzyme (LPL) on endothelial cells lining the blood vessels catalyzes a reaction that ultimately releases glycerol and fatty acids from the chylomicrons.   Glycerol and fatty acids can be absorbed in tissues, especially adipose and muscle, for energy and storage.

Endogenous pathway[15]

The liver is another important source of lipoproteins, principally VLDL. Triglyceride and cholesterol are assembled to form VLDL particles.   VLDL particles are released into the bloodstream.

As in chylomicron metabolism, VLDL particles require proteins from HDL to become mature.   Again like chylomicrons, VLDL particles circulate and encounter LPL on endothelial cells causing hydrolysis of the VLDL particle and the release of glycerol and fatty acids. These products can also be absorbed by peripheral tissues, principally adipose and muscle. The hydrolyzed VLDL particles are now called VLDL remnants or intermediate density lipoproteins (IDLs).   IDL's are hydrolyzed and become LDL which contain a relatively high cholesterol content.

LDL circulates and is absorbed by the liver and peripheral cells.   LDL can bind to cells and release its contents into cells.

LDL and VLDL circulate through the body depositing triglycerides to all cells (muscle, fat, etc.).   These cells also take up cholesterol, fatty acids, and phosphate to build new membranes, make hormones, etc.   Most of the triglycerides are taken up by fat cells, although muscle cells can take up and store small amounts.   The VLDL and LDL remnants are removed by the liver.   High levels of LDL and cholesterol damage arteries and increase risk for CVD.

HDL removes fats that have been released from cells and returns them to the liver for recycling or removal.   High levels of HDL are protective and decrease risk for disease.[2]

To determine disease risk the total cholesterol level is divided by the HDL level. If the ratio is 4.5 or less there is no increased risk for disease.[2]

Example: Total cholesterol is 220 and HDL is 35
220/35 = 6.29 6.29 is considered high risk

Cholesterol
Desirable < 200 mg/dl
Borderline High 200 to 239 mg/dl
high > 240 mg/dl

HDL
40 mg/dl or less indicates risk

RATIO
Total cholesterol/HDL > 4.5 indicates risk

LDL
Desirable < 130 mg/dl
Borderline High 130 to 159 mg/dl
high > 160 mg/dl

Triglyceride
> 200 mg/dl may indicate risk

SUMMARY

Fats consist of a wide group of compounds that are generally soluble in organic solvents and largely insoluble in water. Fats may be either solid or liquid at normal room temperature, depending on their structure and composition.

The major fats found in the foods we eat are triglyceride, phospholipid, and cholesterol (a sterol found only in animal products). Approximately 90% to 95% of the fat in animal products is in the form of triglycerides.[7] The major role of triglycerides is energy. Triglycerides consist of a glycerol molecule and three fatty acids.

Phospholipids (also known as phosphatides) are a second type of fat found in foods. About 5% to 9% of fat in animal products is phospholipid. A phospholipid also has a glycerol molecule, but has only two fatty acids. The third fatty acid is replaced by a phosphate group. The major roles of phospholipids include membrane structure and immune system function.

About 1% of the fat in animal products is cholesterol. Cholesterol is a circular molecule that does not contain fatty acids or glycerol.

Fatty acids can be saturated, monounsaturated, or polyunsaturated. Saturated fatty acids are the simplest of the fatty acids. Saturated fatty acids have no double bonds between the carbon atoms of the fatty acid chain; hence, they are fully saturated with hydrogen atoms. An unsaturated fat is a fat or fatty acid in which there are one or more double bonds in the fatty acid chain. A fat molecule is monounsaturated if it contains one double bond, and polyunsaturated if it contains more than one double bond. Where double bonds are formed, hydrogen atoms are eliminated.

Chemically, trans fats are made of the same building blocks as non-trans fats, but have a different arrangement. In trans fatty acid molecules, the hydrogen atoms bonded to pair(s) of doubly bonded carbon atoms (characteristic of all unsaturated fats) are in the *trans* rather than the *cis* arrangement. Trans fats occur when hydrogen is added to unsaturated fatty acids transforming them from a cis configuration into a trans configuration.

Unlike other dietary fats, trans fats are neither required nor beneficial for health[7] and in fact, the consumption of trans fats increases one's risk of coronary heart disease[8] by raising levels of "bad" LDL cholesterol and lowering levels of "good" HDL cholesterol.[9] Health authorities worldwide recommend that consumption of trans fat be reduced to trace amounts. Trans fats from partially hydrogenated oils are generally considered to be more of a health risk than naturally occurring oils.[10]

Two fatty acids are essential, linoleic and linolenic. The best sources of essential fatty acids are fish, oils of certain seeds and nuts.

A prostaglandin is any member of a group of lipid compounds that are derived enzymatically from fatty acids and have important functions in the human body. A major effect of prostaglandins is control of platelet aggregation. Platelets, along with red cells and plasma, form a major portion of both human and animal blood. Platelets are actually fragments of the cells in bone marrow, called megakaryocytes. Under hormonal control, platelets break off the megakaryocytes and enter the blood stream, where they circulate for about 10 days before ending their short lives in the spleen. Specifically, platelets provide the necessary hormones and proteins for coagulation.[11]   When choosing essential fats for optimum health, one should choose plant products and fish.

Fish and shellfish are an important part of a healthy diet. They also contain high-quality protein, are low in saturated fat, and contain omega-3 fatty acids. A well-balanced diet that includes a variety of fish and shellfish can contribute to heart health. So everyone should include fish or shellfish in their diets due to the many nutritional benefits.[13] But salmon and other fish produced may not be as healthful as was once hoped. News reports and scientific studies vary widely in opinions of the safety of eating farmed salmon vs wild. On one side are the proponents of farmed salmon and on the other are the environmentalist groups.[14] Totally eliminating fish from the diet because of perceived dangers could lead to health consequences that outweigh the alternatives. The facts remain that all salmon is lower in saturated fats than red meat. All salmon are an excellent source of omega-3 fatty acids, too. As with so many other choices in the modern world, a moderate approach to fish consumption is key to reaping the benefits.[14]

According to experts at Tufts University, Center for Science in the Public Interest and University of California Berkeley to reduce your exposure to PCBs, trim fat from fish before cooking. Also, choose broiling, baking, or grilling over frying, as these cooking methods allow the PCB-laden fat to cook off the fish. When possible, choose wild and canned Alaskan salmon instead of farmed, and eat farmed salmon no more than once a month.

Many fish and shellfish are "flash frozen" within hours of harvest. It might take several days for the same seafood to make it to your local seafood dealer as "fresh". With recent technological advances, fishing fleets are able to clean and flash-freeze fish virtually moments after they are caught. There is never a need to ask the questions you would ask about "fresh" seafood: how long it traveled to distributors, whether it was kept cold enough in route to maintain its flavor and safety, or how long it has been on ice.

Absorption of fats requires bile acids which surround the fats and makes them water soluble. Once absorbed, the fats must be reassembled to be transported throughout the body.

Free radicals are indeed formed when vegetable oils are heated. Trans fats are also formed, but the process becomes significant only when the oil is heated at very high temperatures and for prolonged periods (which occurs in some restaurants where the oil is reused). Reheating the oil is especially damaging. Formation of various mutagens occurs in the food being fried, which can damage human DNA and increase cancer risk. When exposed to extreme heating, the highly polyunsaturated oils produce the highest levels of trans fats and free radicals. Olive oil and canola oil are less susceptible to oxidation and are healthier choices when it comes to cooking. It is true that partially hydrogenated oils and highly saturated fats (butter, coconut oil) are damaged less by heating, but they are already heart damaging before heating and are unhealthy choices.[12]

CHAPTER 3 - SAMPLE TEST

1. List two other roles for fats in addition to providing energy.

2. Which form of dietary fat is stored in the fat cell, and which form is part of all cell membranes?

3. What are trans fatty acids?

4. Name the essential fatty acids and discuss their importance in health.

5. Discuss mercury and PCB's in fish.

6. Discuss digestion, absorption, and transportation of fats.

REFERENCES

1. Wikipedia, The Free Encyclopedia, *Fats*. Jan. 2008.

2. Whitney, E, S Rolfes. *Understanding Nutrition,* 8th ed. NY: West Publishing Co., 2005.

3. Shils, et al. *Modern Nutrition in Health & Disease*, 10th ed. Philadelphia PA: Lea & Febiger, 2005.

4. Lehninger, A. *Principles of Biochemistry Fourth Edition,* NY: Worth Publishers, Inc, 2004.

5. http://www.dietaryfiberfood.com/fat-saturated.php.

6. Erasmus,U. *Fats and Oils*, Canada: Alive Books, 1991.

7. Food and nutrition board, institute of medicine of the national academies (2005). *Dietary Reference Intakes for Energy, Carbohydrate, Fiber, Fat, Fatty Acids, Cholesterol, Protein, and Amino Acids (Macronutrients)*. National Academies Press, 423.

8. Food and nutrition board, institute of medicine of the national academies (2005). *Dietary Reference Intakes for Energy, Carbohydrate, Fiber, Fat, Fatty Acids, Cholesterol, Protein, and Amino Acids (Macronutrients)*. National Academies Press, 504.

9. Trans fat: Avoid this cholesterol double whammy. Mayo Foundation for Medical Education and Research (MFMER).. Retrieved on 2007-12-10.

10. Mozaffarian D, Katan MB, Ascherio A, Stampfer MJ, Willett WC (April 2006). "Trans Fatty Acids and Cardiovascular Disease". *New England Journal of Medicine* **354** (15): 1601–1613. PMID 16611951.

11. Wikipedia, The Free Encyclopedia, *Prostaglandins*. Jan. 2008.

12. University of CA, Berkely Wellness Letter, *Heating Oils*, Aug 2000.

13. http://www.epa.gov/waterscience/fishadvice/advice.html.

14. http://www.ewg.org/node/18797, Sept 2006.

15. Wikipedia, The Free Encyclopedia, *Lipoproteins*. Jan. 2008.

16. "America's fish: fair or foul?" Consumer Reports, February 2001.

17. University of California, the United States Department of Agriculture, and the United States Department of Commerce cooperating.

18. Alaska Sea Grant Marine Advisory Program, John P Doyle.

19. The Complete Guide to Buying and Cooking Fish, Bittman, Mark (Macmillan, 1994).

Chapter 4
Proteins

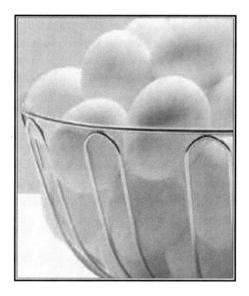

In this chapter we will take a more in depth look at the biochemistry of proteins. We will examine proteins in detail, including digestion, absorption, transport and importance in health.

Objectives

After reading and studying this chapter, you should:

1. Be able to describe digestion, absorption, transport and roles of proteins.

2. Be able to discuss the types of proteins.

3. Be able to discuss amino acids and roles in metabolism.

4. Be able to discuss essential amino acids and their importance in health.

5. Be able to discuss biological consequences of nitrogen toxicity.

6. Be able to discuss protein quality.

INTRODUCTION

Proteins are large organic compounds made of amino acids. Like other biological macromolecules proteins are essential parts of organisms and participate in every process within cells. Through the process of digestion, humans break down ingested protein into free amino acids that are then used in metabolism.

The words protein, polypeptide, and peptide are a little ambiguous and can overlap in meaning. Protein is generally used to refer to the complete biological molecule in a stable conformation, whereas peptide is generally reserved for a short amino acid chain often lacking a stable 3-dimensional structure. However, the boundary between the two is ill-defined and usually lies near 20-30 residues.[1] Polypeptide can refer to any single linear chain of amino acids, usually regardless of length, but often implies an absence of a defined conformation.

Amino acids are the building blocks of proteins. A protein forms via the condensation of amino acids to form a chain of amino acid "residues" linked by peptide bonds. Proteins are defined by their unique sequence of amino acid residues; this sequence is the primary structure of the protein. Just as the letters of the alphabet can be combined to form an almost endless variety of words, amino acids can be linked in varying sequences to form a huge variety of proteins.

Protein Foods

Item	Serving Size	Protein (g)
Meat, poultry, fish	3 oz. cooked	21
Milk	8 oz.	10
Yogurt	8 oz.	8
Cottage cheese	4 oz.	13
Eggs (whites)	1 large	4
Beans, dried peas, lentils	1/2 cup cooked	7

PHYSIOLOGY

Proteins are linear molecules built from 20 different amino acids. All amino acids possess common structural features, including a carbon to which an amino group (NH2) is bonded. The amino acids in a polypeptide chain are linked by peptide bonds. Once linked in the protein chain, an individual amino acid is called a residue, and the linked series of carbon, nitrogen, and oxygen atoms are known as the main chain or protein backbone.[1]

Proteins are assembled from amino acids using information encoded in genes. Each protein has its own unique amino acid sequence that is specified by the nucleotide sequence of the gene encoding this protein.[2]

Proteins are classified according to their structure. Some proteins are large globular compounds and are found in tissue fluids. Enzymes, protein hormones, hemoglobin, myoglobin, globulins and albumins of blood are all globular proteins. Other proteins form long chains bound together in a parallel fashion, and are called fibrous proteins. These consist of long, folded chains of amino acids and are the proteins of connective tissue and elastic tissue including collagen, elastin, and keratin.[2]

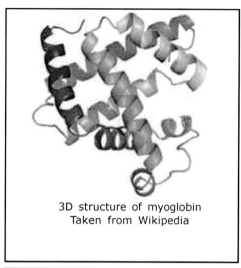

3D structure of myoglobin
Taken from Wikipedia

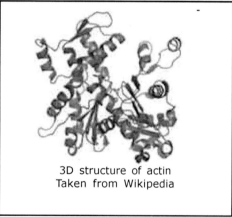

3D structure of actin
Taken from Wikipedia

The extraordinary structures of proteins enable them to play more versatile roles in the body than carbohydrates or lipids.[2] The body uses proteins to build and repair all of its tissues. From the moment of conception the body uses proteins to manufacture its cells. In building bones, cells lay down a matrix of the protein collagen. Collagen also serves as the mending material in torn tissue, forming scars to hold the separated parts together. Ligaments and tendons are also made of collagen.[2] New cells are constantly growing from underneath the skin which requires proteins. The cells that manufacture hair and fingernails are also constantly synthesizing new protein.

GI tract cells live for only three days and must be replaced; the body constantly deposits protein into new cells that replace the lost ones.[3]

Many immune system molecules are proteins. Antibodies are proteins and are produced in response to the presence of foreign particles that invade the body. A foreign particle may be part of a bacterium, a virus, or a toxin. Once the body has manufactured antibodies against an invader, it remembers how to make them. Hence, the next time the body encounters that same invader, it will produce antibodies even more quickly.

Growth hormone, insulin and glucagon are also proteins, as are many other hormones. Hormones are messenger molecules. Various glands in the body secrete hormones in response to changes in the internal environment. The blood carries the hormones to their target tissues, where they elicit the appropriate responses to restore normal conditions. Insulin and glucagon help regulate the concentration of blood glucose. Thyroid hormone, another protein, regulates the body's metabolic rate. The light sensitive pigments in the cells of the retina (of the eyes) are protein molecules called opsin.[3]

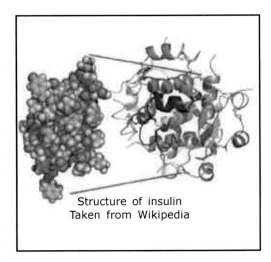

Structure of insulin
Taken from Wikipedia

Some proteins are transport molecules. These proteins specialize in moving molecules into and out of cells. They reside in cell membranes and work to maintain equilibrium in the surrounding fluids. Most of these proteins cannot leave the cell membrane. Almost every water-soluble nutrient has its own transport system in cell membranes; in contrast, lipids can cross membranes without the help of proteins. Other transport proteins not attached to membranes move about in fluids carrying nutrients from one organ to another. The protein hemoglobin carries oxygen to all cells. The protein albumin in the bloodstream carries amino acids. The lipoproteins (proteins and lipids) carry lipids from place to place. Iron is captured by a protein residing in the cell which will not let go unless the body needs the iron (ferritin).[3]

Proteins are involved in blood clotting. When a tissue is injured, a chain of events leads to the production of fibrin. Fibrin is a stringy insoluble mass of protein fibers that form a clot. A scar forms more slowly to replace the clot and permanently heal the cut.[3]

Proteins are enzymes and are involved in the billions of chemical reactions that take place in the body every millisecond. Enzymes not only break down substances, they also build substances, and transform one substance into another. Each reaction requires its own specific enzyme. The shape of the enzyme is critical to it's activity; i.e., when an enzyme loses its shape it can no longer perform its function.[3]

DIGESTION OF PROTEINS

The role of dietary proteins is to provide the body with amino acids that the body can then use to make its own proteins.[4] Proteins in the diet are broken down to amino acid chains in the stomach. Once a protein loses its shape it is no longer functional as that specific protein (because it no longer maintains its shape). Hence proteins in the diet have nothing to do with proteins made in the body, except in providing amino acids for the body to build its own proteins. In the small intestines chains of amino acids are reduced to individual (sometimes two or three) amino acids and absorbed. Once in the bloodstream, these amino acids can reach muscles, other cell, and the liver where they are transaminated (changed to amino acids the body needs).[4]

Mouth: There is no breakdown of proteins in the mouth.

Stomach: Acid in the stomach begins to denature proteins (lose their shape). Enzymes then break the bonds between amino acids and form peptides (chains of amino acids). Another enzyme breaks peptides into smaller chains.

Intestines: When these peptides enter the small intestine, pancreatic enzymes break them further into short peptide chains. What remains are free amino acids, dipeptides, and tripeptides.

ABSORPTION OF AMINO ACIDS

Free amino acids and dipeptides (sometimes tripeptides) are absorbed into the intestinal cells. In the small intestine carrier molecules transport these amino acids and small peptides across the intestinal cells, into the blood and into the body. Once in the bloodstream, amino acids enter cells by different carriers (see Transport).

TRANSPORT OF AMINO ACIDS

Amino Acids can enter cells by several mechanisms. Some amino acids are neutral and enter by a neutral carrier, some amino acids have a charge, and enter the cell by a different carrier. This property becomes important when persons obtain an excess of certain individual amino acids through supplementation. The four types of amino acid carrier systems are:[3]

Neutral	Acidic	Basic	Polar
BCAA*	Aspartic Acid	Lysine*	Threonine*
Methionine*	Glutamic Acid	Arginine	Cystine - sulfur
Phenylalanine*			
Tryptophan*			
Tyrosine			
Histidine*			
Serine			
Cysteine			
Proline			
Glycine			
Asparagine			
Glutamine			
Alanine	* indispensable amino acids		

The neutral amino acids and polar acids enter cells through two transport systems. Since all neutral amino acids are transported across cell membranes via the same transport system, competition for transport sites exists.

The influx of essential amino acids into the brain is a function of the blood brain barrier and plasma amino acid concentrations. Intake of any of the neutral amino acids, in larger than physiological amounts, at the exclusion of the other neutral amino acids can result in changing patterns of neurotransmitter production.[3] The catecholamines (dopamine and norepinephrine) are synthesized by histidine and tyrosine. Hence the synthesis of these neurotransmitters is influenced by the supply of histidine and tryosine to the brain. Tryptophan is involved in the synthesis of serotonin, and the supply of tryptophan influences the synthesis of serotonin. When larger than physiological amounts of BCAA are ingested, in the absence of the other neutral amino acids, neurotransmitter synthesis is disrupted.

The acidic and basic amino acids are the other two carrier systems. Acidic amino acids, as well as the basic amino acids also compete with each other for entry into cells. These transport systems require energy and entry of these amino acids across the blood brain barrier is very limited.

AMINO ACIDS

Twenty standard amino acids are used by cells in protein biosynthesis, and these are specified by the general genetic code. These 20 amino acids are biosynthesized from other molecules, but organisms differ in which ones they can synthesize and which ones must be provided in their diet. The ones that cannot be synthesized by an organism are called *essential amino acids.*[5]

Besides being the building blocks for proteins, amino acids have other roles as well. Tryptophan serves as a precursor to the neurotransmitter serotonin and the vitamin niacin. Tyrosine serves as a precursor for norepinephrine and epinephrine. Tyrosine can also make the pigment melanin.[2]

Amino acids are the basic structural building units of proteins. They form short polymer chains called peptides or longer chains called either polypeptides or proteins.

A small group of amino acids comprised of isoleucine, phenylalanine, threonine, tryptophan, and tyrosine give rise to both glucose and fatty acid precursors and are thus characterized as being glucogenic and ketogenic.

The 20 standard amino acids are either used to synthesize proteins and other biomolecules or oxidized to urea and carbon dioxide as a source of energy.[6] The oxidation pathway starts with the removal of the amino group by a transaminase, the amino group is then fed into the urea cycle. The other product of transamination is a keto acid that enters the citric acid cycle.[6] Glucogenic amino acids can also be converted into glucose, through gluconeogenesis.[5]

During times of starvation, the amino acid is catabolized into a carbon skeleton and nitrogen. The carbon skeleton is then synthesized to glucose and is used for energy production. This is considered a "costly" process since free energy is expended to produce the irreversible process of gluconeogenesis. In the liver, the amino acid combines with water; ammonia is formed and is then converted into urea. The urea is then delivered to the kidneys where it is converted to urine and excreted.

While a cell may need an amino acid to build a vital protein, the need for energy in the form of glucose supersedes protein needs. Without energy cells die; without glucose the brain and nervous system die. Cells are forced to use amino acids for glucose only when glucose is not available. Breakdown of body protein to meet energy and glucose needs can lead to muscle wasting. An adequate intake of carbohydrates spares amino acids from being used for energy.

Amino acids also have other biologically important roles. Glycine, gamma-aminobutyric acid, and glutamate are neurotransmitters. Many amino acids are used to synthesize other molecules, for example:

- Tryptophan is a precursor of the neurotransmitter serotonin.
- Glycine is a precursor of porphyrins such as heme.
- Arginine is a precursor of nitric oxide.
- Carnitine is used in lipid transport within the cell.
- Ornithine and S-adenosylmethionine are precursors of polyamines.
- Homocysteine is an intermediate in S-adenosylmethionine recycling.

Indispensable Amino Acids

Essential amino acids (indispensable) and nonessential (dispensable) amino acids have traditionally been distinguished on the basis of whether the amino acids can or cannot be synthesized by the body. Metabolically, however, the distinctions are less clear because a number of essential amino acids can be formed by transamination. By this criterion, only the amino acids lysine and threonine

Amino Acids	
Essential Amino Acids	Nonessential Amino Acids
Histidine, Leucine, Isoleucine, Lysine, Methionine, Phenylalanine, Threonine, Tryptophan, Valine	Alanine, Arginine, Asparagine, Aspartic Acid, Cystine or Cysteine, Glutamic Acid, Glycine, Glutamine, Proline, Serine, Tyrosine
Indispensable Amino Acids	Dispensable Amino Acids
Histidine, Leucine, IsoLeucine, Lysine, Methionine, *Cysteine,* Phenylalanine, *Tyrosine,* Threonine, Tryptophan, Valine	Alanine, Arginine, Asparagine, Aspartic Acid, Cystine, Glutamic Acid, Glycine, Glutamine, Proline, Serine

appear not to be synthesized by transamination and are therefore indispensable. By this same argument, glutamic acid and serine are the only truly dispensable amino acids because they can be synthesized by reductive amination of ketoacids. A third class, the conditionally essential amino acids, is synthesized from other amino acids.[2] However, this synthesis is confined to particular organs and may be limited by certain physiological factors such as age or disease state.[4]

In 1985, the Food and Agriculture Organization (FAO), World Health Organization (WHO), and United Nations University (UNU) published a report in which recommendations for total indispensable amino acids (IAAs) as a percentage of protein intake is 43% for infants and 11% for adults.[7] Since the FAO/WHO/UNU report, Young and coworkers have presented data that contradict the above mentioned findings.[8]   Young suggests that the adult requirement for total indispensable amino acids is 31% of the protein requirement, or about three times the FAO/WHO/UNU estimate.[21] In 1989 Young, et al, derived The Massachusetts Institute of Technology Amino Acid Requirement Pattern (MIT-AARP).[9,10] In 1999, The Committee on Military Nutrition Research, the Food and Nutrition Board, Institute of

Medicine recommended that amino acid requirements be reexamined but that, in the interim, the MIT pattern be accepted.[11] If indispensable amino acids are not obtained from food, the body will be forced to break down its own proteins (particularly from muscle) to obtain these needed amino acids.

Mix and Match to make Complete Protein*

To make a complete protein combine different foods from any two columns (column one has no limiting amino acids and these foods are considered complete)

No limiting amino acid	Low in lycine	Low in sulfur amino acids	Low in tryptophan
dairy products cheese (except cream cheese) cottage cheese milk, all types including powdered eggs-whole and whites legumes - soybeans, soybean curd (tofu), soy milk grains - wheat germ nuts - black walnuts	legumes - peanuts grains - barley, buckwheat, bulgur wheat, cornmeal, millet, oats, rice, rye, wheat nuts and seeds - almonds, Brazil nuts cashews, coconut, filberts, pecans, pumpkin seeds, sunflower seeds, walnuts, vegetables - asparagus, beet greens, corn, kale, mushrooms, potato, sweet potato, yams	legumes (dried beans) (black, pinto, red, white) dried black eyed peas, garbanzo, lentils, mung beans, peanuts nuts - filberts vegetables - asparagus, green beans, beet greens, broccoli, brussel sprouts, mushrooms, parsley, green peas, potatoes, soybeans, swiss chard	legume (dried beans) (black, pinto, red, white) garbanzo, lima, mung beans, peanuts grain - cornmeal nuts - almonds, Brazil nuts, walnuts, vegetables - corn, beet greens, mushrooms, green peas, swiss chard

* Taken from Sunset Vegetarian Cooking. Menlo Park, Ca: Sunset Publishing Corp, 1991.

NITROGEN

Nitrogen is a chemical element that has the symbol N and atomic number 7 and atomic weight 14. Elemental nitrogen is a colorless, odorless, tasteless and mostly inert diatomic gas at standard conditions, constituting 78.1% by volume of Earth's atmosphere. Nitrogen is a constituent element of amino acids and therefore of all living organisms. Many industrially important compounds, such as ammonia, nitric acid, and cyanides, contain nitrogen.[13] Nitrogen is an essential part of amino acids and nucleic acids, both of which are essential to all life on Earth.[13]

Nitrogen is present in all living organisms in proteins, nucleic acids and other molecules. It is a large component of animal waste, usually in the form of urea, uric acid, ammonium compounds and derivatives of these nitrogenous products, which are essential nutrients for all plants that are unable to fix atmospheric nitrogen.[13] Molecular nitrogen in the atmosphere cannot be used directly by either plants or animals, and needs to be converted into nitrogen compounds, or "fixed," in order to be used by life. Precipitation often contains substantial quantities of ammonium and nitrate, both thought to be a result of nitrogen fixation by lightning and other atmospheric electric phenomena. However, because ammonium is preferentially retained by the forest canopy relative to atmospheric nitrate, most of the fixed nitrogen that reaches the soil surface under trees is in the form of nitrate. Soil nitrate is preferentially assimilated by tree roots relative to soil ammonium. Some plants are able to assimilate nitrogen directly in the form of nitrates which may be present in soil. Humans use nitrogen-containing amino acids from plant sources to manufacture proteins and nucleic acids.[13] Hence, nitrogen cannot be "fixed" (produced) by humans and must be obtained through absorption of amino acids.

Nitrogen is toxic and must be eliminated daily. While amino acids cannot be stored, there does exist a small amino acid pool in the bloodstream and in tissues. The concentration of amino acids in these pools is very small compared to the amino acid pool found in skeletal muscle (skeletal muscle makes up 40% of body weight and contains about 75% of whole-body amino acids).[3] The liver is the major site of nitrogen metabolism in the body. In times of dietary surplus, the potentially toxic nitrogen of amino acids is eliminated via transaminations, deamination, and urea formation. The carbon skeletons are generally conserved as carbohydrate, via gluconeogenesis, or as fatty acid via fatty acid synthesis pathways. In this respect amino acids fall into three categories: glucogenic, ketogenic, or both glucogenic and ketogenic. Glucogenic amino acids are those that give rise to a net production of pyruvate or energy cycle intermediates, all of which are precursors to glucose via gluconeogenesis. All amino acids except lysine and leucine are at least partly glucogenic. Lysine and leucine are the only amino acids that are solely ketogenic, neither of which can bring about net glucose production.

Nitrogen balance is the difference between the dietary intake of nitrogen (mainly protein) and its excretion (as urea and other waste products). Healthy adults excrete the same amount as is ingested, and so are in N equilibrium. During growth and tissue repair the body is in positive N balance, i.e. intake is greater than loss and there is an increase in the total body pool of protein. In fevers, fasting, and wasting diseases the loss is greater than the intake and the individual is in negative balance; there is a net loss of protein from the body.

BCAA, ALANINE, GLUTAMINE

Alanine is a nonessential amino acid and, along with glutamine, is an interorgan nitrogen carrier and an energy producing amino acid.[3] The branched chain amino acids (BCAA) - leucine, isoleucine, and valine - are essential amino acids whose key role is also in the transport of nitrogen.

Only muscles have the complete set of enzymes to fully metabolize the BCAA. The liver can not metabolize the BCAA (can only metabolize branched chain keto acids). After a meal branched chain amino acids are taken up by the muscle and broken down to branched chain keto acids.

The branched chain keto acids have several fates; they can be transaminated in the muscle (changed to other amino acids) or they can be transported to the liver. In fasting the branched chain amino acids entering muscle are broken down to keto acids which are then transaminated to alanine and glutamine.[2] While muscle is made up of 15% BCAA, only 6% is released indicating that much of the BCAAs are transaminated. Alanine and glutamine make up approximately 6% of muscle tissue, but are 60% to 70% of amino acids released in fasting, also indicating that these two amino acids are being produced.[19] The alanine released by muscle is taken up by the liver where it is converted to glucose. The glucose is released into the bloodstream and provides energy for glucose requiring cells. Glutamine released by muscle is transported to the intestines where it is the primary energy source for intestinal cells.

Glutamine is the major transport form of ammonia $(NH4)$[2] and is present in blood in much higher concentrations than other amino acids. Glutamine in the liver combines with water and the ammonia formed from nitrogen is converted into urea. The urea is then delivered to the kidneys where it is converted to urine and excreted. In this pathway, toxic ammonia from amino acid degradation is converted to nontoxic substances and eliminated through urine.

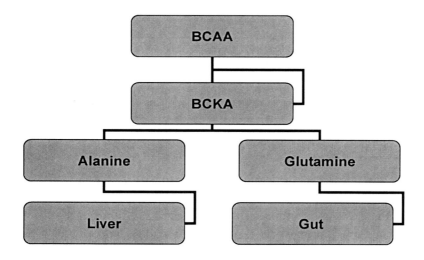

PROTEIN QUALITY

Protein quality refers to the amounts of essential amino acids in certain foods. A complete protein contains all of the essential amino acids in relatively the same amounts as the body requires. The protein from animal products is complete, while plant proteins (vegetables, grains, and legumes) tend to be limiting in one or more essential amino acids. An essential amino acid supplied in less than the amount needed to support protein synthesis is called a limiting amino acid. Food proteins that offer the body an unbalanced assortment of amino acids in which the body cannot make full use of them are said to poor quality proteins. Vegetarians can receive all the essential amino acids if, over the course of a day, they eat a variety of grains, legumes, seeds, nuts, and vegetables. These foods must also be eaten in sufficient quantities. Some of these foods, such as seeds and nuts, contain large amounts of fat, which can also contribute to obesity.

To be regarded as a high quality protein, a protein must be complete, and also digestible. The most complete protein is worthless if it cannot be digested and absorbed. Digestibility depends on the configuration of the protein, other factors in foods eaten with it, and on reactions that influence the release of amino acids. Overcooking (bacon to a crisp) reduces protein bioavailability. The amino acid cysteine is particularly vulnerable to heat destruction. Overcooking also causes lysine and glutamine residues to bond together hampering digestibility. Overcooking can cause sugar molecules to cross-link with proteins (Maillard Reaction) and protein digestibility is reduced by this "browning" effect.[1] Excessive heat due to roasting can also reduce protein availability. The key is not to overcook. In some circumstances, cooking actually improves bioavailability. Cooking improves the absorption of soy protein by inactivating an enzyme inhibitor so that protein value is improved.[14] If the proteins in the diet are of poor quality (missing one or more of the essential amino acids) the body will not be able to build the proteins it needs for all of the varied roles that involve protein. If these amino acids are not obtained from the diet, the body is forced to obtain them from other proteins, particularly muscle tissue.

Percentage of Essential Amino Acids in Ideal Reference Protein					
Isoleucine	4%	Methionine	3.5%	Threonine	4%
Leucine	7%	Cystine	3.5%	Tryptophan	1%
Valine	5%	Phenylalanine	6%		
Lysine	5.5%	Tyrosine	6%		

Measuring Protein Quality

Amino Acid Score is the simplest way to evaluate the protein quality of a food. Amino acid composition of a protein can be determined in a laboratory and its composition compared to that of an ideal reference protein.[4] The amino acid pattern for humans aged 2 to 5 years is used as the ideal standard protein. This age group matches or exceeds amino acid requirements of older children and adults. The amino acids in one gram of the dietary protein are expressed as percentages of the amounts of each essential amino acid in one gram of the ideal standard protein.[14] The amino acid showing the lowest percentage is the limiting amino acid and its percentage determines the chemical score (or amino acid score). For example, the limiting amino acid in cereal protein is lysine (2.4%. The ideal reference protein has 5.5% lysine. The amino acid score is 2.4% divided by 5.5%; the amino acid score for cereal is 44. This measure, however, does not take into account digestibility.

Biological value[14] (another measure of protein quality) attempted to take into account digestibility of the protein. One of the most important complete and digestible proteins available from food is egg protein. Hence, egg protein is a reference protein used as the standard for measuring biological value. The biological value (BV) of proteins is the efficiency of a protein in supporting the needs of the body. Protein synthesis stops when an essential amino acid is missing. Because the remaining amino acids cannot be stored they are dismantled, their nitrogen is removed and excreted. The quality of a given food protein can be tested by feeding it to experimental animals as the sole protein in their diet. Excretion of nitrogen is measured, and the difference is assumed to be retention. The higher the amount of nitrogen retained, the higher the quality of the protein. BV is expressed as a percentage of the nitrogen absorbed that is retained. Egg protein has been given a BV of 100 (by the Food and Agriculture Organization), milk protein 93, beef 75, and fish 75. A BV of 70 or greater can support human growth as long as energy intake is adequate.

Net Protein Utilization (NPU)[14], like BV, measures nitrogen retention. Instead of measuring retention of absorbed nitrogen, NPU measures retention of food nitrogen. The protein efficiency ratio (PER) measures the weight gain of a growing animal and compares that to the animals protein intake. PER was once widely used to compare protein in foods for labeling. Now the protein quality score for labels includes a measure of protein content, amino acid composition, and protein digestibility.

Protein Efficiency ratio (PER)[14] measures the growth of young animals fed a protein source at a standard level and the weight gain per gram of protein eaten provides the PER. Casein has a PER of 2.8 and soy protein 2.4. This means that young animals gained 2.8 grams for every gram of casein eaten, and only 2.4 grams for every gram of soy eaten.

The protein digestibility-corrected amino acid score (PDCAAS)[2] is similar to the amino acid score, but is corrected for digestibility.[2] The amino acid pattern for humans aged 2 to 5 years is also used as the basis for determination of PDCAAS. Corrections for digestibility of protein are taken from human data. PDCAA scores range from 1.0 to 0.0, with 1.0 being the upper limit of protein quality (able to support growth and health).

Discrepancies between PER and PDCAAS are related to the differences between young growing rats and humans. Growing rats have a larger requirement for sulfur-containing amino acids to generate larger amounts of keratin for whole-body coats of hair. Thus soy protein has been added to the list of complete proteins for humans.

SUMMARY

Proteins are large organic compounds made of amino acids. Through the process of digestion, humans break down ingested protein into free amino acids that are then used in metabolism. Amino acids are the building blocks of proteins. A protein forms via the condensation of amino acids to form a chain of amino acid "residues" linked by peptide bonds.

Proteins are defined by their unique sequence of amino acid residues; this sequence is the primary structure of the protein. Just as the letters of the alphabet can be combined to form an almost endless variety of words, amino acids can be linked in varying sequences to form a huge variety of proteins.

Proteins are classified according to their structure. The extraordinary structures of proteins enable them to play more versatile roles in the body than carbohydrates or lipids.[2] The body uses proteins to build and repair all of its tissues. New cells are constantly growing from underneath the skin with requires proteins. The cells that manufacture hair and fingernails are also constantly synthesizing new protein. GI tract cells live for only three days and must be replaced; the body constantly deposits protein into new cells that replace the lost ones.[3]

Antibodies are proteins and are produced in response to the presence of foreign particles that invade the body. Growth hormone, insulin and glucagon are also proteins, as are many other hormones. Some proteins are transport molecules. These proteins specialize in moving molecules into and out of cells. Other transport proteins not attached to membranes move about in fluids carrying nutrients from one organ to another. The protein hemoglobin carries oxygen to all cells. The protein albumin in the bloodstream carries amino acids. The lipoproteins (proteins and lipids) carry lipids from place to place. Iron is captured by a protein residing in the cell which will not let go unless the body needs the iron (ferritin).[3]

Proteins are involved in blood clotting. Proteins are enzymes and are involved in the billions of chemical reactions that take place in the body every millisecond. Enzymes not only break down substances, they also build substances, and transform one substance into another. Each reaction requires its own specific enzyme. The shape of the enzyme is critical to it's activity; i.e., when an enzyme loses its shape it can not longer perform its function.[3]

Proteins in the diet are broken down to amino acid chains in the stomach. In the small intestines chains of amino acids are reduced to individual (sometimes two or three) amino acids and absorbed. Once in the bloodstream these amino acids can reach muscles, other cell, and liver where many are transaminated (changed to amino acids the body needs).[4] Free amino acids and dipeptides (sometimes tripeptides) are absorbed into the intestinal cells. In the small intestines, carrier molecules transport these amino acids and small peptides across the intestinal cells, into the blood and into the body. Once in the bloodstream, amino acids enter cells by different carriers (see Transport).

Twenty standard amino acids are used by cells in protein biosynthesis, and these are specified by the general genetic code. The ones that cannot be synthesized by an organism are called *essential amino acids.* A small group of amino acids comprised of isoleucine, phenylalanine, threonine, tryptophan, and tyrosine give rise to both glucose and fatty acid precursors and are thus characterized as being glucogenic and ketogenic.[5]

Essential amino acids (indispensable) and nonessential (dispensable) amino acids have traditionally been distinguished on the basis of whether the amino acids can or cannot be synthesized by the body. Metabolically, however, the distinctions are less clear because a number of essential amino acids can be formed by transamination. By this criterion, only the amino acids lysine and threonine appear not to be synthesized by transamination and are therefore indispensable. By this same argument, glutamic acid and serine are the only truly dispensable amino acids because they can be synthesized by reductive amination of ketoacids. A third class, the conditionally essential amino acids, is synthesized from other amino acids.[2] However, this synthesis is confined to particular organs and may be limited by certain physiological factors such as age or disease state.[4]

Nitrogen is a chemical element that has the symbol N and atomic number 7 and atomic weight 14. Nitrogen is the largest single constituent of the Earth's atmosphere (78.082% by volume of dry air, 75.3% by weight in dry air). Nitrogen is an essential part of amino acids and nucleic acids, both of which are essential to all life on Earth.[13]

Nitrogen is present in all living organisms in proteins, nucleic acids and other molecules. It is a large component of animal waste (for example, guano), usually in the form of urea, uric acid, ammonium compounds and derivatives of these nitrogenous products, which are essential nutrients for all plants that are unable to fix atmospheric nitrogen.[13]

Some plants are able to assimilate nitrogen directly in the form of nitrates which may be present in soil. Humans use nitrogen-containing amino acids from plant sources in the manufacture of proteins and nucleic acids.[13] Hence, nitrogen cannot be "fixed" (produced) by humans and must be obtained through absorption of amino acids.

Nitrogen is toxic and must be eliminated daily. While amino acids cannot be stored, there does exist a small amino acid pool in the bloodstream and in tissues. The concentration of amino acids in these pools is very small compared to the amino acid pool found in skeletal muscle (skeletal muscle makes up 40% of body weight and contains about 75% of whole-body amino acids).[3]

During times of starvation the amino acid is catabolized into a carbon skeleton and nitrogen. The carbon skeleton is then synthesized to glucose and is used for energy production. This is considered a "costly" process since free energy is expended to produce the irreversible process of gluconeogenesis. In the liver, the amino acid combines with water; ammonia is formed and is then converted into urea. The urea is then delivered to the kidneys where it is converted to urine and excreted.

While a cell may need an amino acid to build a vital protein, the need for energy in the form of glucose supersedes protein needs. Without energy cells die; without glucose the brain and nervous system die. Cells are forced to use amino acids for glucose only when glucose is not available.

Breakdown of body protein to meet energy and glucose needs can lead to muscle wasting. An adequate intake of carbohydrates spares amino acids from being used for energy.

Protein quality refers to the amounts of essential amino acids in certain foods. A complete protein contains all of the essential amino acids in relatively the same amounts as the body requires. The protein from animal products are complete, while plant proteins (vegetables, grains, and legumes) tend to be limiting in one or more essential amino acids.   An essential amino acid supplied in less than the amount needed to support protein synthesis is called a limiting amino acid. Food proteins that offer the body an unbalanced assortment of amino acids in which the body cannot make full use of them are said to poor quality proteins. Vegetarians can receive all the essential amino acids if, over the course of a day, they eat a variety of grains, legumes, seeds, nuts, and vegetables. These foods must also be eaten in sufficient quantities.   Some of these foods, such as seeds and nuts, contain large amounts of fat, which can also contribute to obesity.

To be regarded as a high quality protein, a protein must be complete, and also digestible. The most complete protein is worthless if it cannot be digested and absorbed. Digestibility depends on the configuration of the protein, other factors in foods eaten with it, and on reactions that influence the release of amino acids. Overcooking (bacon to a crisp) reduces protein bioavailability. The amino acid cysteine is particularly vulnerable to heat destruction. Overcooking also causes lysine and glutamine residues to bond together hampering digestibility. Overcooking can cause sugar molecules to cross-link with proteins (Maillard Reaction) and protein digestibility is reduced by this "browning" effect.[1] Excessive heat due to roasting can also reduce protein availability. The key is not to overcook. In some circumstances cooking actually improves bioavailability. Cooking improves the absorption of soy protein by inactivating an enzyme inhibitor so that protein value is improved.

If the proteins in the diet are of poor quality (missing one or more of the essential amino acids) the body will not be able to build the proteins it needs for all of the varied roles that involve protein. If these amino acids are not obtained from the diet, the body is forced to obtain them from other proteins, particularly muscle tissue.

The popular high protein diets are neither the answer for weight loss nor for athletic performance.[14] Humans can store carbohydrates in muscle and liver (glycogen), fat in fat cells, but cannot store proteins. The nitrogen in the amino acids is toxic and must be continuously eliminated. Muscle tissue can provide needed amino acids for gluconeogenesis but only through muscle breakdown. If a person eats excess protein, beyond the needs of the body, the amino acids are deaminated (nitrogen is removed), the nitrogen is excreted, and the remaining carbon fragments are converted to fat and stored for later use. In this way, valuable, energy expensive protein-rich foods can contribute to obesity. (See also Diet).

CHAPTER 4 - SAMPLE TEST

1. List three different food sources of proteins.

2. Define protein classification and list several physiological roles for each classification.

3. Describe digestion and absorption of proteins.

4. Define amino acids and describe their functions in the human body?

5. Define the indispensable amino acids and discuss the physiological effects of excessive and insufficient amounts in the diet.

6. How is nitrogen obtained in the diet; why is it toxic and how does the body eliminate it?

7. Discuss the transport of amino acids into cells.

8. Discuss protein quality as it pertains to digestibility.

REFERENCES

1. Wikipedia, The Free Encyclopedia, *Proteins*. Jan 2008.

2. DiPasquale, M. *Amino acids and Proteins for the Athlete,* NY: CRC Press, 1997.

3. Guyton, A. *Textbook of Medical Physiology*, 8th ed. Phil: W.B. Saunders Co., 1991.

4. Whitney, E, S Rolfes. *Understanding Nutrition,* 10th ed. NY: West Publishing Co., 2005.

5. Wikipedia, The Free Encyclopedia, *Amino Acids*. Jan 2008.

6. Sakami W, Harrington H. "Amino acid metabolism". *Annu Rev Biochem* 32: 355-98. PMID 14144484. Brosnan J (2000). "Glutamate, at the interface between amino acid and carbohydrate metabolism". *J Nutr* 130 (4S Suppl): 988S-90S. PMID 10736367.

7. FAO/WHO/UNU (Food and Agriculture Organization of the United Nations/World Health Organization/United Nations University). 1985. *Energy and protein requirements.* Report of a joint expert consultation. World health Organization Technical Report Series no 724. Geneva: World Health Organization.

8. Young, VR. McCollum Award Lecture: Kinetics of human amino acid metabolism: Nutritional implications and some lessons. *Am. J. Clin Nutr.* 46:709-725, 1987.

9. Young, VR et al. A theoretical basis for increasing current estimates of the amino acid requirements in adult man with experimental support. *Am. J. Clin. Nutr.* 50:80-92, 1989.

10. Young, VR. Adult amino acid requirement: The case for a major revision in current recommendations. *J. Nutr.* 124:1517s-1523s, 1994.

11. Institute of Medicine, Food and Nutrition Board, Committee on Military Nutrition Research, Committee on Body Composition, Nutrition and Health. Washington, DC, 1999.

12. *Tufts University Health & Nutrition Letter,* Dec 1997.

13. Wikipedia, The Free Encyclopedia, *Nitrogen*. Jan 2008.

14. Shils, M, V Young. *Modern Nutrition in Health & Disease*, 7th ed. Philadelphia PA: Lea & Febiger, 1987.

Chapter 5
Energy

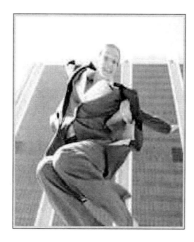

In this chapter we will we will take a more in-depth look at each energy nutrient utilization.

Objectives

After reading and studying this chapter, you should:

1. Be able to discuss the physiology of energy production.

2. Be able to discuss the factors involved in nutrient utilization (food in the diet, rest, exercise intensity, exercise duration, fitness levels, anabolic and catabolic factors).

3. Be able to discuss the effects of stress as it relates to metabolism of the energy nutrients.

4. Discuss nutrient timing and its role in muscle hypertrophy and fat utilization.

5. Be able to provide several examples of cellular control.

6. Determine the recommended ranges for daily energy nutrient intakes and determine the components involved in calculating total energy expenditure.

7. Discuss methods of determining body composition and provide the benefits and limitations of each.

INTRODUCTION

The citric acid cycle is also known as the tricarboxylic acid cycle (TCA cycle) or the Krebs cycle. It is a series of enzyme-catalyzed chemical reactions of central importance in all living cells that use oxygen as part of cellular respiration. In eukaryotes, the citric acid cycle is located in the matrix of the mitochondrion.[1] In aerobic organisms, the citric acid cycle is part of a metabolic pathway involved in the chemical conversion of carbohydrates, fats and proteins into carbon dioxide and water to generate energy.

PHYSIOLOGY

In carbohydrate catabolism, the citric acid cycle is the third step. Glycolysis, the first step, breaks glucose (a six-carbon-molecule) down into pyruvate (a three-carbon molecule). In eukaryotes, pyruvate moves into the mitochondria in the second step. In step 3, it is converted into acetyl-CoA by decarboxylation and enters the citric acid cycle.[1]

The citric acid cycle begins with acetyl-CoA transferring its two-carbon acetyl group to the four-carbon acceptor compound (oxaloacetate) to form a six-carbon compound (citrate). The citrate then goes through a series of chemical transformations, losing first one, then a second carboxyl group as CO_2. The carbons lost as CO_2 originate from what was oxaloacetate, not directly from acetyl-CoA. The carbons donated by acetyl-CoA become part of the oxaloacetate carbon backbone after the first turn of the citric acid cycle. Loss of the acetyl-CoA-donated carbons as CO_2 requires several turns of the citric acid cycle. However, because of the role of the citric acid cycle in anabolism, they may not be lost since many TCA cycle intermediates are also used as precursors for the biosynthesis of other molecules.[1] Most of the energy made available by the oxidative steps of the cycle is transferred as energy-rich electrons to NAD^+, forming NADH. For each acetyl group that enters the citric acid cycle, three molecules of NADH are produced. Electrons are also transferred to the electron acceptor FAD, forming $FADH_2$. At the end of each cycle, the four-carbon oxaloacetate has been regenerated, and the cycle continues.[1]

In protein catabolism, proteins are broken down into their constituent amino acids. The carbon backbone of these amino acids can become a source of energy by being converted to Acetyl-CoA and entering into the citric acid cycle.[1]

In fat catabolism, triglycerides are hydrolyzed into fatty acids and glycerol. In the liver the glycerol can be converted into glucose by way of gluconeogenesis. In many tissues, especially heart tissue, fatty acids are broken down through a process known as beta oxidation which results in acetyl-CoA which can be used in the citric acid cycle.[1]

The citric acid cycle is always followed by oxidative phosphorylation. This process extracts the energy (as electrons) from NADH and $FADH_2$, oxidizing them to NAD^+ and FAD, respectively, so that the cycle can continue. Whereas the citric acid cycle does not use oxygen, oxidative phosphorylation does. The total energy gained from the complete breakdown of one molecule of glucose by glycolysis, the citric acid cycle and oxidative phosphorylation equals about 36 ATP molecules.

Energy Production

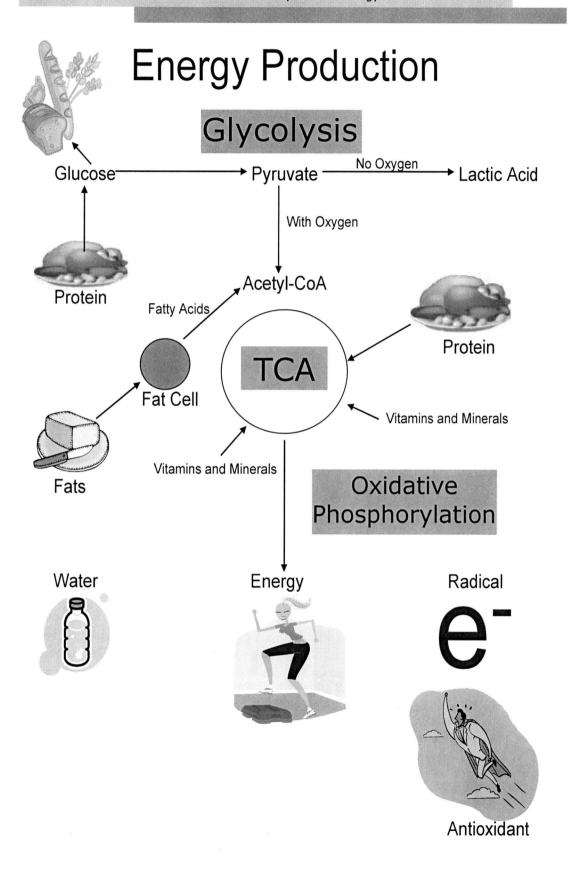

NUTRIENT UTILIZATION

When muscles contract they respond immediately without metabolizing fat or carbohydrate for energy. In the first fraction of a second, muscles use ATP and Phosphocreatine (PC).[2] ATP (adenosine triphosphate) is present in small amounts in all body tissues, and in muscle, is the driving force for contraction. Immediately after the onset of muscle contraction, before muscle ATP pools are depleted, a muscle enzyme begins to break down PC (phosphocreatine). Supplies of ATP and PC last for approximately 30 seconds. To meet prolonged needs, the body must generate ATP from glucose, fatty acids, and amino acids (aerobic metabolism), and this process requires oxygen. Muscles never use just one single fuel. Energy utilization is always a combination of glucose and fat (or fat by-products). How much of which fuels are used depends on an interplay among the fuels available from the diet, the intensity of exercise, duration of the exercise and the fitness level of the individual.[2] Other factors involved in nutrient utilization include anabolic and catabolic factors.

Foods in the Diet

Glycogen storage in muscle and liver depends on diet.[2] The body constantly uses and replenishes its glycogen. How much carbohydrate is eaten, influences how much glycogen is stored, which in turn influences how much will be used during exercise. The more glycogen the muscles store the longer the supply will last during exercise. As a reminder, if muscle cells become depleted of glucose energy ceases. A person who eats a high fat diet with little carbohydrate sacrifices athletic performance and needlessly degrades protein tissues to produce the needed glucose.

Rest

During rest, the body derives slightly more than half of its energy from fatty acids and most of the rest from glucose. In order for fat to be utilized as an energy source, glucose and oxygen must be available. When both oxygen and glucose are available (aerobic metabolism) the muscles will use a combination of fat and glucose. Many other nutrients are involved in production of energy (see ketosis); however such a detailed discussion is beyond the scope of this textbook.

Exercise Intensity

During aerobic exercise the muscles use a combination of energy nutrients for energy.[2] During anaerobic exercise (without oxygen) the body must utilize glucose for energy (since utilization of fat requires oxygen) and lactic acid is produced as a by product. Whenever a person exercises at a rate that exceeds the capacity of the heart and lungs to supply oxygen to the muscles, the muscles must draw more heavily on glucose.

A popular myth suggests that in order to burn greater amounts of fat, individuals should exercise at a lower intensity. However, at the higher intensity more calories are utilized than at a lower intensity resulting in a greater amount of actual fat being utilized.

Wayne Wescott, Fitness Research Director of the South Shore YMCA, Boston, MA, confirmed the following calculation through research:

If a 160 pound male walks for 30 minutes at 3.5 miles/hour he utilizes approximately 240 calories; 40% of those calories would come from fat and 60% from carbohydrates. This results in utilization of 96 calories from fat, or 10.6 grams of fat.

If the same male runs for 30 minutes at a pace of 6.5 miles/hour he utilizes approximately 450 calories; 25% of those calories from fat and 75% from carbohydrates. This results in utilization of 112 calories from fat, or 13.5 grams.

At the higher intensity more calories are utilized. The higher intensity also increases aerobic capacity. Aerobically fit individuals utilize more fat as an energy source during exercise and at rest.

Exercise Duration

How long glycogen stores last depends on the duration of the exercise.[2,3] During the first few minutes of exercise the major source of fuel is glycogen since oxygen is not yet available to the muscle cells. As exercise continues (10 to 20 minutes) more oxygen becomes available and greater fat utilization occurs.

After several hours of exercise, glycogen stores are depleted. When depletion occurs it brings activity to a near halt (what marathon runners refer to as "hitting the wall").[2,3] Maximizing glucose storage requires: Consuming a high carbohydrate diet (as much as 70% of the diet); ingesting glucose periodically during exercise that lasts longer than 90 minutes; training the muscles to store as much glycogen as possible; and remaining as fit as possible since trained muscles store more glycogen.

Fitness

Another critical component to extending glycogen stores is an individuals' fitness level. The more aerobically fit a person is, the more oxygen is delivered to muscles cells. This additional oxygen allows this "fit" individual to utilize more fat in conjunction with glucose, thereby extending the glycogen stores. Conditioned muscles also rely less on glycogen and more on fat so that glycogen breakdown occurs more slowly in these trained athletes. These individuals utilize a greater percentage of fat even at rest.[2]

Anabolic Factors

Muscle hypertrophy is a scientific term for the growth and increase of the size of muscle cells. It differs from muscle hyperplasia, which is the formation of new muscle cells.[9] Muscle hypertrophy is dependent on several factors such as genetics, gender, age and nutrition.

Muscle fiber types are determined genetically. Fiber types affect skeletal muscle hypertrophy. The force generated by a muscle is dependent on its size and the muscle fiber type composition. Skeletal muscle fibers are classified into two major categories; slow-twitch (Type 1) and fast-twitch fibers (Type II). The difference between the two fibers can be distinguished by metabolism, contractile velocity, neuromuscular differences, glycogen stores, capillary density of the muscle, and the actual response to hypertrophy. Type I fibers are primarily responsible for maintenance of body posture and skeletal support. They utilize fats and carbohydrates better because of the increased reliance on oxidative metabolism. Type II fibers require greater amounts of force production for shorter periods of time. These fibers rely on anaerobic metabolism for energy for contraction.[10]

Gender differences occur in muscle hypertrophy due to hormones. During puberty in males, hypertrophy occurs at an increased rate due to increased testosterone levels. Testosterone is an androgen, or a male sex hormone. The primary physiological role of androgens is to promote the growth and development of male organs and characteristics. Testosterone affects the nervous system, skeletal muscle, bone marrow, skin, hair and the sex organs. With skeletal muscle, testosterone, which is produced in significantly greater amounts in males, has an anabolic (muscle building) effect. This contributes to the gender differences observed in body weight and composition between men and women. Testosterone increases protein synthesis, which induces hypertrophy.[10]

Fast twitch muscles decline with age. However, according to Rosenberg and Evans[11] a decline in muscle hypertrophy is not inevitable. Landmark research has shown that muscle hypertrophy occurs through appropriate resistance training in individuals at any age.

Nutrition is also a factor in muscle hypertrophy. Without proper nutrition muscle hypertrophy will not occur. Without adequate caloric intake, along with adequate protein, fat, carbohydrate and micronutrient intake muscle hypertrophy will not occur. Other nutrition factors include adequate hydration, adequate sleep and stress reduction.

Catabolic Factors

Some of the catabolic factors in muscle hypertrophy include fasting, starvation, illness, stress, caffeine, alcohol and inadequate amount of rest.

Fasting

During fasting glycogen stores are depleted and the body must produce glucose from glucogenic amino acids. After twelve to sixteen hours, the liver is depleted of glycogen and must, therefore, make glucose.[2,3] As fasting continues, ketones are produced and provide energy for muscles while brain cells, nerve cells, red blood cells, and other cells still require glucose. The body cannot use fat at this point and must form glucose from non-carbohydrate sources (gluconeogenesis). The body begins to utilize muscle protein as an energy source.[2]

Starvation

After 2 to 3 days of not eating, the process of ketosis increases (the incomplete breakdown of fats). If the body continued the breakdown of muscle at the same rate as in fasting, death would ensue within several days. The body compensates by breaking down fats into molecules that "look like glucose" known as ketones. However, high levels of ketones are toxic to the body. Many brain and nerve cells cannot use ketones and these cells continue to utilize muscle protein for energy.[10] Death occurs when loss of lean body mass is 54% and weight loss is 66% of ideal body weight.

Illness

During periods of infection or illness, the immune system utilizes the amino acids from muscle protein breakdown to make the molecules necessary to fight the illness.

Stress

Cortisol is a steroid hormone which is produced in the adrenal cortex of the kidney. It is a stress hormone that stimulates gluconeogenesis. Cortisol also inhibits the use of glucose by most body cells. This can initiate protein catabolism (break down), thus freeing amino acids to be used to make different proteins, which may be necessary and critical in times of stress. In terms of hypertrophy, an increase in cortisol is related to an increased rate of protein catabolism. Therefore, cortisol breaks down muscle proteins, inhibiting skeletal muscle hypertrophy.[10] The body responds to stress with an elaborate series of physiological steps, using the nervous system and hormone systems to bring about defensive readiness in every body part, i.e. the "fight or flight response".[3] Stress that is chronic will produce a state of constant catabolism - that is, stress can drain the body of its energy reserves and leave it weakened, aged, and vulnerable to disease. The heart beats faster, breathing changes, blood pressure increases, serum cholesterol increases, more acid is secreted in the stomach, and muscle proteins are broken down into their constituent amino acids. Some of these amino acids are transported to the liver and made into glucose which is released into the bloodstream readying the body to run or fight. Liver glycogen is also broken down into glucose. Under chronic psychological stress cells are not able to take up these nutrients in sufficient amounts; these stress products build up in the bloodstream and increase the risk of development of chronic diseases such as diabetes, cardiovascular disease, hypertension, etc.

Caffeine

Caffeine is a stimulant drug. It is a xanthine alkaloid compound that acts as a psychoactive stimulant and diuretic in humans. Caffeine is also called guaranine when found in guarana; theine when found in tea; all of these names are synonyms for the same chemical compound.[5] Caffeine is the world's most widely consumed psychoactive substance, but unlike most other psychoactive substances, it is legal and unregulated in nearly all countries.

In North America, 90% of adults consume caffeine daily. The U.S. Food and Drug Administration lists caffeine as a "Multiple Purpose Generally Recognized as Safe Food Substance".[5] In humans, caffeine is a central nervous system (CNS) stimulant, having the effect of temporarily warding off drowsiness and restoring alertness.[5]

Humans have consumed caffeine since the Stone Age. Early people found that chewing the seeds, bark, or leaves of certain plants had the effects of easing fatigue, stimulating awareness, and elevating mood. Only much later was it found that the effect of caffeine was increased by steeping such plants in hot water. Many cultures have legends that attribute the discovery of such plants to people living many thousands of years ago.[5]

Caffeine is found in varying quantities in the beans, leaves, and fruit of over 60 plants, where it acts as a natural pesticide that paralyzes and kills certain insects feeding on the plants. It is most commonly consumed by humans in infusions extracted from the beans of the coffee plant and the leaves.[5] The world's primary source of caffeine is the coffee bean (the seed of the coffee plant), from which coffee is brewed. Caffeine content in coffee varies widely depending on the type of coffee bean and the method of preparation used. Tea is another common source of caffeine. Tea usually contains about half as much caffeine per serving as coffee, depending on the strength of the brew. Certain types of tea, such as black and oolong, contain somewhat more caffeine than most other teas. Tea contains small amounts of theobromine and slightly higher levels of theophylline than coffee.

Caffeine is also a common ingredient of soft drinks such as cola, originally prepared from kola nuts. Guarana, a prime ingredient of energy drinks, contains large amounts of caffeine with small amounts of theobromine and theophylline. Chocolate derived from cocoa contains a small amount of caffeine. The weak stimulant effect of chocolate may be due to a combination of theobromine and theophylline as well as caffeine. Chocolate contains too little of these compounds for a reasonable serving to create effects in humans that are on par with coffee. A typical 28-gram serving of a milk chocolate bar has about as much caffeine as a cup of *decaffeinated* coffee.[5]

Because caffeine is primarily an antagonist of the central nervous system's receptors for the neurotransmitter adenosine, individuals who regularly consume caffeine adapt to the continual presence of the drug by substantially increasing the number of adenosine receptors in the central nervous system.

This increase in the number of the adenosine receptors makes the body much more sensitive to adenosine, with two primary consequences. First, the stimulatory effects of caffeine are substantially reduced, a phenomenon known as a tolerance adaptation. Second, because these adaptive responses to caffeine make individuals much more sensitive to adenosine, a reduction in caffeine intake will effectively increase the normal physiological effects resulting in unwelcome withdrawal symptoms.[6]

The precise amount of caffeine necessary to produce effects varies from person to person depending on body size and degree of tolerance to caffeine. It takes less than an hour for caffeine to begin affecting the body and a mild dose wears off in three to four hours. Consumption of caffeine does not eliminate the need for sleep: it only temporarily reduces the sensation of being tired.[6]

For years, athletes have been using caffeine in various doses to improve their performance.[6] Everyone knows that a strong cup of Java gives you that alertness and sense of extra energy. Though many professional endurance athletes use caffeine to enhance their performance, the US Olympic Committee, World Anti-Doping Association (WADA) and US Anti-doping association ban certain substances, including caffeine, for safety reasons as well as any unfair advantages those substances may offer. Caffeine is banned at a level of 12mcg/ml in urine, which requires about 1,200 mg of pure caffeine or 8 cups of strong coffee. WADA has lifted this ban starting in January of 2004, although it comes with some controversy since caffeine does have some ergogenic properties and can be dangerous if abused.[6]   See section on caffeine as an ergogenic aid in Chapter 9 for further details.

In large amounts, and especially over extended periods of time, caffeine can lead to a condition known as *caffeinism*. Caffeinism usually combines caffeine dependency with a wide range of unpleasant physical and mental conditions including nervousness, irritability, anxiety, tremulousness, muscle twitching (hyperreflexia), insomnia, headaches, respiratory alkalosis and heart palpitations. Furthermore, because caffeine increases the production of stomach acid, high usage over time can lead to peptic ulcers, erosive esophagitis, and gastroesophageal reflux disease. However, since both "regular" and decaffeinated coffees have been shown to stimulate the gastric mucosa and increase stomach acid secretion, caffeine is probably not the sole component responsible.[5]

An acute overdose of caffeine, usually in excess of 400 milligrams (more than 3–4 cups of brewed coffee), can result in a state of central nervous system overstimulation called caffeine intoxication. The symptoms of caffeine intoxication are not unlike overdoses of other stimulants. It may include restlessness, nervousness, excitement, insomnia, flushing of the face, increased urination, gastrointestinal disturbance, muscle twitching, a rambling flow of thought and speech, irritability, irregular or rapid heart beat, and psychomotor agitation. In cases of much larger overdoses mania, depression, lapses in judgment, disorientation, loss of social inhibition, delusions, hallucinations, psychosis, rhabdomyolysis, and death may occur.[5]

Long-term overuse of caffeine can elicit a number of psychiatric disturbances. Two such disorders recognized by the American Psychiatric Association (APA) are *caffeine-induced sleep disorder* and *caffeine-induced anxiety disorder*. In the case of caffeine-induced sleep disorder, an individual regularly ingests high doses of caffeine sufficient to induce a significant disturbance in his or her sleep, sufficiently severe to warrant clinical attention.[5]

Pure caffeine is a white powder, and can be extracted from a variety of natural sources. Benzene, chloroform, trichloroethylene and dichloromethane have all been used over the years but for reasons of safety, environmental impact, cost and flavor, they have been superseded by the following main methods. In water extraction, coffee beans are soaked in water. The water, which contains not only caffeine but also many other compounds which contribute to the flavor of coffee, is then passed through activated charcoal, which removes the caffeine. The water can then be put back with the beans and evaporated dry, leaving decaffeinated coffee with a good flavor. Coffee manufacturers recover the caffeine and resell it for use in soft drinks and over-the-counter caffeine tablets.[5]

A recent study confirmed the dangers of caffeine in pregnancy.[25]   Pregnant women who drank the equivalent of at least two cups of coffee daily, or five cans of a soft drink with caffeine, were twice as likely to miscarry as women who consumed no caffeine. The study controlled for the confounding effects of nausea and vomiting during pregnancy. Other studies have also reported increased risk of miscarriage with caffeine, which crosses the placenta but is poorly metabolized by the fetus and may influence cell development and decrease placental blood flow. The study removed those doubts, Dr. Li concluded, and strengthened the recommendation for women to avoid caffeine in pregnancy. It may be prudent to stop or reduce caffeine intake during pregnancy," he and colleagues wrote.

Caffeine

Drink/Food	Food	Caffeine
Jolt soft drink	12 ounces	71.2 mg
Mountain Dew	12 ounces	55.0 mg
Coca-Cola	12 ounces	34.0 mg
Diet Coke	12 ounces	45.0 mg
Pepsi 1	2 ounces	38.0 mg
7-Up	12 ounces	0 mg
Brewed coffee (drip method)	5 ounces	115 mg*
Iced tea	12 ounces	70 mg*
Dark chocolate	1 ounce	20 mg*
Milk chocolate	1 ounce	6 mg*
Cocoa beverage	5 ounces	4 mg*
Chocolate milk beverage	8 ounces	5 mg*
Cold relief medication	1 tablet	30 mg*
Vivarin	1 tablet	200 mg

*denotes average amount of caffeine

Source: U.S. Food and Drug Administration and National Soft Drink Association

For a complete list of caffeine in foods and drinks visit http://www.energyfiend.com/huge-caffeine-database.

Alcohol

Alcohol has been shown to have catabolic effects. Skeletal muscle atrophy is a common feature in alcoholism that affects up to two-thirds of alcohol misusers, and women appear to be particularly susceptible. There is also some evidence to suggest that malnutrition exacerbates the effects of alcohol on muscle.[7]

Excessive exposure to alcohol causes damage to skeletal muscle, leading to the development of a specific disease entity called alcoholic myopathy. It is one of the most common skeletal muscle disorders, with a prevalence of 2,000 cases per 100,000 population.[8]   Although principally occurring in men (due to the greater prevalence of alcoholism in this gender) women appear to be particularly susceptible , and there is some evidence to suggest that malnutrition may also exacerbate this disease. Predominant features of alcoholic myopathy include difficulties in gait, cramps, impaired muscle strength, and reduced whole body lean tissue mass. These pathologies are also accompanied by reductions in the relative amounts of specific contractile proteins within the muscle itself, such as myosin, desmin, actin, and troponin. The sequence of events between alcohol exposure and skeletal muscle damage is unknown, although recent evidence suggests that changes may be initiated at the molecular level.

Excessive alcohol ingestion disturbs the metabolism of most nutrients. Although alcohol can lead to severe hypoglycemia, alcoholics are usually glucose intolerant, probably due to a inhibition of glucose-stimulated insulin secretion.   Ethanol intake also leads to negative nitrogen balance and an increased protein turnover.   Alcohol also alters lipid metabolism, causing a profound inhibition of lipolysis. Looking for an association between alcohol intake, nutrition, and alcoholic liver disease, we have observed a higher prevalence of subclinical histologic liver damage among obese alcoholics. The ingestion of polyunsaturated fatty acids can also increase the damaging effects of alcohol on the liver.[8]

Lack of Sleep

Although muscle stimulation occurs in the gym lifting weights, muscle growth occurs afterward during rest. Without adequate rest and sleep, muscles do not have an opportunity to recover and build. About eight hours of sleep a night is desirable to be refreshed, although this varies from person to person.   Training at a high intensity too frequently also stimulates the central nervous system (CNS) and can result in a hyper-adrenergic state that interferes with sleep patterns. To avoid overtraining, intense frequent training must be met with at least an equal amount of purposeful recovery.[12]

NUTRIENT TIMING

Optimizing muscle hypertrophy and body fat utilization requires and understanding of appropriate nutrient timing.

Dr. John Ivy, chairperson of the Department of Kinesiology and Health Education in the College of Education at The University of Texas at Austin, has spent the past thirty years looking at simple, healthy options for building strength, endurance and muscle mass. What he has discovered is that timing is everything.[13]

For decades, serious athletes as well as not so serious athletes have followed one trend after another in an effort to capture the magic formula that increases strength, endurance and lean muscle mass.

Conventional wisdom in the late 1960s and early 1970s pointed to carbo-loading as a way to super-saturate muscles with carbohydrate and fuel cross-country skiers as well as long-distance runners and endurance cyclists. For strength athletes, that paradigm was flipped on its head and protein intake was stressed. With each new wave of information and fad-following, the one element that often seemed to be missing was strong, conclusive scientific substantiation.

When Dr. Ivy began to study the maximization of physical performance, his research concentrated on the cellular level nutrient timing. His goal was to explain, in scientific terms, why an athlete sees particular effects when supplements are ingested at specific times with certain nutrients.[13] "When you exercise," says Ivy, "the muscles become very sensitive to certain hormones and nutrients, and you can initiate many highly desirable training adaptations if you make sure the correct nutrients are present. This increased sensitivity of the muscles only lasts for a limited length of time, so the element of time becomes absolutely crucial. If you miss this window of opportunity, there's no way you can stimulate the muscle adaptations to that extent until after the next bout of exercise."[13]

To understand Ivy's breakthrough findings, it's helpful to understand the fuels required by muscles. A contracting muscle needs fuel. Adenosine triphosphate (ATP) is the only energy source that can drive muscle contraction. Muscles can only store enough ATP for a few seconds of high intensity contraction. If muscle contraction is going to be sustained the muscle needs ATP to be continuously replenished.

Fortunately, the body has ways of generating more ATP and keeping the marathon-runner running and the soccer player blocking goals. Through the anaerobic pathway, glycogen and creatine phosphate rush to provide rapid energy for intense bursts of activity as you speed from third base to home plate. Through the aerobic pathway, fat, carbohydrate and protein fill the void and are used to provide sustained energy with much more efficiency than the anaerobic pathway.[13] "What we found in our studies," says Ivy, "is that you can recover more effectively, work out harder more frequently, increase muscle mass and enhance the physical adaptations through proper nutrition."[13]

Ivy tested distance runners, triathletes and strength athletes between the ages of 19 and 35, hoping to determine what allowed for the fastest recovery of muscle glycogen, a key fuel for contracting, hardworking muscle.[13] When the athletes ingested a carbohydrate supplement immediately after exercise, they had a much higher rate of glycogen recovery, which is fuel for the muscle, than if the supplement was delayed for several hours. Ivy also discovered that once this fuel storage process kicked in it could be maintained at a rapid rate if the individual supplemented at two-hour intervals for up to eight hours after exercise ended.[13]

Although approximately 1.4 grams of carb per kilogram of body weight maximized glycogen storage, Ivy found that more of a seemingly good thing did not end up being better—the rate of glycogen storage could not be increased with an increase in carb intake.[13] The surprising addition of a limited amount of protein, however, sparked a chain reaction. When protein is added to carbohydrate, the insulin concentration in the blood rises. Insulin is a facilitator and stimulates glucose uptake by the muscle and the conversion of glucose into the highly valuable glycogen, as well as increasing the rate of protein synthesis when the supplement is taken immediately after exercise.[13] In one study with cyclists, Ivy discovered that drinking a fluid containing carbohydrate and protein in a 4:1 ratio improved endurance 57 percent compared with water and 24 percent compared with a carbohydrate drink.[13] According to Ivy, because muscle breakdown occurs faster during exercise, consuming a supplement that includes protein while exercising gives muscles some of the protein they need to produce extra energy. The result is less muscle damage. Similarly, maintaining blood glucose levels by ingesting carbohydrates during exercise leads to less depletion of glycogen stores and less fatigue.

With his research findings, Ivy identified a span of time during which exercise and post-exercise nutrition is very important to the athlete who wants to improve endurance, reduce muscle damage, maintain immune function and jumpstart a much quicker recovery.[13] According to Ivy, "nutrient timing" begins 30 minutes before exercise, when one should fully hydrate and raise blood glucose levels by consuming approximately 14-20 ounces of water or electrolyte solution. This delays the development of dehydration, hastens the onset of sweating and moderates the rise in body temperature. [13] During exercise, smart nutrition choices become even more important. In order to spare muscle glycogen, limit cortisol and free radical levels, prevent dehydration and set the stage for faster recovery after a workout, Ivy found that fluids should be replenished every 15 to 20 minutes, if possible. According to Ivy, this is the *most* important time for minding nutrition p's and q's. In the 30 minutes following a workout, a muscle's potential to rebuild peaks, and it is extremely sensitive to insulin. To take full advantage of the muscle rebuilding benefits that can occur in this golden window of opportunity, the right combination of nutrients, such as carbohydrate and high quality protein, should be consumed within 15 to 45 minutes after exercise.

Insulin sensitivity, and the ability of muscle fibers to pack in as much energy as possible, falls significantly one hour after exercise. After two hours, muscles not only lose their sensitivity but actually become insulin resistant and muscle breakdown occurs. Even though activity has stopped, the muscles continue to lose protein and nutrients without supplementation.

"Paying attention to what you eat or drink and when you consume it is a lot easier, cheaper, healthier and safer than using some plant steroids, androstenedione or creatine supplementation, for example," says Ivy." Just following a good basic diet and supplementing at the right time may not sound all that exciting, but solid scientific research says it works and yields increases in muscle mass, strength and endurance. It can even protect your immune system and keep you from getting as many colds and upper respiratory ailments."[13]

ENERGY NUTRIENT NEEDS

Determining the daily caloric intake required for muscle hypertrophy and fat utilization is dependent on three factors. The first is the number of calories due to basal metabolic rate.

Basal metabolic rate (BMR) is the number of calories the body utilizes at rest on a daily basis. This is at total rest. Almost two-thirds of the energy a person spends in a day supports the body's metabolic activities. This rate is quite variable and is dependent on gender, age, height, body composition (muscle mass), fever, stress, and thyroxin (the hormone in the thyroid gland that controls basal metabolism). As estimate of basal metabolic rate for females is body weight times 11; and for males it is body weight times 12.[14]

The second factor in determining daily energy requirements is physical activity. Physical activity can be determined several ways. A classic method is to look at the number of metabolic equivalents for a given activity (METs). In this course we will use another method used in the health professions known as the Paffenbarger scale[15]. This scale takes into account total daily activity rather than the number of calories per activity. This scale however requires a subjective determination. It must be determined whether the client is sedentary, active, or very active. For example, a sedentary person performs no formal exercise during the day, i.e. administrative assistant with two teenage children who walks to and from the car. An active person exercises aerobically at least 3 hours per week, and does not have a sedentary career. A very active person is an athlete who exercises several hours per day. To determine the number of calories for a sedentary person multiply the BMR times 25% (or .25); for an active person multiply the BMR times 50% (.5); and for a very active person multiply the BMR times 75% (.75).[15] The third component in total energy expenditure is thermal effect of food. Thermal effect of food is the number of calories the body expends in digesting foods. This amount is dependent on the composition of the diet. If the diet is high in fat (40%) then the estimate is 5% of the BMR; if the diet is higher in carbohydrates or proteins, then the estimate is 10% of the BMR.[2]
All of the above calculations are based on "average body fat percentages". The total energy expenditure must be adjusted for muscle mass. A female with average percent body fat (22%) will utilize many more calories than a female with 50% body fat. If a client is above this average body fat percentage then the total energy expenditure will be overestimated. The body fat percentage for purposes of these calculations is 22 percent fat for females and 18% for males.

The adjusted total caloric energy expenditure is an estimate; i.e. the number of calories required to begin building muscle and burning fat. It is critically important to understand that his number is an estimate. It is an estimate of the number of calories needed for muscle hypertrophy and fat burning. However, for muscle hypertrophy and fat burning it is not only the amount of calories required per day, but also the types of calories and when eating that will result in successful body composition change.

Discussion will next center on appropriate percentage of energy nutrients required for muscle hypertrophy and body fat utilization along with determining total energy expenditure.

Macronutrient Percentages

<table>
<tr><td colspan="4" align="center"><u>Daily Percentages</u></td></tr>
<tr><td>Nutrient</td><td>Carb</td><td>Fat</td><td>Protein</td></tr>
<tr><td>Percent</td><td>45% to 65%*</td><td>20% to 35%</td><td>15% to 20%
or
1.2 to 1.8 g/kg/BW</td></tr>
</table>

* 45% not recommended for athletes or individuals wishing to optimize energy

Carbohydrates: The recommendations for carbohydrate intake are between 45% to 60% of total caloric intake[16] (note 45% may be too low for optimizing energy)

> fiber: 21 to 35 grams of fiber daily[17]
> sugar: 10% of total caloric intake[18]

Fats: The recommendations for fat intake by the government is 30% of total caloric intake or less. In the past optimum health and fitness recommendations are 20% of total caloric intake.[7] It now appears that the type of fat is the more critical criteria.

Proteins: Protein intake can be determined in several ways:

> 1.   as a percentage of total caloric intake which is 15 to 20%[7]
> 2.   or as a component of body weight (assuming average muscle content):   1.2 to 1.98 grams per kilogram body weight

Much debate exists concerning protein requirements. The RDA for protein is .8 grams per kilogram body weight.   Many fitness authorities believe this value is too low to maintain/increase muscle mass.   Nancy Clark states that protein intake should be in the range of 1.3 to 1.98 grams per kilogram body weight (.6 to .9 grams per pound body weight).[16] Dr. Peter Lemon, an exercise physiologist at Kent State University, advises long distance runners and other endurance athletes to consume 1.2 grams of protein per kilogram of body weight each day.[19]   Strength athletes should consume even more protein - 1.6 to 1.8 grams per kilogram body weight per day.   Dr. Lemon advises that too much protein fills the stomach and will not provide adequate fuel for muscles. Consuming more than 2.0 grams of protein per kilogram body weight stresses the liver and kidneys and leads to dehydration.[19]

The Committee on Military Research, Food and Nutrition Board, Institute of Medicine[20] suggest that protein quality may be the more important question since high quality proteins are used with greater efficiency, resulting in the excretion of less urea and a decreased renal solute load.   Chronic high levels of protein intake may increase amino acid catabolism and foster the body's adaptation to higher protein intakes.   These adaptations may be detrimental in situations where stress increases need or intake is diminished.   Therefore, the Military Recommended Dietary Allowances (100 g/day for men and 80 g/day for women) have not been increased and appear to be adequate provided calories and high quality protein are consumed. The Committee does however acknowledge that clear evidence exists for higher protein intakes for active individuals wishing to increase tissue mass (1.2 to 1.5 g/kg BW/day).

Research at the USDA Human Nutrition Research Center on aging indicates that a range of protein necessary to build muscle in the elderly (over 70 years of age) is 1.0 to 1.2 grams of protein per kilogram body weight per day.[21]

It appears prudent that protein recommendations remain in the range of 1.0 to 1.8 grams per kilogram body weight per day, keeping in mind that there may be adaptive responses at the higher intakes.

Caution: Too much protein fills the stomach and will not provide adequate fuel for muscles.   According-ing to Dr. Lemon, when strength athletes consume more than 2.0 grams of protein per kilogram body weight they are wasting their money and stressing their livers.[19] Excess protein causes the body to urinate more frequently because the excess nitrogen forms the waste product urea. This process burdens the kidneys and could cause dehydration.

Determining Percentages of Energy nutrients

In this section we will look at determining percentages of energy nutrients in the diet. We will begin with several examples of determining percentages of energy nutrients on labels.

% Protein: (grams protein x 4) ÷ total calories
% fat: (grams fat x 9) ÷ total calories
% carbs: (grams carbs x 4) ÷ total calories

Example 1:

If a label states that the product has only 2 grams of fat and that the total caloric content is 30 calories, what is the percentage of fat in this product?

2 grams of fat x 9calories/gram   = 18 calories

18 of the 30 calories are fat

18 ÷ 30 = .60 (60%)

The product is 60% fat

Example 2:

A product claims that it is a high protein product; the product contains 10 grams of protein out of 100 calories. What is the percentage of protein in this product?

10 grams of protein x 4 calories/gram = 40 calories

40 calories of the 100 calories are protein

40 ÷ 100 = .40 (40%)

The product is 40 percent protein - a high protein product.

Example 3:

You buy 1% milk. You believe the product is 99% fat free. You read the label which indicates that the product has 2 grams of fat per 100 calorie serving. You then proceed to determine the percentage of fat:

$$2 \text{ grams of fat} \times 9 \text{ calories/gram} = 18 \text{ calories}$$

$$18 \div \text{ by } 100 = .18 \text{ (18\% fat)}$$

Is the product 1% fat or 18% fat? The answer is both. The 1% fat refers to the percent fat by volume. Milk contains water and other non-caloric constituents. One percent milk is 1% fat by volume and 18% fat by caloric content. Whole milk is 3.3% fat by volume, but is 49% fat by caloric content (8.2 grams of fat per 150 calorie serving).

Example 4:

What is the percentage of nutrients in the following daily food log? The following is an example of a typical food log with the calculation of percentages of energy nutrients.

		Calories	protein (g)	carbs (g)	fat (g)
Breakfast:	1 cup milk	100	10	11	2
	1/2 cup cereal	110	2	23	1
	1/2 banana	50	-	12.5	-
Lunch:	2 slices bread	150	2	31	2
	1 Tbs mayo	50	-	-	5.5
	1 sm can tuna	140	26	-	4.0
	1 apple	50	-	12.5	-
Dinner:	2 slices pizza	300	15	25	15.5
	salad	24	-	6	-
	1 Tbs oil	120	-	-	13.3
	2 beers	200		12**	
Total Calories:		1294	55	133	43.3

Percentages:

Protein	= 55 g x 4 kcal/g = 220 kcal	220 kcal ÷ 1294 kcal = 17%
Carbohydrate	= 133g x 4 kcal/g = 532 kcal	532 kcal ÷ 1294 kcal = 41.1%
Fat	= 43.3g x 9 kcal/g = 390 kcal	390 kcal ÷ 1294 kcal = 30.1%

** Alcohol calories (not carb) from 2 beers = 152 calories which is 11.7% (152 ÷ 1294)

Protein Recommendations

So what figures do you use to determine daily protein intake for your clients? The answer depends on your client. The prudent estimated range is from 1.0 grams per kilogram body weight (low end for individuals over 70) to 1.8 grams per kilogram body weight (high end).

Protein Recommendations[19]	
Teenagers	.4 to 1.0 g/kg BW/day
General Adults	.8 g/kg/ BW/day
During Training	1.2 to 1.8 g/kg/ BW/day
Strength Training	1.4 to 1.8 g/kg/ BW/day
Endurance Athletes	1.2 to 1.4 g/kg/ BW/day

Example 1: Your client is a 45 year old male weighing 220 pounds (100 kilograms) and is just beginning an exercise program. This 45 man is not elderly (over 70, at least not yet). You do his Total Energy Expenditure and his caloric intake should be around 3000 calories. The goal is to determine adequate protein intake that will allow for muscle building, but not excessive intake that can produce adaptation, dehydration and add to body fat.

Step 1   Protein intake determination by calories:
              Twenty percent of 3000 calories is 600 calories (3000 X .20 = 600 calories)
              600 calories ÷ by 4 calories per gram = 150 grams of protein per day
Step 2   Protein intake determination by weight:
              Range is 1.2 to 1.8 grams of protein per kilogram body weight
              1.2 x 100 kilograms = 120 grams protein per day
              1.8 x 100 kilograms = 180 grams protein per day
              The average protein intake in step 2 is 150 grams of protein per day.
Step 3:   Our 45 year old male (100 kilograms body weight) does not require 180
              grams of protein per day. A more reasonable estimate would be between
              140 to 160 grams per day. If this 100 kilogram male were a teenage athlete then
              180 grams of protein per day might be a reasonable estimate.

Example 2: Your client is a 35 year old female who weighs 130 pounds (59.09 kilograms); she does not need to lose weight, but does need to build muscle. You do her Total Energy Expenditure and her caloric intake should be around 2000 calories.
Step 1   Protein intake determination by calories:
              Twenty percent of 2000 calories is 400 calories (2000 x .20 = 400)
              400 calories ÷ 4 calories per gram = 100 grams protein per day
Step 2   Protein intake determination by weight:
              1.2 x 59.1 kilograms = 71 grams protein per day
              1.8 x 59.1 kilograms = 106 grams protein per day
Step 3:   This woman would not require 106 grams of protein per day. A reasonable
              estimate would be in the range of 80 to 100 grams of protein per day.

As you can see, the range for determining protein intake is large and requires a subjective decision on your part. If the protein intake is too high, your client will complain of frequent urination and will exhibit signs of dehydration. If the protein intake is too low your client may not be able to build muscle. The man in example 1 and the woman in example 2 will build muscle on the suggested protein intakes and will not exhibit signs of dehydration.

Total Energy Expenditure

How many calories a person expends on a daily basis, total energy expenditure (TEE), consists of three components: basal metabolic rate (BMR),[2] physical activity (PA),[15] and thermal effect of food (TEF).[2] Each will be explained individually.

$$TEE = BMR + PA + TEF$$

Metabolism is the chemical process in the body that builds and destroys tissue and releases energy, thereby generating heat. Basal metabolic rate (BMR) is the number of calories the body utilizes at rest on a daily basis. This is at total rest. Almost two-thirds of the energy a person spends in a day supports the body's metabolic activities. This rate is quite variable and is dependent on gender, age, height, body composition (muscle mass), fever, stress, and thyroxin (the hormone in the thyroid gland that controls basal metabolism). The largest determining factor is muscle mass. An estimate of basal metabolic rate for females is their weight times 11; and for males it is their weight times 12.[14]

Physical activity can be determined several ways. A classic method is to look at the number of metabolic equivalents for a given activity (METs). In this course we will use another method used in the health professions known as the Paffenbarger scale.[15] This scale takes into account total daily activity rather than the number of calories per activity. This scale however requires a subjective determination. It must be determined whether the client is sedentary, active, or very active. For example, a sedentary person performs no formal exercise during the day, i.e. administrative assistant with two teenage children who walks to and from the car. An active person exercises aerobically at least 3 hours per week, and does not have a sedentary career. A very active person is an athlete who exercises several hours per day. To determine the number of calories for a sedentary person multiply the BMR times 25% (or .25); for an active person multiply the BMR times 50% (.5); and for a very active person multiply the BMR times 75% (.75).[15]

Thermal effect of food is the number of calories the body expends in digesting foods. This amount is dependent on the composition of the diet. If the diet is high in fat (40%) then the estimate is 5% of the BMR; if the diet is higher in carbohydrates or proteins, then the estimate is 10% of the BMR. Total energy expenditure is determined by adding BMR, plus physical activity, plus thermal effect of food.

All of the above calculations are based on "average body fat percentages". The total energy expenditure must be adjusted for muscle mass. A female with average percent body fat (22%) will utilize many more calories than a female with 50% body fat. If a client is above this average body fat percentage then the total energy expenditure will be overestimated. The average body fat percentage for a female is 22 percent fat, and for a male is 18% fat. Hence the TEE has to be adjusted for percentage of body fat.

The adjusted total caloric energy expenditure is an estimate; i.e. the number of calories required to begin building muscle and burning fat.

Determining Total Energy Expenditure

Below details the steps involved in determining total energy expenditure.

$$\text{TEE} = \text{BMR} + \text{PA} + \text{TEF}$$

Step 1:

Metabolism is the chemical process in the body that builds and destroys tissue and releases energy, thereby generating heat. Basal metabolic rate (BMR)[2] is the number of calories the body utilizes at rest on a daily basis. This is at total rest. Almost two-thirds of the energy a person spends in a day supports the body's metabolic activities. This rate is quite variable and is dependent on gender, age, height, body composition (muscle mass), fever, stress, and thyroxin (the hormone in the thyroid gland that controls basal metabolism). The largest determining factor is muscle mass. The following equation is used to estimate basal metabolic rate:[14]

FEMALES: BMR = Weight x 11   MALES: BMR = Weight x 12
Example: A female weighs 150 pounds   Example: Male weighs 150 pounds
150 x 11 = 1650 calories   150 x 12 = 1800 calories

Step 2:

Physical activity can be determined several ways. A classic method is to look at the number of metabolic equivalents for a given activity (METs). In this course we will use another method used in the health professions known as the Paffenbarger scale.[15] This scale takes into account total daily activity rather than the number of calories per activity. This scale however requires a subjective determination on your part. You must determine whether your client is sedentary, active, or very active and then take a percentage of that client's basal metabolic rate. For example, a sedentary person performs no formal exercise during the day, i.e. secretary with two teenage children who walks to and from the car. An active person exercises aerobically at least 3 hours per week, and does not have a sedentary career. A very active person is an athlete who exercises several hours per day. The following guidelines are to be used when determining the caloric expenditure due to exercise:[11]

Sedentary = BMR x .25   Active = BMR x .50   Very Active = BMR x .75
Example: The same female in the previous example for BMR (1650 calories)
who lives a sedentary lifestyle.
1650 calories x .25 = 412.5 calories

Step 3:

Thermal effect of food is the number of calories the body expends in digesting foods. This amount is dependent on the composition of the diet. If the diet is high in fat (40%) then the estimate is 5% of the BMR; if the diet is high in carbohydrates, then the estimate is 10% of the BMR.

High fat diet: BMR x .05   High Carb diet: BMR x .10
Example: Same female in the previous example that eats a diet high in fat
1650 calories x .05 = 82.5 calories

Step 4:
Add BMR and PA and TEF to determine total energy expenditure.

TEE = 1650 calories + 412.5 calories + 82.5 calories = 2145 calories

2145 calories is the Total Energy Expenditure for this client

Step 5:
The total energy expenditure must be adjusted for muscle mass. A female with average percent body fat (22%) will utilize many more calories than a female with 50% body fat.

All of the above calculations are based on "average body fat percentages". If a client is above this average body fat percentage then the total energy expenditure will be overestimated. The average body fat percentage for a female is 22 percent fat, and for a male is 18% fat.   The adjustment is as follows:

1. Adjusted % of TEE = 100% - (actual % fat - average % fat)

2. Adjusted TEE = TEE X Adjusted % of TEE
Example: Same female who is 30% body fat
step 1.   100% - (30% - 22%) = 92%
step 2.   2145 calories x .92 = 1973 calories

This is the adjusted total caloric energy expenditure and is an estimate. This number represents the estimated number of calories an individual needs to eat to build muscle and burn fat . A reasonable goal for this client would be 1900 to 2000 calories. We will discuss in detail in the next session why a low calorie diet should not be recommended.

BODY COMPOSITION

Three important measures of body composition are Body Mass Index, percent body fat, and waist to hip ratio.

Body Mass Index

Body mass index is a way to judge weight in relation to height. Researchers and health professionals use this index as a predictor of chronic disease.[14,22] This measure is dependent on mass, not body fat. The calculation provides a figure that is sometimes difficult to interpret; but, nonetheless, important. Body Mass Index can determine a persons risk of dying before reaching full life expectancy and can give an estimate of how much weight a person needs to lose. While not taking into account body fat percentage, it is an important predictor of disease.

Body Mass Index is determined by the following equation:

$$\frac{weight \div 2.2}{(height_{(inches)} \times .0254)^2}$$

Example: weight is 220 pounds and height is 6 feet 4 inches

step 1 - 220 ÷ 2.2 = 100

step 2 - 76 inches x .0254 = 1.93

step 3 - 1.93 x 1.93 = 3.72

step 4 - 100 ÷ 3.72 = 26.88

Body Mass Index is 26.88

The norms on page 133 indicate that this person is overweight.

Percent Body Fat

Percent body fat can be determined by several methods. Underwater weighing can be a very accurate method of body fat determination if done properly.

Another method is Bioelectric Impedance Analysis. This method relies on the principle that fat and water conduct electricity differently. Electrodes are placed on the hand and foot and a small electrical current, similar to an EKG current, flows through the body. Total body water is determined and an equation based on the principle that fat contains very little water is then used to estimate percent body fat. The problem with this method is that the results are quite variable if the person is dehydrated, has eaten, or has exercised. For these reasons this method is not recommended unless these variables can be controlled.

A new method depends on sound waves that penetrate the skin and relies on the same principle as above, i.e. total body water. This method can also be variable. To many clients this method appears more "scientific". We need to make persons aware of the large margin of error associated with this method.

The old standby method is calipers.[23] Calipers measure the subcutaneous fat underneath the skin. The amount of fat under the skin is correlated to total body fat using a "standard measure". There is also a margin of error associated with this method. However, while not totally accurate, this method offers precision, i.e., consecutive readings over months will be consistent. Therefore, if someone is losing fat this method measures that reduction. Whether the actual percentage of fat is 25 or 26% is not as important as knowing that the percentage is going down over time.

Waist to hip ratio

Waist to hip ratio indicates where the fat is distributed. Body fat distribution is also an important factor in disease prediction. Fat distributed around the waistline is an independent risk factor for heart disease, stroke, and diabetes.[24] A person who is not overweight but most of their fat is stored around the waist, will have a greater risk for developing one of these diseases.

The waist is measured at the narrowest point, and the hips are measured at the widest point. The waist measurement is then divided by the hip measurement and the ratio determines risk. Increased risk is indicated if a female has a ratio above .8 and if a male has a ratio above .9.

Example: A man has a waist of 39 inches, and a hip measurement of 40 inches.
step 1:   39 ÷ 40 = .98
This man is at increased risk for the chronic
diseases mentioned above.

Body Composition

1. Percent Body Fat
2. Body Mass Index   = $\dfrac{\text{weight} \div 2.2}{(\text{height}_{(inches)} \times .0254)^2}$

3. Waist to hip ratio = waist/hip

                Increased risk is indicated if ratio is greater than:

                        .8 for females

                        .9 for males

Energy Expenditure

Adjusted Total Energy Expenditure = (BMR + PA + TEF) x (Body Fat Adjustment)

Basal Metabolic Rate = weight x 11 (if female)   Basal Metabolic Rate = Weight x 12 (if male)

Physical Activity** = .25 x BMR sedentary   .50 x BMR active   .75 x BMR very active

Thermal Effect of Food = .05 x BMR (high fat diet)   .10 x BMR (high carb diet)

Body Fat Adjustment   Adjusted percentage = (actual % body fat - average % body fat)

Adjusted TEE = TEE x adjusted %

    **   sedentary = less than 3 hours cv exercise per week and sedentary job

      active = at least 3 hours per week of cv exercise and moving during the day

      very active = more than 7 hours cv exercise and very active during the day

             Easier calculation but not as accurate:

         Female: weight x16 if sedentary   Male: weight x 17 if sedentary

         weight x 17 if active   weight x 19 if active

         weight x 20 if very active   weight x 23 if very active

Body Mass Index Norms*

emaciated	less	than	15
severely underweight	15.0	to	16.9
underweight	17.0	to	18.9
normal weight	19.0	to	24.9
overweight	25.0	to	29.9
obese	30.0	to	39.9
severely overweight	40.0	or	more

*Information taken from: Whitney E, S Rolfes, Understanding Nutrition, 6th ed. NY: West Publishing Co.,2005

SUMMARY

In carbohydrate catabolism, the citric acid cycle is the third step. Glycolysis, the first step, breaks glucose (a six-carbon-molecule) down into pyruvate (a three-carbon molecule). In eukaryotes, pyruvate moves into the mitochondria in the second step. In step 3, it is converted into acetyl-CoA by decarboxylation and enters the citric acid cycle.[1]

In protein catabolism, proteins are broken down into their constituent amino acids. The carbon backbone of these amino acids can become a source of energy by being converted to Acetyl-CoA and entering into the citric acid cycle.

In fat catabolism, triglycerides are hydrolyzed into fatty acids and glycerol. In the liver the glycerol can be converted into glucose by way of gluconeogenesis. In many tissues, especially heart tissue, fatty acids are broken down through a process known as beta oxidation which results in acetyl-CoA which can be used in the citric acid cycle.

When muscles contract they respond immediately without metabolizing fat or carbohydrate for energy. In the first fraction of a second, muscles use ATP and Phosphocreatine (PC).[2] ATP (adenosine triphosphate) is present in small amounts in all body tissues and in muscle is the driving force for contraction. Immediately after the onset of muscle contraction, before muscle ATP pools are depleted, a muscle enzyme begins to break down PC (phosphocreatine). Supplies of ATP and PC last for approximately 30 seconds. To meet prolonged needs, the body must generate ATP from glucose, fatty acids, and amino acids (aerobic metabolism), and this process requires oxygen. Muscles never use just one single fuel. Energy utilization is always a combination of glucose and fat (or fat by-products). How much of which fuels are used depends on an interplay among the fuels available from the diet, the intensity of exercise, duration of the exercise and the fitness level of the individual.[2] Other factors involved in nutrient utilization include anabolic and catabolic factors such as fasting, starvation, illness, stress, caffeine, alcohol, sleep and recovery.

Nutrient timing is "everything" according to Dr. Ivy. "When you exercise," says Ivy, "the muscles become very sensitive to certain hormones and nutrients, and you can initiate many highly desirable training adaptations if you make sure the correct nutrients are present. This increased sensitivity of the muscles only lasts for a limited length of time, so the element of time becomes absolutely crucial. If you miss this window of opportunity, there's no way you can stimulate the muscle adaptations to that extent until after the next bout of exercise.

To view metabolism as what one eats is simplistic. Metabolism is defined as the complex set of physical and chemical processes occurring within a living cell or organism that are necessary for the maintenance of life; i.e., provide energy for maintaining life. There are many factors that control metabolism.[3] Some of these factors are enzymatic, others are hormonal, while still others are controlled at the cellular level through concentration and compartmentalization.

Determining the daily caloric intake required for muscle hypertrophy and fat utilization is dependent on three factors. The first is the number of calories due to basal metabolic rate.

Recommended Daily Values for the energy nutrients are approximately 45% to 65% or total caloric intake for carbohydrates, 15% to 20% for proteins, and 20% to 35% for fats. These nutrients should, whenever possible, be obtained from the diet.

Much debate exists concerning protein requirements. The RDA for protein is .8 grams per kilogram body weight. Many fitness authorities believe this value is too low to maintain/increase muscle mass. The Committee on Military Research, Food and Nutrition Board, Institute of Medicine (2000) suggest that protein quality may be the more important question since high quality proteins are used with greater efficiency, resulting in the excretion of less urea and a decreased renal solute load. Chronic high levels of protein intake may increase amino acid catabolism and foster the body's adaptation to higher protein intakes. These adaptations may be detrimental in situations where stress increases need or intake is diminished. Therefore, the Military Recommended Dietary Allowances (100 g/day for men and 80 g/day for women) have not been increased and appear to be adequate provided calories and high quality protein are consumed. The Committee does however acknowledge that clear evidence exists for higher protein intakes for active individuals wishing to increase tissue mass (1.2 to 1.5 g/kg BW/day). Research at the USDA Human Nutrition Research Center on aging indicates that a range of protein necessary to build muscle in the elderly (over 70 years of age) is 1.0 to 1.2 grams of protein per kilogram body weight per day. It appears prudent that protein recommendations remain in the range of 1.0 to 1.8 grams per kilogram body weight per day, keeping in mind that there may be adaptive responses at the higher intakes.

The adjusted total caloric energy expenditure is an estimate; i.e. the number of calories required to begin building muscle and burning fat. It is critically important to understand that his number is an estimate. It is an estimate of the number of calories needed for muscle hypertrophy and fat burning. However, for muscle hypertrophy and fat burning it is not only the amount of calories required per day, but also the types of calories and when eating that will result in successful body composition change.

Three important measure of body composition are body mass index, percent body fat, and waist to hip ratio.

CHAPTER 5 - SAMPLE TEST

1. What are the three steps in energy production? Provide details of each step.

2. What are the factors involved in nutrition utilization? Provide example of each.

3. What are the anabolic and catabolic factors involved in muscle hypertrophy and fat utilization? Provide details of each.

4. What is the benefit of nutrient timing in regards to muscle hypertrophy and fat utilization?

5. What are 3 levels of metabolic control? Provide examples.

REFERENCES

1. Wikipedia, The Free Encyclopedia, *Citric Acid Cycle*. Jan 2008.

2. Whitney, E, S Rolfes. *Understanding Nutrition,* 8th ed. NY: West Publishing Co., 2005.

3. Shils, et al. *Modern Nutrition in Health & Disease*, 10th ed. Philadelphia PA: Lea & Febiger, 2005.

4. Lehninger, A. *Principles of Biochemistry Fourth Edition,* NY: Worth Publishers, Inc, 2004.

5. Wikipedia, The Free Encyclopedia, *Caffeine.* Jan 2008.

6. http://www.trifuel.com/triathlon/nutrition/caffeine-and-endurance-000402.php.+

3. University of California, *Berkeley Wellness Letter,* Aug, 2000.

4. University of California, *Berkeley Wellness Letter,* Aug 1998.

5. Consumer Reports on Health, April 1999.

6. New England Journal of Medicine 333:276-282, 1995.

7. http://ajpendo.physiology.org/cgi/content/full/285/6/E1273.

8. Nutrition, Volume 15, Issue 7, Pages 583-589.July 1999.

9. Wikipedia, The Free Encyclopedia, *Muscle Hypertrophy*. Jan 2008.

10. The Mystery of Skeletal Muscle HypertrophyRichard Joshua Hernandez, B.S. and Len Kravitz, Ph.D.http://www.unm.edu/~lkravitz/Article%20folder/hypertrophy.html.

11. Evans, W, IH Rosenberg. Biomarkers. NY: Simon & Schuster, 1991.

12. Wikipedia, The Free Encyclopedia, Muscle Recovery, Jan 2008.

13. http://www.utexas.edu/features/archive/2004/nutrition.html.

14. Howley, E. *Health Fitness Instructor Handbook,* 2nd ed. Champaign, Il: Human Kinetics Books, 1992.

15. Paffenbarger, R Jr, Al Wing, R Hyde. Physical Activity as an index of heart attack risk in college alumni. *Am J Epidemiology. 30:*10-15, 1983.

16. Clark, N. *Sports Nutrition* Guidebook, Ill: Leisure Press, 1990.

17. Position of the American Dietetic Association: Health implications of dietary fiber, *Journal of the American Dietetic Association* 88:216, 1988.

18. 2005 Dietary Guidelines. www.mypyramid.gov.

19. Lemon, PWR. Do athletes need more dietary protein and amino acids? *Int J Sports Nutr*, s:S39-S61, 1995.

20. Reeds, PJ, PR Becket. *Protein and amino acids in Present Knowledge in Nutrition*, 7th Zeegler and Filer, eds. Washington, DC: ILSI Press, 1996.

21. Williams, M H. *Ergogenic Aids in Sports.* Champaign Il: Human Kinetics Publishers, 1983.

22. Sudy, M. *Personal Trainer Manual. San Diego:* American Council on Exercise, 1991

23. Nieman, D. *Fitness and Sports Medicine.* Palo Alto: Bull Publishing Co., 1991.

24. Donahue, R.P., et al. Central obesity and coronary heart disease in men. *Lancet,* April 11: 821-824, 1987.

25. Weng X, et al "Maternal caffeine consumption during pregnancy and the risk of miscarriage: a prospective cohort study" *Am J Obstet Gynecol* 2008; DOI: 10.1016/j.ajog.2007.10.803.

Chapter 6
Nutrition and Disease

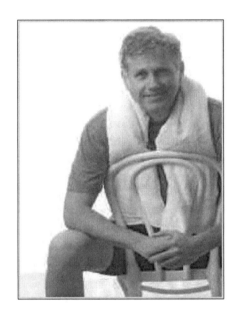

In this chapter we will take a more in-depth look at reduction of disease risk through adequate nutrient intake.

Some micronutrients, such as antioxidants, have been shown to reduce risk for cancer. Other micronutrients have been shown to reduce risk for heart disease, while still others are known to reduce blood pressure.

Objectives

After reading and studying this session you should:

1. Be able to discuss the factors associated with diabetes.

2. Be able to discuss the nutritional components of reducing hypertension.

3. Be able to describe the DASH diet.

4. Be able to discuss factors involved with stroke.

5. Be able to discuss the lifestyle components necessary to reduce cancer risk.

6. Be able to discuss other related nutrition and disease states.

INTRODUCTION

During the past decade, research in population-based epidemiological studies has helped to clarify the role of diet in preventing and controlling death and disease relating to dietary and lifestyle changes.   A Joint WHO/FAO Expert Consultation on Diet, Nutrition and the Prevention of Chronic Diseases met in Geneva in 2002.

The FAO group undertook the task of reviewing the scientific data. Their findings were not surprising. While many of the diseases associated with age and gender are modifiable, the growing epidemic of chronic diseases is related to dietary and lifestyle changes. Population based studies indicate increased consumption of energy-dense diets high in fat, particularly saturated fat, and low in unrefined carbohydrates. These patterns were found to be in combination with a decline in energy expenditure associated with a sedentary lifestyle — motorized transport, labor-saving devices in the home, the phasing out of physically demanding manual tasks in the workplace, and leisure time that is preponderantly devoted to physically undemanding pastimes. Because of these changes in dietary and lifestyle patterns, chronic diseases — including diabetes mellitus, cardiovascular disease (CVD), hypertension and stroke, and some types of cancer — are becoming increasingly significant causes of death and disease both in developing and newly developed countries, placing additional burdens on already overtaxed national health budgets. In order to achieve the best results in preventing these chronic diseases, national policies must fully recognize the essential role of diet, nutrition and physical activity.

Diet has been known for many years to play a key role as a risk factor for chronic diseases. What is apparent at the global level is that great changes have swept the entire world since the second half of the twentieth century, inducing major modifications in diet, first in industrial regions and more recently in developing countries.

It has been calculated that, in 2001, chronic diseases contributed approximately 60% of the 56.5 million total reported deaths in the world and approximately 46% of the global burden of disease. The proportion of this burden is expected to increase to 57% by 2020. Almost half of the total chronic disease deaths are attributable to cardiovascular diseases; obesity and diabetes are also showing worrying trends, not only because they already affect a large proportion of the population, but also because they have started to appear earlier in life.   It has been projected that, by 2020, chronic diseases will account for almost three-quarters of all deaths worldwide, with 71% of deaths due to ischemic heart disease (IHD), 75% of deaths due to stroke, and 70% of deaths due to diabetes.[4]

DIABETES

Diabetes is widely recognized as one of the leading causes of death and disability in the United States.   About 65 percent of deaths among those with diabetes are attributed to heart disease and stroke. There are 20.8 million adults and children diagnosed with diabetes in the U.S.   "Age, race, and educational level all are associated with diabetes; however obesity is by far the best predictor of being newly diagnosed with diabetes. The inability of the body to control blood glucose levels leads to life threatening health problems.[1]

Diabetes is a disease in which the body does not produce or properly use insulin.[2]   Diabetes is associated with long-term complications that affect almost every part of the body. The disease often leads to blindness, heart and blood vessel disease, stroke, kidney failure, amputations, and nerve damage.   Uncontrolled diabetes can complicate pregnancy, and birth defects are more common in babies born to women with diabetes. Increases in diabetes among US adults continue in both sexes, all ages, all races, all educational levels, and all smoking levels.

Initially, cells may be starved for energy because the glucose can not enter insulin dependent cells. The buildup of sugar in the blood can cause an increase in urination (to try to clear the sugar from the body). When the kidneys lose the glucose through the urine, a large amount of water is also lost, causing dehydration. When a person with type 2 diabetes becomes severely dehydrated and is not able to drink enough fluids to make up for the fluid losses, they may develop this life-threatening complications.[2]

Over time, the high glucose levels in the blood may damage red blood cells, nerve cells, cells involved in vision, kidney cells or heart cells. After a meal, the pancreas automatically produces the correct amount of insulin to move glucose from blood into cells. In people with diabetes, however, the pancreas either produces little or no insulin, or the cells do not respond appropriately to the insulin that is produced. Glucose builds up in the blood, overflows into the urine, and passes out of the body. Thus, the body loses its main source of fuel even though the blood contains large amounts of glucose.[2]

The three main types of diabetes are: type 1 diabetes; type 2 diabetes; and gestational diabetes.[2]

Type 1 Diabetes

Type 1 diabetes is usually diagnosed in children and young adults, and was previously known as juvenile diabetes. In type 1 diabetes, the body does not produce insulin. Type 1 diabetes is an autoimmune disease. An autoimmune disease results when the body's system for fighting infection (the immune system) turns against a part of the body. In diabetes, the immune system attacks the insulin-producing beta cells in the pancreas and destroys them. The pancreas then produces little or no insulin. A person who has type 1 diabetes must take insulin daily to live.

At present, scientists do not know exactly what causes the body's immune system to attack the beta cells, but they believe that autoimmune, genetic, and environmental factors, possibly viruses, are involved. Type 1 diabetes accounts for about 5 to 10 percent of diagnosed diabetes in the United

States. It develops most often in children and young adults, but can appear at any age. Symptoms of type 1 diabetes usually develop over a short period, although beta cell destruction can begin years earlier. Symptoms include increased thirst and urination, constant hunger, weight loss, blurred vision, and extreme fatigue. If not diagnosed and treated with insulin, a person with type 1 diabetes can lapse into a life-threatening diabetic coma, also known as diabetic ketoacidosis.

Type 2 Diabetes

The most common form of diabetes is type 2 diabetes. About 90 to 95 percent of people with diabetes have type 2. In type 2 diabetes, either the body does not produce enough insulin or the cells ignore the insulin. Glucose builds up in the blood instead of going into cells and can cause serious problems. This form of diabetes is associated with older age, obesity, family history of diabetes, previous history of gestational diabetes, physical inactivity, and ethnicity. About 80 percent of people with type 2 diabetes are overweight. Type 2 diabetes is increasingly being diagnosed in children and adolescents. However, nationally representative data on prevalence of type 2 diabetes in youth are not available. When type 2 diabetes is diagnosed, the pancreas is usually producing enough insulin, but for unknown reasons, the body cannot use the insulin effectively, a condition called insulin resistance. After several years, insulin production decreases. The result is the same as for type 1 diabetes—glucose builds up in the blood and the body cannot make efficient use of its main source of fuel. The symptoms of type 2 diabetes develop gradually. Their onset is not as sudden as in type 1 diabetes. Symptoms may include fatigue or nausea, frequent urination, unusual thirst, weight loss, blurred vision, frequent infections, and slow healing of wounds or sores. Some people have no symptoms.

Gestational Diabetes

Gestational diabetes develops only during pregnancy.[2] Like type 2 diabetes, it occurs more often in African Americans, American Indians, Hispanic Americans, and among women with a family history of diabetes. Women who have had gestational diabetes have a 20 to 50 percent chance of developing type 2 diabetes within 5 to 10 years.

Diagnosing Diabetes

The fasting plasma glucose test is the preferred test for diagnosing type 1 or type 2 diabetes. It is most reliable when done in the morning. However, a diagnosis of diabetes can be made after positive results on any one of three tests, with confirmation from a second positive test on a different day: A random (taken any time of day) plasma glucose value of 200 mg/dL or more, along with the presence of diabetes symptoms; A plasma glucose value of 126 mg/dL or more after a person has fasted for 8 hours; An oral glucose tolerance test (OGTT) plasma glucose value of 200 mg/dL or more in a blood sample taken 2 hours after a person has consumed a drink containing 75 grams of glucose dissolved in water. This test taken in a laboratory or the doctor's office, measures plasma glucose at timed intervals over a 3-hour period. Gestational diabetes is diagnosed based on plasma glucose values measured during the OGTT. Glucose levels are normally lower during pregnancy, so the threshold values for diagnosis of diabetes in pregnancy are lower. If a woman has two plasma glucose values meeting or exceeding any of the following numbers, she has gestational diabetes: a fasting plasma glucose level of 95 mg/dL, a 1-hour level of 180 mg/dL, a 2-hour level of 155 mg/dL, or a 3-hour level of 140 mg/dL. People with pre-diabetes, a state between "normal" and "diabetes," are at risk for developing diabetes, heart attacks, and strokes. However, studies suggest that weight loss and increased physical activity can prevent or delay diabetes, as weight loss and physical activity make the body more sensitive to insulin.

Impaired Glucose

A person has impaired fasting glucose (IFG) when fasting plasma glucose is 100 to 125 mg/dL. This level is higher than normal but less than the level indicating a diagnosis of diabetes. Impaired glucose tolerance (IGT) means that blood glucose during the oral glucose tolerance test is higher than normal but not high enough for a diagnosis of diabetes. IGT is diagnosed when the glucose level is 140 to 199 mg/dL 2 hours after a person drinks a liquid containing 75 grams of glucose. About 35 million people ages 40 to 74 have impaired fasting glucose and 16 million have impaired glucose tolerance. Because some people have both conditions, the total number of U.S. adults ages 40 to 74 with pre-diabetes comes to about 41 million. These recent estimates were calculated using data from the 1988-1994 National Health and Nutrition Examination Survey and projected to the 2000 U.S. population.

Preventing Diabetes

Studies show that people at high risk for diabetes can prevent or delay the onset of the disease by losing 5 to 7 percent of their weight, if they are overweight—that's 10 to 14 pounds for a 200-pound person. Getting at least 30 minutes of moderate-intensity physical activity five days a week and eating a variety of foods that are low in fat can produce the wanted results.[3]

Small Steps for Big Rewards provides 50 steps for reducing diabetes risk:[2]
1. Reduce Portion Sizes
2. Less on your plate
3. Keep meat, poultry and fish servings to about 3 ounces (about the size of a deck of cards)
4. Make less food look like more by serving your meal on a salad or breakfast plate.
5. Try not to snack while cooking or cleaning the kitchen.
6. Try to eat sensible meals and snacks at regular times throughout the day.
7. Make sure you eat breakfast every day.
8. Use broth and cured meats (smoked turkey and turkey bacon) in small amounts. They are high in sodium. Low sodium broths are available in cans and powder.
9. Share your desserts.
10. When eating out, have a big vegetable salad, then split an entre with a friend or have the other half wrapped to go.
11. Stir fry, broil or bake with non-stick spray or low sodium broth and try to cook with less oil and butter.
12. Drink a glass of water or other "no-calorie" beverage 10 minutes before your meal to take the edge off your appetite.
12. Select the healthier choice at fast food restaurants. Try grilled chicken instead of the cheeseburger. Skip the french fries or replace the fries with a salad.
13. Listen to music while you eat instead of watching TV (people tend to eat more while watching TV).
14. Eat slowly.
15. Eat a small meal
16. Teaspoons, salad forks, or child-size utensils may help you take smaller bites and eat less.

17. You don't have to cut out the foods you love to eat. Just cut down on your portion size and eat it less often.
18. Dance.
19. Show your kids the dances you used to do when you were their age.
20. Turn up the music and jam while doing household chores.
21. Deliver a message in person to a co-worker instead of e-mailing.
22. Take the stairs to your office. Or take the stairs as far as you feel comfortable, and then take the elevator.
23. Make a few less phone calls. Catch up with friends during a regularly scheduled walk.
24. March in place while you watch TV.
25. Park as far away as possible from your favorite store at the mall.
26. Select an exercise video from the store or library.
27. Get off the bus one stop earlier and walk the rest of the way home or to work at least two days a week.
28. Snack on a veggie
29. Try getting at least one new fruit or vegetable every time you grocery shop.
30. Macaroni and low-fat cheese can be a main dish. Serve it with your favorite vegetable dish and a salad.
31. Try eating foods from other countries. International dishes feature more vegetables, whole grains and beans and less meat.
32 Cook with a variety of spices instead of salt.
33. Find a water bottle you really like (church or club event souvenir, favorite sports team, etc.) and drink water from it wherever and whenever you can.
34. Always keep a healthy snack with you.
35. Choose veggie toppings like spinach, broccoli and peppers for your pizza.
36. Try different recipes for baking or broiling meat, chicken, and fish.
37. Try to choose foods with little or no added sugar.
38. Gradually work your way down from whole milk to 2% milk to 1% milk until you're drinking and cooking with fat free (skim) milk.
39. Try keeping a written record of what you eat for a week. It can help you see when you tend to overeat or eat foods high in fat or calories.
40. Eat foods made from a variety of whole grains-such as whole wheat bread, brown rice, oats, and whole grain corn-every day. Use whole grain bread for toast and sandwiches; substitute brown rice for white rice for home-cooked meals and when dining out.
41. Don't grocery shop on an empty stomach and make a list before you go.
42. Read food labels. Choose foods with lower fat, saturated fat, calories, and salt.
43. Fruits are colorful and make a welcoming centerpiece for any table. Have a nice chat while sharing a bowl of fruit with family and friends.
44. Slow down at snack time. Eating a bag of low-fat popcorn takes longer than eating a slice of cake. Peel and eat an orange instead of drinking orange juice.
45. You can exhale, Gail.
46. Don't try to change your entire way of eating and exercising all at once. Try one new activity or food a week.
47. Find mellow ways to relax—try deep breathing, take an easy paced walk, or enjoy your favorite easy listening music.
48. Give yourself daily "pampering time" and honor this time like any other appointment you make... whether it's spending time reading a book, taking a long bath, or meditating.
49. Try not to eat out of boredom or frustration. If you're not hungry, do something else.
50. Honor your health as your most precious gift.

CARDIOVASCULAR DISEASE

Cardiovascular disease refers to the class of diseases that involve the heart or blood vessels (arteries and veins). While the term technically refers to any disease that affects the cardiovascular system, it is usually used to refer to those related to atherosclerosis (arterial disease). These conditions have similar causes, mechanisms, and treatments.[6]

Each year, heart disease kills more Americans than cancer. Diseases of the heart alone caused 30% of all deaths, with other diseases of the cardiovascular system causing substantial further death and disability. By the time that heart problems are detected, the underlying cause (atherosclerosis) is usually quite advanced, having progressed for decades. The major injurious factors that promote atherogenesis — cigarette smoking, hypertension, atherogenic lipoproteins, and hyperglycemia — are well established.[6]

Attempts to prevent cardiovascular disease are more effective when they remove and prevent causes, and they often take the form of modifying risk factors. Some factors, such as gender, age, and family history, cannot be modified. Smoking cessation (or abstinence) is one of the most effective and easily modifiable changes. Regular cardiovascular exercise (aerobic exercise) complements the healthful eating habits. According to the American Heart Association, build up of plaque on the arteries (atherosclerosis), partly as a result of high cholesterol and fat diet, is a leading cause for cardiovascular diseases. The combination of healthy diet and exercise is a means to improve serum cholesterol levels and reduce risks of cardiovascular diseases; if not, a physician may prescribe "cholesterol-lowering" drugs, such as the statins.[6]

Eating oily fish at least twice a week may help reduce the risk of sudden death and arrhythmias. A 2005 review of 97 clinical trials by Studer et al. noted that omega-3 fats gave lower risk ratios than did statins. Olive oil is said to have benefits.[6]

Nutrition and Atherosclerosis

Atherosclerosis is the accumulation of lipids and other materials in the arteries. No one is free from atherosclerosis; the important questions become how far advanced is it and what can be done to slow or reverse its progression. Atherosclerosis usually begins with the accumulation of soft fatty streaks along the inner arterial walls, especially at branch points. These fatty streaks gradually enlarge and become hardened with minerals forming plaques. Plaques stiffen the arteries and narrow them. Most people have well-developed plaques in their arteries by the age of 30.[2] As the arteries harden, blood flows less freely through the kidneys. The kidneys respond by raising the blood pressure. Clots normally form and dissolve in the blood all the time. When these processes are balanced, the clots do not harm. Platelets cause clots to form whenever they encounter injuries in blood vessels. In atherosclerosis, platelets form and aid in the formation of clots.[7]

The underlying cause of these deposits is under intense investigation. A popular theory indicates that free radicals may be the underlying cause of damage to arterial walls, and that cholesterol deposits are a part of the mechanism causing damage.[7]

Most heart attacks occur in individuals where there is less than 50% blockage of the vessel lumen and unstable plaques burst, triggering formation of an intraluminal clot. A number of nutritional factors including obesity, increased fat intake, reduced fiber intake, and reduced intake of fruits and vegetables have all been associated with an increased risk of heart disease. In fact, many of these factors have occurred together in modern diets making it difficult to separately evaluate each of these nutritional entities.[7]

Cholesterol

Cholesterol levels correlate with risk of heart disease, with two fold increase in risk between patients with cholesterol levels <180 mg/dl compared to individuals with cholesterol levels > 240 mg/dl. There are 37 million Americans with cholesterol > 240 mg/dl, and 56 million individuals with cholesterol levels greater than 200 mg/dl.[7]

Three to four million individuals are taking cholesterol-lowering drugs, and debates on the effectiveness of these medications continue. An article published in Business Week (Jan. 17, 2008) reported the results from of research completed by Dr. James M. Wright, a professor at the University of British Columbia and director of the government-funded Therapeutics Initiative. Dr. Wright was very surprised when he looked at the data for the majority of patients who don't have heart disease. He found no benefit in people over the age of 65, no matter how much their cholesterol levels declined, and no benefit in women of any age. He did see a small reduction in the number of heart attacks for middle-aged men taking statins in clinical trials. But even for these men, there was no overall reduction in total deaths or illnesses requiring hospitalization—despite big reductions in "bad" cholesterol.[8] (See "Integrity in Science" for more details concerning the controversy over cholesterol-lowering drugs.)

According to Dr. Wright, perhaps urging people to switch to a Mediterranean diet or simply to eat more fish is the healthiest choice. In several studies, both lifestyle changes brought greater declines in heart attacks than statins, though the trials were too small to be completely persuasive. Being physically fit is also important. "The things that really work are lifestyle, exercise, diet, and weight reduction," says UCLA's Hoffman.[8]

Other ways to reduce cholesterol levels include:[9]
1. Reduce total dietary fat: Saturated fat is a bigger culprit than dietary cholesterol. Reducing total daily fat intake to 20% of caloric intake, with at least 10% unsaturated, appears to be ideal (although very difficult). Dr. Dean Ornish of the University at San Francisco School of Medicine has had excellent results in reducing the risk of heart disease with only 10% total fat intake. His results actually indicate a reversal of heart disease with this very low fat diet. Dr. Ornish's diet contains no animal products, except egg whites and nonfat dairy products. The regimen contains no added oils, eliminates caffeine totally, incorporates moderate exercise and stress management. For someone who has already had a heart attack, Dr. Ornish's program, with its severely restrictive diet, may be a much more attractive option than surgery.

2. Reduce dietary cholesterol: Reducing cholesterol intake from 500 to 200 milligrams a day will lower total blood cholesterol by an average of 10 milligrams. This response is very variable; some people have little response while others have much greater responses.

3. Include lots of fiber (oats, beans, fruits and vegetables): Oats have a fiber-rich bran layer that effectively lowers cholesterol; beans, fruits, and vegetables have also been shown to have cholesterol lowering properties (they also contain folic acid and phytochemicals).

4. Eat more fish: The oilier fish, such as salmon, mackerel, albacore, and herring, guard against heart disease and hypertension. Eating 2 to 3 meals of fish per week will reduce your risk of heart disease.

5. Add small amounts of unsaturated fats to your diet: Unsaturated fatty acids, in small amounts, has been shown to be heart healthy. Small amounts of these fats can decrease LDL cholesterol, while preserving HDL. Cooking with oils, however, may destroy essential fatty acid activity, and is not as heart healthy as adding uncooked sources to your foods.

6. Eat your fruits and veggies: A meta analysis of the latest studies concluded that individuals who consumed the most fruits and vegetables reduced risk of heart disease by 15%. A lower risk of stroke is also associated with higher intake of fruits and vegetables. The lowest risks were associated with consumption of cruciferous vegetables (broccoli, cabbage, cauliflower, brussel sprouts), green leafy vegetables, citrus fruits, and vitamin C rich fruit and vegetables.

7. Decrease caffeine in your diet: Caffeine has been shown to increase cholesterol levels; however, accumulated research indicates that this effect is minimized when coffee is brewed from drip coffee makers using filters. The older version of "percolating" coffee for long periods of time produces chemicals known to increase lipid cholesterol levels.

8. Minimize concentrated simple sugars. Concentrated simple sugar intake—sugar and other concentrated sweeteners like fructose, corn syrup, and honey—produce a liver enzyme (HMG-CoA reductase) that causes the liver to make more cholesterol (from acetate). Hence, eating sugar can increase your blood cholesterol levels.

Homocysteine

Over half of the people that get heart attacks do not have elevated cholesterol levels. The latest research is centered on several other molecules known to be involved in the process of plaque formation. A molecule called homocysteine is under intense investigation.[7] Homocysteine is an amino acid from protein-rich foods, which may be a better predictor of CVD. Homocysteine may combine with LDL cholesterol to form plaque on arterial walls. A B vitamin, folic acid, reduces levels of homocysteine. Folic acid is involved in the reaction that converts homocysteine back to another amino acid, methionine. Vitamin B6 and B12 are also involved in the reaction. Initial research indicates that as little as 150 micrograms of folic acid (20 ounces of orange juice) daily can reduce homocystine levels by 11% within one month.[10]

High-Sensitivity C-Reactive Protein

"Inflammation" is the process by which the body responds to injury or an infection. Laboratory evidence and findings from clinical and population studies suggest that inflammation is important in atherosclerosis This is the process in which fatty deposits build up in the inner lining of arteries.[11]

C-reactive protein (CRP) is one of the acute phase proteins that increase during systemic inflammation. It's been suggested that testing CRP levels in the blood may be an additional way to assess cardiovascular disease risk. A more sensitive CRP test, called a highly sensitive C-reactive protein (hs-CRP) assay, is available to determine heart disease risk.[11]

A growing number of studies have examined whether hs-CRP can predict recurrent cardiovascular disease, stroke and death in different settings. High levels of hs-CRP consistently predict recurrent coronary events in patients with unstable angina and acute myocardial infarction (heart attack). Higher hs-CRP levels also are associated with lower survival rates in these patients. Many studies have suggested that after adjusting for other prognostic factors, hs-CRP is useful as a risk predictor.[11] These studies have found that the higher the hs-CRP levels, the higher the risk of having a heart attack. In fact, the risk for heart attack in people in the upper third of hs-CRP levels has been determined to be twice that of those whose hs-CRP level is in the lower third. Studies have also found an association between sudden cardiac death, peripheral arterial disease and hs-CRP.[11]

Reducing CRP
Antioxidants – Vitamin A,C,E
Reduce weight if overweight, Aerobic exercise
Reduce/Eliminate Trans fats
Mediterranean diet (DASH), including olive oil and fish, fiber and walnuts and flaxseed
Brushing and flossing teeth
Aspirin, Statin Drugs

The major injurious factors that promote atherogenesis — cigarette smoking, hypertension, atherogenic lipoproteins, and hyperglycemia — are well established. These risk factors give rise to a variety of noxious stimuli that cause the release of chemicals and the activation of cells involved in the inflammatory process. These events are thought to contribute not only to the formation of plaque but may also contribute to its disruption resulting in the formation of a blood clot. Thus, virtually every step in atherogenesis is believed to involve substances involved in the inflammatory response and cells that are characteristic of inflammation.[11]

Blood levels of hs-CRP include:[11]
- If hs-CRP level is lower than 1.0 mg/L, a person has a low risk of developing cardiovascular disease.
- If hs-CRP is between 1.0 and 3.0 mg/L, a person has an average risk.
- If hs-CRP is higher than 3.0 mg/L, a person is at high risk.

If, after repeated testing, patients have persistently unexplained, markedly elevated hs-CRP, they should be evaluated to exclude noncardiovascular causes. Patients with autoimmune diseases or cancer, as well as other infectious diseases, may also have elevated CRP levels.[11]

Reducing hs-CRP include ingesting foods with antioxidants, reduce weight if overweight, incorporate cardiovascular disease, eliminate trans fats, eat a DASH type diet (see Hypertension), brush and floss teeth, and possibly aspirin and statin drugs.[11]

HYPERTENSION

The initial Dash study (Dietary Approaches to Stop Hypertension, 1997)[12] looked at the effects of entire diet, not supplements, on hypertension. The eight-week study consisted of 459 adults with normal, high-normal, or high blood pressure. Each was randomly assigned to eat one of three diets prepared by DASH dieticians. The usual diet (similar to the average American diet) had average levels of fat and cholesterol, and below-average levels of potassium, magnesium, and calcium; the Fruit and vegetable diet was identical except that eight to ten servings of fruits and vegetables a day replaced most snacks and sweets which increased potassium, magnesium, and fiber. The third diet, *the combination diet*, cut fat, saturated fat, and cholesterol while upping not only fruits and vegetables, but low-fat dairy foods which increased protein and calcium in addition to potassium, magnesium, and fiber. Calories, alcohol and sodium were the same in all three diets. The results reported in 1997 were indisputable. The combination diet reduced systolic blood pressure by 5.5 points and diastolic blood pressure by 3.0 points. Researchers indicated that there was no way of "teasing out" which nutrients were responsible. But from a public health perspective, it didn't matter. What does matter is that a diet rich in fruits and vegetables, with low fat dairy foods, seafood, and only lean meats and poultry, lowers blood pressure dramatically.

Dash-Sodium Diet

The same researchers published results from a second study known as the Dash-Sodium study[10]. The study consisted of 412 men and women. Participants were randomly assigned to either the DASH diet or a usual diet for 12 weeks. The sodium in both diets was changed every four weeks to one of three levels; a higher intake of 3,300 mg a day, an intermediate intake of 2,400 mg a day, or a lower intake of 1,500 mg a day. The results were startling. On both the DASH and the usual diets, the lower the sodium fell, the lower blood pressures fell. The DASH diet with lowest sodium intake cut blood pressure by an impressive 8.9 points in systolic pressure and 4.5 points in diastolic pressure when compared to the usual diet with the higher sodium intake. This is roughly twice the impact of the usual DASH diet alone. As expected, blood pressure fell more in the people with hypertension (11.5 systolic) than in individuals without hypertension (7.1 points).

Hundreds of other studies on animals and people, along with the startling results of the DASH-Sodium study have convinced most experts that sodium is a blood pressure booster. "This study unequivocally shows how important it is for people with or without hypertension to cut salt," says J. Stamler, professor emeritus at Northwestern University.

Cutting back to 1,500 mg of sodium a day isn't just about throwing out the salt shaker, it's about avoiding the large amounts that manufacturers dump into prepackaged foods. Salt in processed foods and restaurants accounts for more than 75% of the sodium we consume. Taste is not a good indicator of just how much salt is in these foods. A McDonald's burger has more sodium than its super size french fries. Even bread can contain large amounts of sodium without tasting salty. The lowest you can expect in a restaurant meal is 1000 mg (even if it is only grilled chicken breast, salad and a baked potato). Buffalo wings or fried mozzarella sticks contain approximately 1,800 mg of sodium. Meals in Chinese or Mexican restaurants will supply at least 2,000 mg of sodium; and an order of cheese fries contains 4,000 mg of sodium. The key to decreasing salt in the diet is to begin. While 1,500 mg appears to be ideal, cutting out even small amounts in the diet can add up to big health benefits.

According to the experts, here's how to begin:
1. Make it yourself. Most unprocessed foods are low in sodium;
2. Look for lower sodium-brands. Many pasta sauces contain well over 1,300 mg of sodium, but a cup of Healthy Choice Traditional sauce has 780 mg - a much healthier choice;
3. Look for low-sodium or reduced-sodium on the label. Low-sodium means less that 140 mg, and reduced-sodium means that the food must have at least 25% less sodium than the usual food.

For more menus, recipes, and eating tips visit the following Web sites: www.nhlbi.nih.gov/hbp/consumer/hearthealth/eating.html; www.dash.bwh.harvard.edu/[11]. Keep in mind to look for recipes and menus that indicate DASH-Sodium study since menus and recipes from the original DASH study may still appear on those sites. Or you can write: Dash Study, NHLBI Information Center, P.O. Box 30105, Bethesda, Maryland 20824-0105.[12]

Count the Nutrients

The DASH Combination Diet - which lowered blood pressure dramatically - is low in total fat, saturated fat, cholesterol, and sweets; high in fiber, potassium, calcium, and magnesium; and moderately high in protein. The following is a comparison of the DASH Combination diet and the DASH usual diet (which is closer to the typical American diet).

Nutrient	DASH Combination Diet	DASH Usual Diet
Total Fat (% of calories)	27	37
Saturated fat (% of calories)	6	16
Monounsaturated fat (% of calories)	13	13
Polyunsaturated fat (% of calories)	8	8
Carbohydrates (% of calories)	55	48
Protein (% of calories)	18	15
Cholesterol (mg per day)	150	300
Fiber (grams per day)	31	9
Potassium (mg per day)	4,700	1,700
Magnesium (mg per day)	500	165
Calcium (mg per day)	1,240	450

Source: Appel LJ, et al. A Clinical trial of the effects of dietary patterns on blood pressure. DASH Collaborative Research Group. N Eng J Med 336:1117, 1997.

Sample menu from the DASH-Sodium Study

		Sodium (mg)	Servings
Breakfast	Shredded wheat cereal (1/2 cup)	2	1 grain
	Skim milk (1 cup)	130	1 dairy
	Orange juice (1 cup	5	1 fruit
	Banana	1	1 fruit
	100% Whole-Wheat bread (1 slice)	150	1 grain
Lunch	Chicken Salad (3/4 cup)	150	1 poultry
	100% Whole-Wheat bread (2 slice)	300	2 grains
	Dijon mustard (1 tsp)	130	
	Tomato (2 large slices)	5	(1/2 veetable)
	Mixed cooked vegetables (1 cup)	25	2 vegetables
	Fruit cocktail, juice pack (1/2 cup)	5	1 fruit
Dinner	Baked Cod (3 oz.)	90	1 fish
	Green snap beans, from frozen, no salt (1 cup)	10	2 vegetables
	Baked potato (1 large)	20	1 vegetable
	Fat-free cheddar cheese (3 Tbs)	170	1 dairy
	Tossed salad with mixed greens (1 1/2 cups)	30	1.5 vegetables
	Olive-oil-and-vinegar dressing	0	1 oil
Snacks	Orange juice (1/2 cup)	3	1 fruit
	Almonds, diced, blanched, no salt	3	1 nuts, seeds, etc.
	Raisins, seedless (1/4 cup)	5	1 fruit
	Yogurt, fat-free with sugar (1 cup)	100	1 dairy

This one day menu provides: 2010 calories, 5 servings of fruits, 7 servings of vegetables, 3 servings of dairy, 59 grams of fat, 120 milligrams of cholesterol, and 1360 milligrams of sodium. (Calculated grams of protein using Nutrition Analysis Software is approximately 100 grams). The sodium was kept low by limiting processed foods. Source: National Heart, Lung, and Blood Institute (as taken from Nutrition Action Health Letter, December 2000).

STROKE

Stroke is the third leading cause of death in America and the No. 1 cause of adult disability. Eighty percent of strokes are preventable.[16]

A stroke occurs when a blood clot blocks an artery (a blood vessel that carries blood from the heart to the body) or a blood vessel (a tube through which the blood moves through the body) breaks, interrupting blood flow to an area of the brain. When either of these things happen, brain cells begin to die and brain damage occurs.[16]

When brain cells die during a stroke, abilities controlled by that area of the brain are lost. These abilities include speech, movement and memory. How a stroke patient is affected depends on where the stroke occurs in the brain and how much the brain is damaged.[16]

Anyone can have a stroke. But your chances of having a stroke increase if you meet certain criteria. Some of these criteria, called risk factors, are beyond your control — such as being over age 55, being male, being African American, Hispanic or Asian/Pacific Islander, or having a family history of stroke. Other stroke risk factors are controllable.[16]

The Stroke Prevention Guidelines were established by National Stroke Association's Stroke Prevention Advisory Board, an elite group of the nation's leading experts on stroke prevention. They were first published in a 1999 issue of Journal of the American Medical Association (JAMA) and have been updated to reflect current medical standards. National Stroke Association suggests you ask your doctor for advice on how to best use these guidelines.[16]

> Know your blood pressure.
> Find out if you have atrial fibrillation.
> If you smoke, stop.
> If you drink alcohol, do so in moderation.
> Find out if you have high cholesterol
> If you are diabetic...
> Exercise.
> Enjoy a lower sodium (salt), lower fat diet.
> Circulation (movement of the blood through the heart and blood vessels) problems.
> Know the Symptoms of Stroke.

It is important to recognize stroke symptoms and act quickly.[16]

> Common stroke symptoms seen in both men and women:
> · Sudden numbness or weakness of face, arm or leg — especially on one side of the body
> · Sudden confusion, trouble speaking or understanding
> · Sudden trouble seeing in one or both eyes
> · Sudden trouble walking, dizziness, loss of balance or coordination
> · Sudden severe headache with no known cause

Women may report unique stroke symptoms:

· sudden face and limb pain

· sudden hiccups

· sudden nausea

· sudden general weakness

· sudden chest pain

· sudden shortness of breath

· sudden palpitations

A new National Stroke Association study shows most Americans do not treat stroke as an emergency. When a stroke first hits, many people don't even recognize the symptoms. In fact, a recent National Stroke Association survey reports 1 in 3 Americans cannot name a single symptom a person might experience while having a stroke.[16]

Every minute counts for stroke patients and acting F.A.S.T. can lead patients to the stroke treatments they desperately need. The most effective stroke treatments are only available if the stroke is recognized and diagnosed within the first three hours of the first symptoms. Actually, many Americans are not aware that stroke patients may not be eligible for stroke treatments if they arrive at the hospital after the three-hour window.[16]

FACE	Ask the person to smile. Does one side of the face droop?
ARMS	Ask the person to raise both arms. Does one arm drift downward?
SPEECH	Ask the person to repeat a simple sentence. Are the words slurred? Can he/she repeat the sentence correctly?
TIME	If the person shows any of these symptoms, time is important. Call 911 or get to the hospital fast. Brain cells are dying.

CANCER

The studies linking a particular vitamin or mineral to good health could fill a small library.[17,18,19] But studies of the isolated nutrient, plucked out if its fruit or vegetable context, have backfired. For example, while antioxidants like vitamin C are widely believed to play a role in the cancer-fighting properties of fruits and vegetables, randomized controlled trials of vitamin C supplements haven't shown much benefit.[14] Isolating a particular vitamin has even proven to do more harm than good. In a famous 1994 study, smokers who took a 20mg supplement of beta-carotene every day had a higher incidence of lung cancer than those who didn't.[18] It appears that beta-carotene must work in concert with other substances to exert its effects.

A significant body of epidemiologic evidence associates certain dietary patterns with an increased risk of cancer.[20] A diet rich in fat and meat, and low in cereals, fiber, fruits, and vegetables is associated with an increased risk of colorectal, mammary, and other common forms of cancer. Limited diets in some countries with evident micronutrient deficiencies are also associated with an increased risk for certain forms of cancer. While population studies such as these cannot establish a cause-effect relationship between nutrition and cancer, a number of studies in animals support the concept that cancer results from a gene-nutrient interaction. In animals with well-defined mutations affecting cell signaling, such as the p53 mutation, tumor development can be affected by diet.

The final common mechanism believed to mediate the effects of different diets on cancer and aging is the oxidation of the genome and other cellular and subcellular structures. Mutations induced by oxidative damage may then lead to increased cellular proliferation, reduced apoptosis or both. Therefore, genes confer susceptibility to oxidative damage through absence or malfunction of the extensive antioxidant defense and DNA repair mechanisms, while the diet can affect whether and to what extent that oxidative damage occurs.

In aging, oxidative damage is increased and aging is the predominant risk factor for cancer. The demonstration of the effects of nutrition on cancer requires using age-adjusted incidences. Furthermore, dietary restriction with vitamin and antioxidant supplementation can extend maximum lifespan significantly in rodents. In epidemiologic studies in humans, the intake of 400 to 600 grams per day of fruits and vegetables is associated with a reduced risk of gastric and other cancers. The most common cancers in developed societies are breast, prostate and colon cancer. Obesity, high fat diets, and reduced intake of fiber from cereals, grains, fruits and vegetables comprise a high risk dietary pattern. For each of the most common cancers, there is extensive evidence of a variation in incidence as individuals move from low risk to high risk countries. For prostate cancer, there is an equal incidence of latent prostate cancer in the U.S. and Japan, but clinical cancer is five times more frequent in the U.S. In animal experiments, nutrition affects the growth, progression and metastasis of established tumors as well as the incidence of new tumors.[18]

Up to one third of all cancer cases may be prevented through healthy diets and exercise, notes FANSA.[18] Healthy diets and exercise may prevent as many cases of cancer in the United States as not smoking, according to a recent statement by the Food and Nutrition Science Alliance (FANSA). Cancer kills more than 500,000 Americans every year. In a review of cancer research, FANSA found overwhelmingly conclusive evidence that the risk of several types of cancer can be dramatically lowered through healthy dietary practices and exercise.[18]

Says Dennis Savaiano, PhD, Professor of Foods and Nutrition at Purdue University and Chair of the FANSA Committee, "In terms of cancer prevention, a healthy diet and exercise are as important as not smoking.[21] Approximately one-third of cancer cases are attributed to smoking, one-third to poor diet and lack of exercise, and one-third to genetic or other factors. Most Americans are already aware of the detrimental effects of smoking, but poor diet is cause for alarm. We need to initiate changes in behavior now, in order to reduce the number of cancer-related deaths in the years to come."

A large number of anticarcinogenic agents have been found in fruits and vegetables (antioxidants, fiber, dithiolthiones, glucosinolates and indoles, isothiocyanates, flavonoids, phenols, protease inhibitors, plant sterols and others).[17] A review by the University of Minnesota researchers of more than 100 studies indicated that these agents are indeed associated with a reduced risk of cancer, particularly in the gastrointestinal tract and respiratory tract, and a weaker association with the hormone related cancers.[22]

The FANSA Statement on Diet and Cancer Prevention in the United States specifically urges Americans to take the following steps to reduce their cancer risk:
- Eat plenty of fruits, vegetables, whole grain, and legumes
- Avoid empty calories from highly processed foods that are high in fat or sugar.
- Choose activities that involve moderate or vigorous exercise.
- Limit or abstain from alcohol.

The FANSA statement, which can be viewed at http://www.faseb.org/ascn/fansa12-99.htm,[21] is the first step in a nationwide call for action. In order to effect a change, all food, nutrition, fitness, health, and government organizations must strive to create consumer demand for a healthy lifestyle.

The Food and Nutrition Science Alliance is a partnership of four professional societies who have joined forces to speak with one voice on food and nutrition issues. Member organizations are The American Dietetics Association, The American Society for Clinical Nutrition, Inc., The American Society for Nutritional Sciences, and the Institute of Food Technologists.

Visit the following website to learn more about cancer risk for men and women: www.health.harvard.edu.

OTHER

Diseases associated with nutrient deficiencies are discussed in the corresponding chapters. This section will focus on several other nutritional disorders.

Celiac Disease

Celiac disease is a chronic inflammatory condition caused by ingestion of dietary gluten. This inflammation can cause malabsorption of several nutrients, which in turn is related to several deficiency disorders, such as anemia, cancer, and osteoporosis. Gluten is a protein found in wheat, rye, and barley.[22,23] It is broken down into smaller proteins and certain portions of these smaller proteins are what are thought to be toxic in celiac disease[24,25,26]. People who have celiac disease have specific genetic markers which elicit an autoimmune inflammatory cascade of events[24,27,28]. When individuals with celiac disease ingest foods containing gluten, the gluten is broken down into the smaller proteins. An enzyme in the small intestine alters part of the smaller proteins which initiates an inflammatory response which causes damage to the intestinal villi. There are 4 stages of tissue damage, progressing from inflammation to eventual complete villous atrophy.[24,25,26,27] This damage to the intestinal villi is responsible for the malabsorption of many nutrients and requisite signs and symptoms characteristic of the disease.

Symptoms include chronic diarrhea, anemia, fatigue, abdominal pain and bloating, weakness, bone pain, osteoporosis, spontaneous abortions and low birth weight babies in untreated pregnant women, and other vitamin-associated deficiencies. The prevalence of the disease appears to be increasing which may be due to increased awareness and better screening techniques.[19] The prevalence of the disease has grown from 1 in 1,000 ten years ago to estimates of between 1 in 300 to 1 in 100 today.[20,21] Individual sensitivity varies greatly among individuals. One person may become extremely ill from eating "gluten-free" food cooked on the same grill as gluten-containing food, while another individual may be able to eat a piece of bread and not have any symptoms.

The short term and long term adverse effects of the disease can be improved and even completely reversed with strict adherence to a gluten-free diet. A gluten-free diet is the only current treatment for celiac disease. Dietary restriction is difficult because gluten is not only in wheat, barley and rye, it is also used in many other foods. Careful attention to constantly changing ingredients in commercially prepared foods is necessary, along with careful cooking habits and extremely careful scrutiny while dining out. Currently, the regulations regarding products that are "gluten-free" are those that contain no more than 0.3% wheat protein, or 40-60 milligrams of gluten per 100 grams of product.[30,31,32] It is important to note that even if the claim "gluten-free" is on the label it does not necessarily mean that the product is totally gluten-free.

The following is a list of resources for individuals diagnosed with celiac disease: www.celiac.com; www.csaceliacs.org; www.glutenfree.com; *The Gluten-Free Gourmet* series of cookbooks by Bette Hagman.

GI Disorders

Gastrointestinal Disorders (GI) is a digestive disorder that interferes with the workings of the intestine. GI generally falls into two categories — functional and inflammatory.[34] Functional GI disorders, such as Irritable Bowel Syndrome (IBS), chronic diarrhea, constipation and intestinal pain, are characterized by symptoms and not by a visible sign of disease or injury. Inflammatory GI disorders include Inflammatory Bowel Disease (IBD), Crohn's Disease and ulcerative colitis.[34]

IBS known as functional gastrointestinal disorders is one of the most common chronic gastrointestinal illnesses. Although a gastrointestinal disorder, IBS has long been dismissed as a psychosomatic condition because a person's psychological disposition, such as anxiety and stress, may induce a feeling of constipation or diarrhea. Other symptoms of IBS, besides diarrhea and constipation, and abdominal pain, are bloating, gas, urgency to defecate, and a feeling of incomplete evacuation after a bowel movement. Studies have shown that IBS affects 3 to 22 percent of persons worldwide and its symptoms are reported by 12 percent of Americans. Women are three times more likely than men to develop IBS, and most IBS sufferers experience their first symptoms before their mid-thirties. The chronic discomfort and embarrassment of IBS besets the lives of millions of Americans every day, hindering social outings, regular work schedules, and family time. Americans spend $ 8 billion each year on medical costs related to IBS.[34]

All GI disorders can lead to anorexia because patients associate eating with unpleasant symptoms and so eat less. Adequate intake of a balanced diet is the goal of patients with IBD. Foods valuable to the diet such as dairy products may have been avoided, as some patients find their symptoms worsened, resulting in deficiency of calcium, protein and vitamin D. For IBS, certain foods and beverages may aggravate symptoms. Some common instigators are fried, fatty and spicy foods; alcohol and caffeine; chocolate; carbonated liquids; dairy products with lactose; sweeteners like sorbitol; wheat products; beans, broccoli and cabbage. Medications and vitamins can also be irritants. Doctors recommend increasing fiber or taking supplements like psyllium.[34]

Gastrointestinal Reflux Disease

Gastroesophageal reflux disease, or GERD, affects at least an estimated 5% to 7% of the global population – men, women, and children. Heartburn and/or acid regurgitation experienced weekly has been found to occur in 19.8% of individuals.[35]

Although common, GERD often is unrecognized – its symptoms misunderstood. This is unfortunate because GERD is generally a treatable disease. Serious complications can result if it is not treated properly.[35]

Persistent heartburn is the most frequent – but not the only – symptom of GERD. (The disease may be present even without apparent symptoms.) Heartburn is so common that it often is not associated with a serious disease, like GERD. All too often, GERD is either self- treated or mistreated.[34] Treatment usually must be maintained on a long-term basis, even after symptoms have been brought under control. Issues of daily living, and compliance with long-term use of medication need to be addressed as well. This can be accomplished through follow-up, support, and education.[34] Various methods to effectively treat GERD range from lifestyle measures to the use of medication or surgical procedures.   It is essential for individuals who suffer persistent heartburn or other chronic and recurrent symptoms of GERD to seek an accurate diagnosis, to work with their physician, and to receive the most effective treatment available.[35]

Crohn's Disease

Crohn's disease may also be called ileitis or enteritis.   Crohn's disease is an ongoing disorder that causes inflammation of the digestive tract, also referred to as the gastrointestinal (GI) tract.   Crohn's disease can affect any area of the GI tract, from the mouth to the anus, but it most commonly affects the lower part of the small intestine, called the ileum.   The swelling extends deep into the lining of the affected organ.   The swelling can cause pain and can make the intestines empty frequently, resulting in diarrhea.[34]

Because the symptoms of Crohn's disease are similar to other intestinal disorders, such as irritable bowel syndrome and ulcerative colitis, it can be difficult to diagnose.   Ulcerative colitis causes inflammation and ulcers in the top layer of the lining of the large intestine. In Crohn's disease, all layers of the intestine may be involved, and normal healthy bowel can be found between sections of diseased bowel.[34]

Crohn's disease affects men and women equally and seems to run in some families.   About 20 percent of people with Crohn's disease have a blood relative with some form of inflammatory bowel disease, most often a brother or sister and sometimes a parent or child.   Crohn's disease can occur in people of all age groups, but it is more often diagnosed in people between the ages of 20 and 30.[34]

Although the cause of Crohn's disease is not known, it is believed to be an autoimmune disease that is genetically linked. The highest relative risk occurs in siblings, affecting males and females equally. Smokers are three times more likely to get Crohn's disease.[34]

Scientists do not know if the abnormality in the functioning of the immune system in people with Crohn's disease is a cause, or a result, of the disease.   Research shows that the inflammation seen in the GI tract of people with Crohn's disease involves several factors: The genes the patient has inherited, the immune system itself, and the environment.   Foreign substances, also referred to as antigens, are found in the environment.   One possible cause for inflammation may be the body's reaction to these antigens, or that the antigens themselves are the cause for the inflammation. Some scientists think that a protein produced by the immune system, called anti-tumor necrosis factor (TNF), may be a possible cause for the inflammation associated with Crohn's disease.[34]

The most common symptoms of Crohn's disease are abdominal pain, often in the lower right area, and diarrhea. Rectal bleeding, weight loss, arthritis, skin problems, and fever may also occur. Bleeding may be serious and persistent, leading to anemia. Children with Crohn's disease may suffer delayed development and stunted growth. The range and severity of symptoms varies.[34]

Nutritional complications are common in Crohn's disease.   Deficiencies of proteins, calories, and vitamins are well documented.   These deficiencies may be caused by inadequate dietary intake, intestinal loss of protein, or poor absorption, also referred to as malabsorption.   Other complications associated with Crohn's disease include arthritis, skin problems, inflammation in the eyes or mouth, kidney stones, gallstones, or other diseases of the liver and biliary system. Some of these problems resolve during treatment for disease in the digestive system, but some must be treated separately.[34]

Treatment may include drugs, nutrition supplements, surgery, or a combination of these options. The goals of treatment are to control inflammation, correct nutritional deficiencies, and relieve symptoms like abdominal pain, diarrhea, and rectal bleeding.[34]   The doctor may recommend nutritional supplements, especially for children whose growth has been slowed. Special high-calorie liquid formulas are sometimes used for this purpose. A small number of patients may need to be fed intravenously for a brief time through a small tube inserted into the vein of the arm. This procedure can help patients who need extra nutrition temporarily, those whose intestines need to rest, or those whose intestines cannot absorb enough nutrition from food. There are no known foods that cause Crohn's disease. However, when people are suffering a flare in disease, foods such as bulky grains, hot spices, alcohol, and milk products may increase diarrhea and cramping.[34] People with Crohn's disease often experience a decrease in appetite, which can affect their ability to receive the daily nutrition needed for good health and healing. In addition, Crohn's disease is associated with diarrhea and poor absorption of necessary nutrients. No special diet has been proven effective for preventing or treating Crohn's disease, but it is very important that people who have Crohn's disease follow a nutritious diet and avoid any foods that seem to worsen symptoms. There are no consistent dietary rules to follow that will improve a person's symptoms.[34]

There is no evidence showing that stress causes Crohn's disease. However, people with Crohn's disease sometimes feel increased stress in their lives from having to live with a chronic illness. Some people with Crohn's disease also report that they experience a flare in disease when they are experiencing a stressful event or situation. There is no type of person that is more likely to experience a flare in disease than another when under stress. For people who find there is a connection between their stress level and a worsening of their symptoms, using relaxation techniques, such as slow breathing, and taking special care to eat well and get enough sleep, may help them feel better.[34]

Ulcerative Colitis

Ulcerative colitis is a form of inflammatory bowel disease (IBD). It is systemic disease and is a form of colitis, a disease of the intestine specifically the large intestine or colon, that includes characteristic ulcers, or open sores, in the colon. The main symptom of the disease is usually diarrhea mixed with blood. Because of the name, IBD is often confused with irritable bowel syndrome ("IBS"), a troublesome, but much less serious condition. Ulcerative colitis has similarities to Crohn's disease, another form of IBD.[6]

SUMMARY

The FAO group undertook the task of reviewing the scientific data. Their findings were not surprising. While many of the diseases associated with age and gender are modifiable. The growing epidemic of chronic diseases is related to dietary and lifestyle changes. Population based studies indicate increased consumption of energy-dense diets high in fat, particularly saturated fat, and low in unrefined carbohydrates. These patterns were found to be in combination with a decline in energy expenditure associated with a sedentary lifestyle — motorized transport, labor-saving devices in the home, the phasing out of physically demanding manual tasks in the workplace, and leisure time that is preponderantly devoted to physically undemanding pastimes. Because of these changes in dietary and lifestyle patterns, chronic diseases — including diabetes mellitus, cardiovascular disease (CVD), hypertension and stroke, and some types of cancer — are becoming increasingly significant causes of death and disease both in developing and newly developed countries, placing additional burdens on already overtaxed national health budgets.

It has been calculated that, in 2001, chronic diseases contributed approximately 60% of the 56.5 million total reported deaths in the world and approximately 46% of the global burden of disease. The proportion of this burden is expected to increase to 57% by 2020. Almost half of the total chronic disease deaths are attributable to cardiovascular diseases; obesity and diabetes are also showing worrying trends, not only because they already affect a large proportion of the population, but also because they have started to appear earlier in life. It has been projected that, by 2020, chronic diseases will account for almost three-quarters of all deaths worldwide, with 71% of deaths due to ischaemic heart disease (IHD), 75% of deaths due to stroke, and 70% of deaths due to diabetes will occur in developing countries.

Diabetes is widely recognized as one of the leading causes of death and disability in the United States. About 65 percent of deaths among those with diabetes are attributed to heart disease and stroke. There are 20.8 million adults and children diagnosed with diabetes in the U.S. "Age, race, and educational level all are associated with diabetes; however obesity is by far the best predictor of being newly diagnosed with diabetes. The inability of the body to control blood glucose levels leads to life threatening health problems.

Diabetes is associated with long-term complications that affect almost every part of the body. The disease often leads to blindness, heart and blood vessel disease, stroke, kidney failure, amputations, and nerve damage. Uncontrolled diabetes can complicate pregnancy, and birth defects are more common in babies born to women with diabetes. Increases in diabetes among US adults continue in both sexes, all ages, all races, all educational levels, and all smoking levels.

Diabetes is a disease in which the body does not produce or properly use insulin.[2] Type 1 diabetes is usually diagnosed in children and young adults, and was previously known as juvenile diabetes. In type 1 diabetes, the body does not produce insulin. Type 2 diabetes is the most common form of diabetes. In type 2 diabetes, either the body does not produce enough insulin or the cells ignore the insulin. Glucose builds up in the blood instead of going into cells and can cause serious problems.

The three main types of diabetes are: type 1 diabetes; type 2 diabetes; and gestational diabetes.

Studies show that people at high risk for diabetes can prevent or delay the onset of the disease by losing 5 to 7 percent of their weight, if they are overweight—that's 10 to 14 pounds for a 200-pound person. Getting at least 30 minutes of moderate-intensity physical activity five days a week and eating a variety of foods that are low in fat can produce the wanted results.

Cardiovascular disease refers to the class of diseases that involve the heart or blood vessels (arteries and veins). While the term technically refers to any disease that affects the cardiovascular system, it is usually used to refer to those related to atherosclerosis (arterial disease). These conditions have similar causes, mechanisms, and treatments. Each year, heart disease kills more Americans than cancer. Diseases of the heart alone caused 30% of all deaths, with other diseases of the cardiovascular system causing substantial further death and disability. By the time that heart problems are detected, the underlying cause (atherosclerosis) is usually quite advanced, having progressed for decades. There is therefore increased emphasis on preventing atherosclerosis by modifying risk factors, such as healthy eating, exercise and avoidance of smoking.

Atherosclerosis is the accumulation of lipids and other materials in the arteries. No one is free from atherosclerosis; the important questions become how far advanced is it and what can be done to slow or reverse its progression. Atherosclerosis usually begins with the accumulation of soft fatty streaks along the inner arterial walls, especially at branch points. These fatty streaks gradually enlarge and become hardened with minerals forming plaques. Plaques stiffen the arteries and narrow them. Most people have well-developed plaques in their arteries by the age of 30.[2] As the arteries harden, blood flows less freely through the kidneys. The kidneys respond by raising the blood pressure. Clots normally form and dissolve in the blood all the time. When these processes are balanced, the clots do not harm. Platelets cause clots to form whenever they encounter injuries in blood vessels. In atherosclerosis, platelets form and aid in the formation of clots.

Most heart attacks occur in individuals where there is less than 50% blockage of the vessel lumen and unstable plaques burst, triggering formation of an intraluminal clot. A number of nutritional factors including obesity, increased fat intake, reduced fiber intake, and reduced intake of fruits and vegetables have all been associated with an increased risk of heart disease. In fact, many of these factors have occurred together in modern diets making it difficult to separately evaluate each of these nutritional entities separately. It is clear that cholesterol intake, when considered separately from high fat foods, has a lesser effect on cholesterol levels than dietary fat and calories.

Cholesterol levels correlate with risk of heart disease, with two fold increase in risk between patients with cholesterol levels <180 mg/dl compared to individuals with cholesterol levels > 240 mg/dl. There are 37 million Americans with cholesterol > 240 mg/dl, and 56 million individuals with cholesterol levels greater than 200 mg/dl.

Three to four million individuals are taking cholesterol-lowering drugs, and debates on the effectiveness of these medications continue. An article published in Business Week (Jan. 17, 2008) reported the results from of research completed by Dr. James M. Wright, a professor at the University of British Columbia and director of the government-funded Therapeutics Initiative. Dr. Wright was very surprised when he looked at the data for the majority of patients who don't have heart disease. He found no benefit in people over the age of 65, no matter how much their cholesterol levels declined, and no benefit in women of any age. He did see a small reduction in the number of heart attacks for middle-aged men taking statins in clinical trials. But even for these men, there was no overall reduction in total deaths or illnesses requiring hospitalization—despite big reductions in "bad" cholesterol. (See "Integrity in Science" for more details concerning the controversy over cholesterol-lowering drugs.)

The initial Dash study (Dietary Approaches to Stop Hypertension, 1997)[9] looked at the effects of entire diet, not supplements, on hypertension. The eight-week study consisted of 459 adults with normal, high-normal, or high blood pressure. Each was randomly assigned to eat one of three diets prepared by DASH dieticians. The usual diet (similar to the average American diet) had average levels of fat and cholesterol, and below-average levels of potassium, magnesium, and calcium; the Fruit and vegetable diet was identical except that eight to ten servings of fruits and vegetables a day replaced most snacks and sweets which increased potassium, magnesium, and fiber. The third diet, *the combination diet*, cut fat, saturated fat, and cholesterol while upping not only fruits and vegetables, but low-fat dairy foods which increased protein and calcium in addition to potassium, magnesium, and fiber. Calories, alcohol and sodium were the same in all three diets. The results reported in 1997 were indisputable. The combination diet reduced systolic blood pressure by 5.5 points and diastolic blood pressure by 3.0 points. Researchers indicated that there was no way of "teasing out" which nutrients were responsible. But from a public health perspective, it didn't matter. What does matter is that a diet rich in fruits and vegetables, with low fat dairy foods, seafood, and only lean meats and poultry, lowers blood pressure dramatically. The same researchers have now published results from a new study known as the Dash-Sodium study[10]. The study consisted of 412 men and women. Participants were randomly assigned to either the DASH diet or a usual diet for 12 weeks. The sodium in both diets was changed every four weeks to one of three levels; a higher intake of 3,300 mg a day, an intermediate intake of 2,400 mg a day, or a lower intake of 1,500 mg a day. The results were startling. On both the DASH and the usual diets, the lower the sodium fell, the lower blood pressures fell.   The DASH diet with lowest sodium intake cut blood pressure by an impressive 8.9 points in systolic pressure and 4.5 points in diastolic pressure when compared to the usual diet with the higher sodium intake. This is roughly twice the impact of the usual DASH diet alone. As expected, blood pressure fell more in the people with hypertension (11.5 systolic) than in individuals without hypertension (7.1 points).

Stroke is the third leading cause of death in America and the No. 1 cause of adult disability. 80% of strokes are preventable; you can prevent a stroke! A stroke occurs when a blood clot blocks an artery (a blood vessel that carries blood from the heart to the body) or a blood vessel (a tube through which the blood moves through the body) breaks, interrupting blood flow to an area of the brain. When either of these things happen, brain cells begin to die and brain damage occurs. When brain cells die during a stroke, abilities controlled by that area of the brain are lost. These abilities include speech, movement and memory. How a stroke patient is affected depends on where the stroke occurs in the brain and how much the brain is damaged.

Up to one third of all cancer cases may be prevented through healthy diets and exercise, notes FANSA.[18] Healthy diets and exercise may prevent as many cases of cancer in the United States as not smoking, according to a recent statement by the Food and Nutrition Science Alliance (FANSA). Cancer kills more than 500,000 Americans every year. In a review of cancer research, FANSA found overwhelmingly conclusive evidence that the risk of several types of cancer can be dramatically lowered through healthy dietary practices and exercise.

Celiac disease is a chronic inflammatory condition caused by ingestion of dietary gluten. This inflammation can cause malabsorption of several nutrients, which in turn is related to several deficiency disorders, such as anemia, cancer, and osteoporosis. Gluten is a protein found in wheat, rye, and barley.[22,23]   When individuals with celiac disease ingest foods containing gluten, the gluten is broken down into the smaller proteins. An enzyme in the small intestine alters part of the smaller proteins which initiates an inflammatory response which causes damage to the intestinal villi. There are 4 stages of tissue damage, progressing from inflammation to eventual complete villous atrophy.[24,25,26,27] This damage to the intestinal villi is responsible for the malabsorption of many nutrients and requisite signs and symptoms characteristic of the disease. A gluten-free diet is the only current treatment for celiac disease. Dietary restriction is difficult because gluten is not only in wheat, barley and rye, it is also used in many other foods. Careful attention to constantly changing ingredients in commercially prepared foods is necessary, along with careful cooking habits and extremely careful scrutiny while dining out. Currently, the regulations regarding products that are "gluten-free" are those that contain no more than 0.3% wheat protein, or 40-60 milligrams of gluten per 100 grams of product.

Gastrointestinal Disorders (GI) is a digestive disorder that interferes with the workings of the intestine. GI generally falls into two categories — functional and inflammatory. Functional GI disorders, such as Irritable Bowel Syndrome (IBS), chronic diarrhea, constipation and intestinal pain, are characterized by symptoms and not by a visible sign of disease or injury. Inflammatory GI disorders include Inflammatory Bowel Disease (IBD), Crohn's Disease and ulcerative colitis. Gastroesophageal reflux disease, or GERD, affects at least an estimated 5% to 7% of the global population – men, women, and children. (Prevalence based on once per day heartburn.) Heartburn and/or acid regurgitation experienced weekly has been found to occur in 19.8% of individuals. Although common, GERD often is unrecognized – its symptoms misunderstood. This is unfortunate because GERD is generally a treatable disease. Serious complications can result if it is not treated properly. Persistent heartburn is the most frequent – but not the only – symptom of GERD. (The disease may be present even without apparent symptoms.) Heartburn is so common that it often is not associated with a serious disease, like GERD. All too often, GERD is either self- treated or mistreated. Various methods to effectively treat GERD range from lifestyle measures to the use of medication or surgical procedures. It is essential for individuals who suffer persistent heartburn or other chronic and recurrent symptoms of GERD to seek an accurate diagnosis, to work with their physician, and to receive the most effective treatment available.

Crohn's disease is an ongoing disorder that causes inflammation of the digestive tract, also referred to as the gastrointestinal (GI) tract. Crohn's disease can affect any area of the GI tract, from the mouth to the anus, but it most commonly affects the lower part of the small intestine, called the ileum. About 20 percent of people with Crohn's disease have a blood relative with some form of inflammatory bowel disease, most often a brother or sister and sometimes a parent or child. Crohn's disease can occur in people of all age groups, but it is more often diagnosed in people between the ages of 20 and 30.

CHAPTER 6- SAMPLE TEST

1. Discuss cardiovascular disease and the role of lifestyle in prevention of the disease.

2. Discuss the role of diet in the reduction of hypertension

3. Discuss the factors involved in stokes and prevention guidelines

5. List and discuss ways to reduce cancer risk.

6. Detail the factors involved in celiac disease.

7. Discuss functional and inflammatory GI disorders and provide details of each.

REFERENCES

1. WHO Library Cataloguing-in-Publication Data Joint WHO/FAO Expert Consultation on Diet, Nutrition and the Prevention of Chronic Diseases (2002 : Geneva, Switzerland) Diet, nutrition and the prevention of chronic diseases: report of a joint WHO/FAO expert consultation, Geneva, 2002.

2. http://www.diabetes.org/about-diabetes.jsp. Jan, 2008.

3. http://diabetes.webmd.com/guide/diabetes-overview. Jan, 2008.

4. http://ndep.nih.gov/diabetes/prev/prevention.htm. Jan, 2008.

5. http://diabetes.webmd.com/more-than-50-ways-prevent-diabetes. Jan, 2008.

6. Wikipedia, The Free Encyclopedia, *Cardiovascular Disease*, Jan, 2008.

7. http://www.mayoclinic.com/health/arteriosclerosis-atherosclerosis/DS00525. Jan, 2008.

8. http://www.businessweek.com/magazine/content/08_04/b4068052092994.htm. Jan, 2008.

9. Tufts University health & Nutrition Letter, Latest Heory on Heart Disease, May 2000.

10. http://www.homocysteine.net/what-is-it.asp?lang=EN. Jan, 2008.

Sources:

11. Inflammation, Heart Disease and Stroke: The Role of C-Reactive Protein. http://www.americanheart.org/presenter.jhtml?identifier=4648. Jan, 2008.

12. Appel, LJ, et al. Clinical trial of the effects of dietary patterns on blood pressure. DASH Collaborative Research Group. *N Eng J Med,* 336:1117, 1997.

13. Conlin PR, et al. The effect of dietary patterns on blood pressure control in hypertensive patients. *Am J Hyperten:* 13(9): 945, 2000.

14. Web sites for more information on DASH Diet: www.nhlbi.nih.gov/hbp/consumer/hearthealth/eating.html; www.dashbwh.harvard.edu/.

15. To write for more information on Dash diet: DASH Study, NHLBI Information Center, P.O.Box 30105, Bethesda, MD 20824-0105.

16. http://www.stroke.org/site/PageNavigator/HOME. Jan, 2008.

17. Steinmertz, KA, et al. Vegetable, fruit and cancer prevention: A review. *J of the Am Dietetic Assoc,* 96, 1027-39, 1996.

18. Tufts University, 2000. New questions about the safety of vitamin C pills. In S. Gershoff (Ed), *Tufts University Health & Nutrition Letter,* 18(2), 1.

19. Liebman, B., Center for Science in the Public Interest. Antioxidants, report sets ceilings. in M Jacobson (Ed), *Nutrition Action Health Letter,* 27(5),9-11,2000.

20. Liebman, B. Center for Science in the Public Interest. Solving the diet and disease puzzle. In M. Jacobson (ed.), *Nutrition Action Health Letter,* 26(4), 1,1999.

21. FANSA Statement on cancer risk: http://www.faseb.org/ascn/fansa12-99.htm.

22. Ciclitiria, P.J. "Recent advances in coeliac disease". Clinical Medicine. 3(2); March-April,2003. 166-169.

23. Abdulkarim, AS & Murray, JA. "Review article: the diagnosis of coeliac disease". Aliment Pharmacol Ther. 17;2003. 987-995.

24. Schuppan, D. "Current concepts of celiac disease pathogenesis". Gastroenterology. 119(1); 2000.234-242.

25. Mowat Amc I. "Dietary modifications: food dependent autoimmunity in coeliac disease". Gut. 43(5); 1998.599-600.

26. Feighery CF. "Coeliac disease: how much of what is toxic to whom?". Gut.43(2);Aug 1998.164-5.

27. Barera G et al. "Body composition in children with celiac disease and the effects of a gluten-free diet: a prospective case-control study". Am J Clin Nutr. 72; 2000.71-5.

28. Bateson MC. "Advances in gastroenterology and hepatology". Postgrad Med J. 7; 2000.328-332.

29. Mustalahti K, Collin P, Sievanen H, Salmi J and Maki M. "Osteopenia in patients with clinically silent celiac disease warrants screening". The Lancet. 354(9180); Aug 28, 1999.744-5.

30. Capristo E et al. "Changes in body composition, substrate oxidation, and resting metabolic rate in adult celiac disease patients after a 1-year gluten-free diet treatment". Am J Clin Nutr. 72; 2000.76-81.

31. Celiac.com: http://www.celiac.com,_www.celiac.com/frequent.html.

32. Kaukinen K, Collin P, Holm K, Rantala I, Vuolteenaho N, Reunala T, Maki M. "Wheat starch-containing gluten-free flour products in the treatment of coeliac disease and dermatitis herpetiformis". Scand J Gastroenterol. 34(2); Feb 1999.163-9.

33. Thompson T. "Questionable foods and the gluten-free diet: survey of current recommendations". JADA. 100(4);Apr 2000.463-5.

34. Crohn's and Colitis Foundation of America, Inc. 1996-2002.

35. http://www.aboutgerd.org/. Jan, 2008.

35. Wilkinson, Donna "Among This Ailment's Symptoms: Acute Embarrassment", June 22, 2003, The New York Times.

36. http://digestive.niddk.nih.gov/ddiseases/pubs/crohns/#what.

Chapter 7
Micronutrients - Vitamins

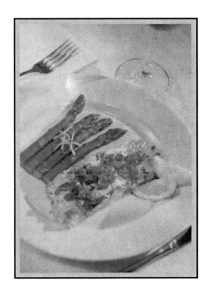

In this chapter we will take a more in-depth look at vitamins. Some vitamins are involved in energy metabolism; some are antioxidants; while others have roles in vision, reproduction, etc. Vitamin C plays a role in immune function and collagen formation. Vitamin D plays a role in bone remodeling.

Please do not feel that you must memorize all the information in this chapter. Some of the information presented here is meant to be a resource for future reference. The goal of this textbook is to have you become familiar with the major roles of each micronutrient and with foods containing substantial amounts of each nutrient.

Objectives

After reading and studying this chapter you should:

1. Be able to discuss the water soluble vitamins: roles, food sources, deficiencies, Dietary Reference Intakes, and toxicities.

2. Be able to discuss the fat soluble vitamins: roles, food sources, deficiencies, Dietary Reference Intakes, and toxicities.

INTRODUCTION

The term vitamin is derived from the root word "vita" meaning essential to life. As discussed in Chapter 1, the RDA's are standards set by scientists studying the individual nutrients and published by the government. These standards include a safety margin and are not "minimum" standards.[1] Many of the diseases occurring during deficiency states are the same diseases manifested during toxic states.

Vitamins are a group of organic compounds other than protein, carbohydrates, or fats that cannot be manufactured by the body and are required in small amounts for specific functions of growth, main-tenance, reproduction and repair and include: vitamin A, vitamin C, vitamin D, vitamin E, vitamin K, vitamin B1 (thiamine), vitamin B2 (riboflavin, vitamin B3 (niacin), pantothenic acid, biotin, vitamin B6, vitamin B12, folate (folic acid). Vitamins differ from the energy nutrients in that they are needed in smaller amounts. The energy nutrients are required in gram amounts, while the micronutrients are needed in milligram, microgram and picogram amounts. Vitamins do not provide energy, and they act singly, not as macromolecules. Vitamins are vital to life, are organic, and are available in all foods. They require no digestion and are absorbed intact into the bloodstream.[1]

The two major categories of vitamins are the water soluble vitamins and the fat soluble vitamins. The water soluble vitamins include all the B vitamins and vitamin C. The fat soluble vitamins are vitamin A, vitamin D, vitamin E, and vitamin K. The body absorbs water soluble vitamins directly into the blood, whereas fat soluble vitamins must be packaged and transported in lipoproteins. In the cells, water soluble vitamins freely circulate while fat soluble vitamins tend to become trapped in the cells associated with fat. Hence, the fat soluble vitamins tend to remain in fat storage sites, are less readily excreted, and more likely to reach toxic levels when consumed in excess.[2]

Because vitamins are organic, they are susceptible to destruction by oxygen. The water soluble vitamins, thiamine, riboflavin, and vitamin C are the most vulnerable. Prolonged heating destroys much of these nutrients.

Dietary Reference Intakes were discussed in Chapter 1. The latest DRI's included a new category. For the first time, the National Academy of Sciences issued Tolerable Upper Intake Levels, or ULs, to tell people how much is a safe upper limit for nearly two dozen nutrients.[3] The UL is the highest level of a vitamin or mineral that can be safely taken without any risk of adverse effect. Just going a little bit above the UL is not going to produce harm, but as you get higher and higher, you're increasing your risk of side effects. ULs are based on the earliest side effects to occur—not necessarily the most serious ones. But that doesn't mean that there are no serious side effects. For example, flushing is the most sensitive indicator of niacin excess. But if people take a much higher dose—like 3,000 to 5,000 mg of niacin a day—to lower their cholesterol, they can get severe liver disease. To protect the population as much as possible, experts do not advise taking more than the UL on a daily basis.[3]

The Center for Science in the Public Interest, publisher of Nutrition Action, wants the Food and Drug Administration to require ULs on at least some supplement labels over the next few years.[3]

WATER SOLUBLE VITAMINS

Water soluble vitamins consist of the B vitamins and Vitamin C.

B Vitamins

The B vitamins are thiamine, riboflavin, pantothenic acid, niacin, biotin, folate (folic acid), B6, and B12. Each of these vitamins have different roles in metabolism. It is beyond the scope of this course to examine each B vitamin individually in great depth. However, more details have been added in the *reference notes*.

Thiamine, riboflavin, niacin, pantothenic acid, and biotin serve as coenzymes. These vitamins are indispensable in the breakdown of foods. In the metabolism of glucose, these coenzymes "hop" onto enzymes; this process activates the enzymes. Remember, enzymes are proteins involved in facilitating chemical reactions. While B vitamins do not, themselves, provide energy, a deficiency will cause inefficient breakdown of carbohydrate resulting in exhaustion. Each of the vitamin B coenzymes is involved, directly or indirectly, in energy metabolism. Some are involved in the energy releasing reactions themselves. Others help build new cells to deliver oxygen and nutrients which permits the energy pathways to run.[2]

Folate, B6, and B12 are involved in the formation of new cells. Folate deficiency impairs cell division and protein synthesis, a process critical to growing tissues. Deficiency of folate during pregnancy can lead to birth defects. Vitamin B12 is required to convert folate to its active form. Hence both vitamins become critical during pregnancy.[2]

Vitamin B12 is unique among the nutrients in that it is found almost exclusively in animal products. For persons over 50 a supplement containing 25 micrograms of vitamin B12 is considered a good idea since many persons over this age have a condition called atrophic gastritis. In this condition not enough stomach acid is secreted to cleave the vitamin from the protein in food. The supplement form is easily absorbed whether or not stomach acid is available.[6]

Food Sources[2]

Thiamine: brewer's yeast, sunflower seeds, wheat germ, asparagus, potatoes, black-eyed peas, mushrooms, green leafy vegetables

Riboflavin: mushrooms, green leafy vegetables, brewer's yeast, milk, yogurt, cheeses, beef

Pantothenic acid: meat, fish, poultry, whole grain cereals, legumes

Niacin: beef, fish, chicken, brewer's yeast, mushrooms, green leafy vegetables

Biotin: widespread in foods in small amounts
There is no RDA for biotin. Biotin is synthesized in the GI tract by bacteria, but it is not known how much is available for absorption. Biotin appears to be resistant to light and heat. Egg yolks are rich sources of biotin.

Vitamin B6:   banana, brewer's yeast, fish, turkey, green leafy vegetables, chicken, dairy products, whole grain foods

Folate: Brewer's yeast, lentils, green leafy vegetables, cauliflower, dairy products, fruits

Vitamin B12:   exclusively found in animal products
Fermented soy products (miso) or sea algae do not provide B12. Vegans need a reliable source such as B12 fortified soy products. It may take fifteen to twenty years to develop deficiencies because the body recycles B12, reabsorbing it over and over again.

Deficiency

The B vitamins are indispensable to metabolism. They are involved in every crucial step. If the body becomes deficient in one of these vitamins, a domino effect occurs, which literally affects all of metabolism. These nutrients are interdependent; they affect one another's absorption, metabolism, and excretion. A deficiency of one may reflect a deficiency or abnormality in the action of another, i.e. deficiencies of single B vitamins seldom show up in isolation. Studies have shown that deficiencies are eliminated by supplying foods not pills.

Dietary Reference Intakes[10]

> *Thiamine* - men 1.2 mg/day, women 1.1 mg/day;   No Tolerable Upper Limit established
> *Riboflavin* - men 1.3 mg/day, women 1.1 mg/day; No Tolerable Upper Limit established
> *Pantothenic Acid* (Estimated safe and adequate intake) - 4 to 7 mg/day for adults; No Tolerable Upper Limit established
> *Biotin* (Estimated safe and adequate intake) - 20 to 35 micrograms/day; No Tolerable Upper Limit established
> *Niacin* - men 16 mg NE/day, women 14 mg NE/day; Tolerable Upper Limit is 35 mg/day for adults
> *Folate* - 400 mcg/day for men, 400 mcg/day women; Tolerable Upper Limit is 1000 mcg per day for adults.
> *Vitamin B6* - 1.3 mg/day for men and women (1.7 men over 50 and 1.5 women over 50); Tolerable Upper Limit is 100 mg/day
> *Vitamin B12* is 2.4 micrograms/day for adults (25 mcg over 50); No Tolerable Upper Limit established

Toxicity

Toxicities of the B vitamins is uncommon, but do occur in individuals taking large amounts through the use of supplements. When the cells become oversaturated with a vitamin, they must work to reduce the excess. Parts of the cell actually see this excess as a "drug" and organelles inside the cell begin to destroy the vitamin. Studies have shown that when pharmacological doses of these vitamins are stopped, the same problems seen in deficiency develop. Hence, large amounts of these vitamins can lead to exhaustion.[2]

Reference notes

Thiamin (vitamin B1) is part of a coenzyme known at thiamin pyrophosphate-TPP. TPP promotes the conversion of pyruvate to acetyl-CoA. Thiamine is also part of nerve cell membranes. Consequently nervous and muscle tissue require thiamin.[2]

Riboflavin, also known as vitamin B2, like thiamin helps enzymes facilitate the release of energy from carbohydrates. The coenzyme forms of riboflavin are FMN (flavin mononucleotide) and FAD (flavin adenine dinucleotide) and are also involved in the energy cycle. Riboflavin also helps support vision and skin health.

Pantothenic acid is important as part of CoA. Acetyl CoA is a crossroad molecule of several metabolic pathways, including glucose, and fatty acid metabolism. Pantothenic acid is involved in more than 100 different steps in the synthesis of lipids, neurotransmitters, steroid hormones, and the molecule that transports oxygen-hemoglobin.[2]

Niacin consists of 2 other chemical structures; nicotinic acid and nicotinamide. Nicotinamide is the major form of niacin in the blood and the body can easily convert nicotinic acid to nicotinamide. The two coenzyme forms of niacin are NAD (nicotinamide adenine dinucleotide) and NADP (the phosphate form of NAD). Both coenzyme forms are involved in the metabolism of glucose, fat, and alcohol. Niacin is unique among the B vitamins because the body can make niacin from the amino acid tryptophan. To make 1 milligram of niacin requires 60 milligrams of dietary tryptophan. This is why niacin requirements are stated in "niacin equivalents", reflecting the body's ability to convert tryptophan to niacin (1 mg niacin = 60 mg tryptophan). The disease seen in niacin deficiency is pellagra. The symptoms of pellagra are diarrhea, dermatitis, and dementia. Other deficiency symptoms include irritability, loss of appetite, weakness, dizziness, mental confusion which can progress to dementia. Large doses of niacin are dangerous. Niacin in large doses (10 times the RDA) dilates the capillaries and causes a tingling effect known as "niacin flush". Physicians sometimes treat high blood cholesterol by prescribing high doses of niacin. Large doses are not supplements, but are drugs and may cause liver damage, peptic ulcers, and possibly diabetes. Symptoms of niacin toxicity include diarrhea, flushing, itching, headaches, nausea, heartburn, fainting, dizziness, and abnormal liver function.[2]

Biotin plays an important role in metabolism as a coenzyme that serves as a carbon dioxide carrier. This role is critical in the energy cycle (TCA). It is involved in the reaction from pyruvate to acetyl-CoA (delivering a carbon). This coenzyme also serves crucial roles in gluconeogenesis, fatty acid synthesis, and the breakdown of certain fatty acids and amino acids. Biotin deficiencies are rarely seen. Deficiencies can be induced by eating lots of raw eggs. A protein in raw egg white binds biotin and thus prevents its absorption. Studies have shown that more than two dozen egg whites must be consumed daily to produce a deficiency. Cooking denatures the protein and does not bind the biotin. Deficiency symptoms would include abnormal heart function, nausea, depression, muscle pain, weakness, fatigue, and hair loss.[2]

Folate occurs naturally in foods and folic acid or folacin is the form found in supplements. Folate (and folic acid) is part of the coenzyme forms DHF (dihydrofolate) and THF (tetrahydrofolate). THF helps convert vitamin B12 to one of its coenzyme forms and helps synthesize the DNA required for all rapidly growing cells (as in pregnancy). Foods deliver folate in bound form (folate bound to amino acids). Enzymes in the intestines must hydrolyze the bound folate to folate with one amino acid (monoglutamate form). The complicated system of transporting and converting folates is vulnerable to GI problems. For instance, in alcohol abuse, a folate deficiency rapidly develops and impairs the GI tract further. Folic acid and vitamin B12 help cells to multiply. This function is especially important in cells that have short life spans and must replace themselves rapidly. Cells such as red blood cells and the cells that line the GI tract are especially vulnerable to deficiency of these vitamins. The first symptoms of a deficiency are a type of anemia and GI tract deterioration. Other symptoms include frequent infections, depression, confusion and fatigue. Deficiency during pregnancy can cause birth defects, specifically neural tube defects.[2]

Folic acid supplementation has been shown to reduce the risk of neural tube defects and fortifying the nation's food supply with folic acid is under consideration. Toxicity symptoms include many of the same symptoms seen in deficiency, including birth defects and masking of B12 deficiency symptoms; hence overdosing the nation's food supply could be just as damaging.[2]

Vitamin B6 assists enzymes that metabolize amino acids. Vitamin B6 occurs in three forms-pyridoxal, pyridoxine, and pyridoxamine. All three forms can be converted to the coenzyme, pyridoxal phosphate (PLP). This coenzyme has the ability to transfer amino groups which allows the body to synthesize nonessential amino acids from essential amino acids. PLP is also involved in the conversion of tryptophan to niacin and the conversion of tryptophan to the neurotransmitter serotonin; and is involved in the synthesis of heme.[2] B6 also influences immune function and steroid hormone activity. Unlike other water soluble vitamins, B6 is stored in muscle tissue. Deficiency symptoms include weakness, irritability, insomnia, cracked corners of the mouth, and dermatitis. Advanced symptoms include growth failure, impaired motor function, and convulsions. Toxicity symptoms include depression, fatigue, irritability, headaches, numbness, nerve damage, and difficulty walking.[2]

The roles of B6 and B12 intertwine because each depends on the other for activation. Vitamin B12 (also known as cobalamin) regenerates the folate coenzyme. The regeneration of an amino acid, methionine and the synthesis of genetic material (DNA and RNA) depend on the folate coenzyme and so depends on both folate and B12. Vitamin B12 is also involved in bone cell activity and metabolism, as well as nerve fiber promotion and normal growth. B12 requires an intrinsic factor for absorption which is synthesized in the stomach. In the stomach this intrinsic factor binds to B12 and the complex is then absorbed by the small intestines. Most B12 deficiencies are due to inadequate absorption, not intake. Some people inherit a defective gene for the intrinsic factor producing a deficiency. A deficiency can also develop if the stomach has been injured and the intrinsic factor can not be produced. One of the first symptoms of B12 deficiency is the anemia due to folate deficiency. Either folate or B12 will clear up the anemia, but if folate is given when B12 is needed, the results are disastrous with devastating neurological symptoms because B12 is the vitamin involved in maintaining and protecting nerve cell fibers and promoting their normal growth. Folate cures the blood symptoms but not the nerve symptoms. Since B12 is found exclusively in animal products, strict vegetarians could become deficient in this nutrient. Also, high folate intakes in this group could mask a B12 deficiency. It is therefore essential that strict vegetarians obtain a reliable source of B12.[10]

Vitamin C

Throughout history, the benefit of plant food to survive long sea voyages has been occasionally recommended by authorities. John Woodall, the first appointed surgeon to the British East India Company, recommended the preventive and curative use of lemon juice in his book "The Surgeon's Mate", in 1617. The Dutch writer, Johann Bachstrom, in 1734, gave the firm opinion that "scurvy is solely owing to a total abstinence from fresh vegetable food, and greens; which is alone the primary cause of the disease."[11]

While the earliest documented case of scurvy was described by Hippocrates around the year 400 BC, the first attempt to give scientific basis for the cause of this disease was by a ship's surgeon in the British Royal Navy, James Lind. Scurvy was common among those with poor access to fresh fruit and vegetables, such as remote, isolated sailors and soldiers. While at sea in May 1747, Lind provided some crew members with two oranges and one lemon per day, in addition to normal rations, while others continued on cider, vinegar, sulfuric acid or seawater, along with their normal rations. In the history of science this is considered to be the first occurrence of a controlled experiment comparing results on two populations of a factor applied to one group only with all other factors the same. The results conclusively showed that citrus fruits prevented the disease. Lind published his work in 1753 in his *Treatise on the Scurvy*.[11]

It was 1795 before the British navy adopted lemons or lime as standard issue at sea. Limes were more popular as they could be found in British West Indian Colonies, unlike lemons which weren't found in British Dominions, and were therefore more expensive. This practice led to the American use of the nickname "limey" to refer to the British. Captain James Cook had previously demonstrated and proven the principle of the advantages of carrying fresh foods on board, by taking his crews to the Hawaiian Islands and beyond without losing any of his men to scurvy. For this otherwise unheard of feat, the British Admiralty awarded him a medal.[11]

The name "antiscorbutic" was used in the eighteenth and nineteenth centuries as general term for those foods known to prevent scurvy, even though there was no understanding of the reason for this. These foods included but were not limited to: lemons, limes, and oranges; sauerkraut, cabbage, malt, and portable soup.[11]

In 1907, Axel Holst and Theodor Frølich, two Norwegian physicians studying beriberi contracted aboard ship's crews in the Norwegian Fishing Fleet, wanted a small test mammal to substitute for the pigeons they used. They fed guinea pigs their test diet, which had earlier produced beriberi in their pigeons, and were surprised when scurvy resulted instead. Until that time scurvy had not been observed in any organism apart from humans, and had been considered an exclusively human disease.[11]

In 1912, the Polish-American biochemist Casimir Funk, while researching deficiency diseases, developed the concept of vitamins to refer to the nutrients which are essential to health. Then, from 1928 to 1933, the Hungarian research team of Joseph L Svirbely and Albert Szent-Györgyi and, independently, the American Charles Glen King, first isolated vitamin C and showed it to be ascorbic acid. For this, Szent-Györgyi was awarded the 1937 Nobel Prize in Medicine.[11]

Vitamin C has many varied roles. Vitamin C (ascorbic acid) is generally known as an antioxidant. An antioxidant is any substance that can donate electrons to another substance. Substances that have an "unpaired electron" are toxic to the cell. Antioxidants have the capacity to pair with the unpaired electron, thereby rendering it nontoxic to the cell. (You can think of antioxidants as a type of pac-man eating up radicals).[12] In other roles vitamin C helps specific enzymes perform their functions. Vitamin C helps to form the fibrous, structural protein collagen. Collagen strengthens blood vessel walls, forms scar tissue, and is a matrix for bone growth. Vitamin C also helps in the absorption or iron.[12]

Food sources

Fruits (papaya, oranges, cantaloupe, grapefruit, strawberries), vegetables (broccoli, brussel sprouts, cauliflower, green pepper, asparagus)[2]

Deficiency

Two of the earliest signs of a deficiency relate to its role in maintaining the integrity of blood vessels. The gums around teeth bleed easily, and capillaries under the skin break producing pinpoint hemorrhages. Plaques grow in the arteries and eventually the disease scurvy develops. In scurvy muscles degenerate, promotion of normal collagen ceases, further hemorrhaging occurs, skin becomes rough, brown, and scaly. Other symptoms include pinpoint hemorrhages, bone fragility, joint pain, rough skin, blotchy patches, and failure of wounds to heal. Too little vitamin C can lead to signs and symptoms of deficiency, including:[12]Dry and splitting hair; gingivitis (inflammation of the gums); bleeding gums; rough, dry, scaly skin; decreased wound-healing rate; easy bruising; nosebleed; Weakened tooth enamel; swollen and painful joints; anemia; decreased ability to fight infection; possible weight gain because of slowed metabolism'

Dietary Reference Intakes[12]

United States vitamin C recommendations include:

Infants 0-6 months 40	
7-12 months 50	
Children 1-3 years 15	
4-8 years 25	
Males	Females
9-13 years 45	9-13 years 45
4-18 years 75	4-18 years 65
19-30 years 90	19-30 years 75
31-50 years 90	31-50 years 75
51-70 years 90	51-70 years 75
>70 years 90	>70 years 75

Toxicity

As with the B vitamins, toxicity is seen only in persons consuming huge amounts through supplements. Doses larger than 200 mg cause suppression of the immune system.[12] Persons taking large pharmacological doses (3000 mg) over an extended time period have an adaptive response. If the person then suddenly reduces intake to normal levels the same disease seen in deficiency - scurvy - develops. The body may adapt by limiting absorption or destroying and excreting more of the vitamin than usual. By suddenly reducing intake the accelerated disposal system may not be able to avoid destroying too much of the vitamin. Toxic symptoms include nausea, abdominal cramps, hot flashes, rashes, and diarrhea.

Reference Notes

Cells are largely held together by collagen. When a person is wounded, collagen glues the separated tissue faces together, forming scar tissue. This is especially important in the artery walls which must expand and contract with each beat of the heart.

In collagen, the amino acids proline and lysine are abundant. These amino acids are hydroxylated to hydroxyproline or hydroxylysine. The enzyme involved in the hydroxylation process requires both vitamin C and iron. Hydroxyproline and hydroxylysine facilitate the binding together of collagen fibers to make strong structures. Vitamin C also assists in the metabolism of several amino acids that are converted to hormones—epinephrine and thyroxin. Epinephrine is the hormone involved in the "fight or flight" reaction, while thyroxin is a thyroid hormone involved in basal metabolism. Thyroxin regulates metabolic rate. Under physiological stress (fever or extreme cold weather), metabolic rate increases, thereby increasing vitamin C needs. The role of vitamin C in the prevention of cancer and other diseases is under investigation. There is a large growing body of evidence that vitamin C is protective against certain types of cancer.

FAT SOLUBLE VITAMINS

The fat soluble vitamins A, D, E, and K are found in the fat and oily parts of foods. Because they are insoluble in water, they require bile for digestion and are transported in lipoproteins. If taken in excess of need, they move into the liver and fat tissue and remain there instead of being excreted. The risk of toxicity is greater than with water soluble vitamins. The four fat soluble vitamins are involved in growth and maintenance of the body. They are involved in the health and functioning of the eyes, skin, GI tract, lungs, bones, teeth, nervous system and blood. They also interact with minerals.

Vitamin A

Vitamin A is a group of compounds that play an important role in vision, bone growth, reproduction, cell division, and cell differentiation (in which a cell becomes part of the brain, muscle, lungs, blood, or other specialized tissue.[14,15,16] Vitamin A helps regulate the immune system, which helps prevent or fight off infections by making white blood cells that destroy harmful bacteria and viruses.[10,15,16] Vitamin A also may help lymphocytes (a type of white blood cell) fight infections more effectively. Vitamin A promotes healthy surface linings of the eyes and the respiratory, urinary, and intestinal tracts.[17] When those linings break down, it becomes easier for bacteria to enter the body and cause infection. Vitamin A also helps the skin and mucous membranes function as a barrier to bacteria and viruses.[15,16,18]

In general, there are two categories of vitamin A, depending on whether the food source is an animal or a plant.   Vitamin A found in foods that come from animals is called preformed vitamin A. Vitamin A has three different active forms: retinol, retinal, and retinoic acid. Together they are called retinoids. It is one of the most usable forms of vitamin A is retinol. Sources include liver, whole milk, and some fortified food products. Retinol can be made into retinal and retinoic acid (other active forms of vitamin A) in the body.[17]

Vitamin A that is found in colorful fruits and vegetables is called provitamin A carotenoid. They can be made into retinol in the body. Common provitamin A carotenoids found in foods that come from plants are beta-carotene, alpha-carotene, and beta-cryptoxanthin.[22] Among these, beta-carotene is most efficiently made into retinol.[19,20,21] Alpha-carotene and beta-cryptoxanthin are also converted to vitamin A, but only half as efficiently as beta-carotene.[18] Of the 563 identified carotenoids, fewer than 10% can be made into vitamin A in the body.[19] Lycpene, lutein, and zeaxanthin are carotenoids that do not have vitamin A activity but have other health promoting properties.[10] The Institute of Medicine (IOM) encourages consumption of all carotenoid-rich fruits and vegetables for their health-promoting benefits.[10] Dietary intake studies suggest an association between diets rich in beta-carotene and vitamin A and a lower risk of many types of cancer.[23] A higher intake of green and yellow vegetables or other food sources of beta carotene and/or vitamin A may decrease the risk of lung cancer.[14,33,34] However, a number of studies that tested the role of beta-carotene supplements in cancer prevention did not find them to protect against the disease. In the Alpha-Tocopherol Beta-Carotene (ATBC) Cancer Prevention Study, more than 29,000 men who regularly smoked cigarettes were randomized to receive 20 mg beta-carotene alone, 50 mg alpha-tocopherol alone, supplements of both, or a placebo for 5 to 8 years. Incidence of lung cancer was 18% higher among men who took the beta-carotene supplement. Eight percent more men in this group died, as compared to those receiving other treatments or placebo.[25] Similar results were seen in the Carotene and Retinol Efficacy Trial (CARET), a lung cancer chemoprevention study that provided subjects with supplements of 30 mg beta-carotene and 25,000 IU retinyl palmitate (a form of vitamin A) or a placebo. This study was stopped after researchers discovered that subjects receiving beta-carotene had a 46% higher risk of dying from lung cancer.[26,27] The IOM states that "beta-carotene supplements are not advisable for the general population," although they also state that this advice "does not pertain to the possible use of supplemental beta-carotene as a provitamin A source for the prevention of vitamin A deficiency in populations with inadequate vitamin A".[10]

Osteoporosis, a disorder characterized by porous and weak bones, is a serious health problem for more than 10 million Americans, 80% of whom are women. Another 18 million Americans have decreased bone density which precedes the development of osteoporosis. Many factors increase the risk for developing osteoporosis, including being female, thin, inactive, at advanced age, and having a family history of osteoporosis. An inadequate dietary intake of calcium, cigarette smoking, and excessive intake of alcohol also increase the risk.[28,29,30] Researchers are now examining a potential new risk factor for osteoporosis: an excess intake of vitamin A. Animal, human, and laboratory research suggests an association between greater vitamin A intake and weaker bones.[31,32] Worldwide, the highest incidence of osteoporosis occurs in northern Europe, a population with a high intake of vitamin A.[32] However, decreased biosynthesis of vitamin D associated with lower levels of sun exposure in this population may also contribute to this finding.

Food Sources

Retinol is found in foods that come from animals such as whole eggs, milk, and liver. Most fat-free milk and dried nonfat milk solids sold in the United States are fortified with vitamin A to replace the amount lost when the fat is removed. Fortified foods such as fortified breakfast cereals also provide vitamin A. Provitamin A carotenoids are abundant in darkly colored fruits and vegetables. The 2000 National Health and Nutrition Examination Survey (NHANES) indicated that major dietary contributors of retinol are milk, margarine, eggs, beef liver and fortified breakfast cereals, whereas major contributors of provitamin A carotenoids are carrots, cantaloupes, sweet potatoes, and spinach.[33]

Deficiency

Deficiency symptoms do not appear until stores are depleted which may take up to a year. Vitamin A deficiency is common in developing countries but rarely seen in the United States. A deficiency is most often associated with strict dietary restrictions and excess alcohol intake.[34] Severe zinc deficiency, which is also associated with strict dietary limitations, often accompanies vitamin A deficiency. Zinc is required to make retinol binding protein (RBP) which transports vitamin A. Therefore, a deficiency in zinc limits the body's ability to move vitamin A stores from the liver to body tissues.[30] Night blindness is one of the first signs of vitamin A deficiency. Vitamin A deficiency contributes to blindness by making the cornea very dry and damaging the retina and cornea. Vitamin A deficiency diminishes the ability to fight infections. In countries where such deficiency is common and immunization programs are limited, millions of children die each year from complications of infectious diseases such as measles. In vitamin A-deficient individuals, cells lining the lungs lose their ability to remove disease-causing microorganisms. This may contribute to the pneumonia associated with vitamin A deficiency.

A deficiency can occur when vitamin A is lost through chronic diarrhea and through an overall inadequate intake, as is often seen with protein-energy malnutrition.[15] Low blood retinol concentrations indicate depleted levels of vitamin A. This occurs with vitamin A deficiency but also can result from an inadequate intake of protein, calories, and zinc, since these nutrients are needed to make RBP.[30] Iron deficiency can also affect vitamin A metabolism, and iron supplements provided to iron-deficient individuals may improve body stores of vitamin A and iron.[10] Excess alcohol intake depletes vitamin A stores. Also, diets high in alcohol often do not provide recommended amounts of vitamin A.[10] It is very important for people who consume excessive amounts of alcohol to include good sources of vitamin A in their diets. Vitamin A supplements may not be recommended for individuals who abuse alcohol, however, because their livers may be more susceptible to potential toxicity from high doses of vitamin A.   A medical doctor will need to evaluate this situation and determine the need for vitamin A supplements. Deficiency symptoms include cessation of bone growth, change in shapes of bones, development of cracks in teeth and tendency to decay, anemia, plugging of hair follicles forming white lumps. Vitamin A deficiency in pregnancy can lead to birth defects. Deficiency of vitamin A is the major cause of childhood blindness (xerophthalmia) in the world. Blindness progresses first appearing as night blindness. If left untreated, this disease quickly progresses to irreversible blindness. Vitamin A deficiency also increases susceptibility to infectious disease. Children in third world countries given vitamin A supplements recovered faster from pneumonia and other respiratory infections. Vitamin A supplementation also reduces the risk of dying from measles by at least 50%.

Dietary Reference Intakes[6]

Recommended Dietary Allowances (RDAs) for vitamin A (mcgRAE)					
Age	Children	Males	Females	Pregnancy	Lactation
1-3	300				
4-8	400				
9-13	600				
14-18		900	700	750	1,200
19+		900	700	770	1,300

Recommended Dietary Allowances (RDAs) for vitamin A (IU)					
Age	Children	Males	Females	Pregnancy	Lactation
1-3	1,000 IU				
4-8	1,320 IU				
9-13	2,000 IU				
14-18		3,000	2,310 IU	2,500 IU	4,000 IU
19+		3,000	2,310 IU	2,565 IU	4,300 IU

Toxicity

There are four major adverse effects of too much vitamin A: birth defects, liver abnormalities, reduced bone mineral density that may result in osteoporosis, and central nervous system disorders[10]. Toxic symptoms can also arise after consuming very large amounts of preformed vitamin A over a short period of time. Signs of acute toxicity include nausea and vomiting, headache, dizziness, blurred vision, and muscular uncoordination.[10]   Tolerable Upper Intake Levels (ULs) have been established for vitamin A.[10]   The UL does not apply to malnourished individuals receiving vitamin A either periodically or through fortification programs as a means of preventing vitamin A deficiency. It also does not apply to individuals being treated with vitamin A by medical doctors for diseases such as retinitis pigmentosa.

The UL for vitamin A from retinol is 10,000 IU. You can find single-nutrient supplements with 25,000 IU of vitamin A in any health-food store. You can put yourself in danger by taking those on a daily basis. And children are better off with a daily multi that has no more than the UL for vitamin A, which is 3,000 IU for 4- to 8-year-olds and 2,000 IU for younger children.[10] In women who are capable of becoming pregnant, the risk is birth defects. In the rest of the population, it's irreversible liver disease. We're talking about severe, fibrotic, cirrhotic liver disease, not just elevated liver enzymes. When the elderly consume vitamin A, they clear it from the blood and store it in the liver less efficiently than younger people. And we have customarily taken those higher blood levels as a sign of overload, so it makes sense that the elderly would be more prone to toxicity. But we don't have evidence that they actually develop liver toxicity more often.[10]

The ULs for Vitamin A assume that all of the vitamin A in the supplement comes from retinyl palmitate or other forms of retinol, not from beta-carotene or other carotenoids, which have no UL because there is insufficient evidence of toxicity.[10] Provitamin A carotenoids such as beta-carotene are generally considered safe because they are not associated with specific adverse health effects. Their conversion to vitamin A decreases when body stores are full. A high intake of provitamin A carotenoids can turn the skin yellow, but this is not considered dangerous to health.

Reference Notes

The cells that reside in the retina of the eye contain about 30 million molecules or retinal containing visual pigment. Visual activity leads to repeated small losses of retinal and necessitates its constant replenishment from retinol in the blood. Vitamin A and its relatives are the source of all the retinal in the pigments of the eye. Seeing a sudden bright light when the eyes are accustomed to dark destroys much more retinal than seeing light by day. Hence if the body's vitamin A stores are low night blindness can result. Most of the vitamin A in the body is found in the body's skin and linings (only about 1000th is found in the retina). All body surfaces, both inside and out, are covered by layers of cells known as epithelial cells (skin, linings of the mouth, stomach, intestines, lungs, urinary tract, bladder, eyelids, mucous membranes of the GI tract). Vitamin A helps maintain the integrity of all these cells by promoting cell differentiation. Vitamin A also plays an important role in immunity by maintaining healthy epithelial tissues which aid in the prevention of invasion of bacteria and viruses.

Vitamin A is involved in bone remodeling; specifically this vitamin is involved in the process of dismantling of bone, removing the parts that are not needed as the bone grows longer. A human fetus also has a tail and loses it, a process that depends on vitamin A. Vitamin A is also involved in the regulation of steroid and thyroid hormones that regulate metabolism, grown, cell differentiation, and embryonic development.

Vitamin D

Vitamin D is a fat soluble vitamin that is found in food and can also be made in your body after exposure to ultraviolet (UV) rays from the sun. Sunshine is a significant source of vitamin D because UV rays from sunlight trigger vitamin D synthesis in the skin.[36,37] Vitamin D exists in several forms, each with a different level of activity. Calciferol is the most active form of vitamin D. Other forms are relatively inactive in the body. The liver and kidney help convert vitamin D to its active hormone form.[38] Once vitamin D is produced in the skin or consumed in food, it requires chemical conversion in the liver and kidney to form 1,25 dihydroxyvitamin D, the physiologically active form of vitamin D. Active vitamin D functions as a hormone because it sends a message to the intestines to increase the absorption of calcium and phosphorus.[38] The major biologic function of vitamin D is to maintain normal blood levels of calcium and phosphorus.[38,39] By promoting calcium absorption, vitamin D helps to form and maintain strong bones. Vitamin D also works in concert with a number of other vitamins, minerals, and hormones to promote bone mineralization. Without vitamin D, bones can become thin, brittle, or misshapen. Vitamin D sufficiency prevents rickets in children and osteomalacia in adults, two forms of skeletal diseases that weaken bones.[40,41] Research also suggests that vitamin D may help maintain a healthy immune system and help regulate cell growth and differentiation, the process that determines what a cell is to become.[38,42,43]

Food Sources

Fortified foods are common sources of vitamin D.[39] In the 1930s, rickets was a major public health problem in the United States (U.S.). A milk fortification program was implemented to combat rickets, and it nearly eliminated this disorder in the U.S.[39,40] About 98% to 99% of the milk supply in the U.S. is fortified with 10 micrograms (ìg) (equal to 400 International Units or IU) of vitamin D per quart. One cup of vitamin D fortified milk supplies one-half of the recommended daily intake for adults between the ages of 19 and 50, one-fourth of the recommended daily intake for adults between the ages of 51 and 70, and approximately 15% of the recommended daily intake for adults age 71 and over. Although milk is fortified with vitamin D, dairy products made from milk, such as cheese and ice creams, are generally not fortified with vitamin D and contain only small amounts. Some ready-to-eat breakfast cereals may be fortified with vitamin D, often at a level of 10% to 15% of the Daily Value*. For a complete list of foods refer to the U.S. Department of Agriculture's Nutrient Database Web site: http://www.nal.usda.gov/fnic/cgi-bin/nut_search.pl.

Sun exposure is perhaps the most important source of vitamin D because exposure to sunlight provides most humans with their vitamin D requirement .[48] UV rays from the sun trigger vitamin D synthesis in skin.[48,49] Season, geographic latitude, time of day, cloud cover, smog, and sunscreen affect UV ray exposure and vitamin D synthesis.[49] For example, sunlight exposure from November through February in Boston is insufficient to produce significant vitamin D synthesis in the skin. Complete cloud cover halves the energy of UV rays, and shade reduces it by 60%. Industrial pollution, which increases shade, also decreases sun exposure and may contribute to the development of rickets in individuals with insufficient dietary intake of vitamin D.[50] Sunscreens with a sun protection factor (SPF) of 8 or greater will block UV rays that produce vitamin D, but it is still important to routinely use sunscreen to help prevent skin cancer and other negative consequences of excessive sun exposure. An initial exposure to sunlight (10 -15 minutes) allows adequate time for Vitamin D synthesis and should be followed by application of a sunscreen with an SPF of at least 15 to protect the skin. Ten to fifteen minutes of sun exposure at least two times per week to the face, arms, hands, or back without sunscreen is usually sufficient to provide adequate vitamin D.[49] It is very important for individuals with limited sun exposure to include good sources of vitamin D in their diet.

Deficiency

Nutrient deficiencies are usually the result of dietary inadequacy, impaired absorption and utilization, increased requirement, or increased excretion. A deficiency of vitamin D can occur when usual intake is below recommended levels when there is limited exposure to sunlight when the kidney cannot convert vitamin D to its active hormone form when someone cannot adequately absorb vitamin D from the digestive tract Vitamin D deficient diets are associated with milk allergy, lactose intolerance, and strict vegetarianism.[44] Infants fed only breast milk also receive insufficient amounts of vitamin D unless they also receive appropriate levels of vitamin D supplementation.[52] The classic vitamin D deficiency diseases are *rickets and osteomalacia*. In children, vitamin D deficiency causes rickets. Rickets is a bone disease characterized by a failure to properly mineralize bone tissue. Rickets results in soft bones and skeletal deformities.[50] Rickets was first described in the mid-17th century by British researchers.[50,53]

In the late 19th and early 20th century, German physicians noted that consuming 1 to 3 teaspoons (3 teaspoons is equal to 1 tablespoon) of cod liver oil per day could reverse rickets.[53] The most common causes of rickets are vitamin D deficiency from a vitamin D deficient diet, lack of sunlight, or both. The recommendation to fortify milk with vitamin D made rickets a rare disease in the U.S. for many years. However, rickets has recently reemerged, in particular among African American infants and children.[50,53] In 2003, a report from Memphis, Tennessee, described 21 cases of rickets among infants, 20 of whom were African-American.[53] Prolonged exclusive breastfeeding without vitamin D supplementation is one of the most significant causes of the reemergence of rickets. Additional causes include extensive use of sunscreens and increased use of day-care, resulting in decreased outdoor activity and sun exposure among children.[50,53] Rickets is more prevalent among immigrants from Asia, Africa, and Middle Eastern countries for a variety of reasons.[50] Among immigrants, vitamin D deficiency has been associated with iron deficiency, leading researchers to question whether or not iron deficiency may impair vitamin D metabolism.[50] Immigrants from these regions are also more likely to follow dress codes that limit sun exposure. In addition, darker pigmented skin converts UV rays to vitamin D less efficiently than lighter skin.[50] In adults, vitamin D deficiency can lead to osteomalacia, which results in muscular weakness in addition to weak bones.[40,41] Symptoms of bone pain and muscle weakness may indicate vitamin D deficiency, but symptoms may be subtle and go undetected in the initial stages. A deficiency is accurately diagnosed by measuring the concentration of a specific form of vitamin D in blood.[44,49]

It can be difficult to obtain enough vitamin D from natural food sources. For many people, consuming vitamin D fortified foods and adequate sunlight exposure are essential for maintaining a healthy vitamin D status. In some groups, dietary supplements may be needed to meet the daily need for vitamin D. In infants, vitamin D requirements cannot be met by human (breast) milk alone,[39,54] which usually provides approximately 25 IU vitamin D per liter. Sunlight is a potential source of vitamin D for infants, but the American Academy of Pediatrics (AAP) advises that infants be kept out of direct sunlight and wear protective clothing and sunscreen when exposed to sunlight.[56] The American Academy of Pediatrics (AAP) recommends a daily supplement of 200 IU vitamin D for breastfed infants beginning within the first 2 months of life unless they are weaned to receive at least 500 ml (about 2 cups) per day of vitamin D-fortified formula.[55] Children and adolescents who are not routinely exposed to sunlight and do not consume at least 2, 8-fluid ounce servings of vitamin D-fortified milk per day are also at higher risk of vitamin D deficiency and may need a dietary supplement containing 200 IU vitamin D. Formula fed infants usually consume recommended amounts of vitamin D because the 1980 Infant Formula Act requires that infant formulas be fortified with vitamin D. The minimal level of fortification required is 40 IU vitamin D per 100 calories of formula. The maximum level of vitamin D fortification allowed is 100 IU per 100 calories of formula. This range of fortification produces a standard 20 calorie per ounce formula providing between 265 and 660 IU vitamin D per liter.

Americans age 50 and older are believed to be at increased risk of developing vitamin D deficiency.[49] As people age, skin cannot synthesize vitamin D as efficiently and the kidney is less able to convert vitamin D to its active hormone form. It is estimated that as many as 30% to 40% of older adults with hip fractures are vitamin D insufficient.[48] Therefore, older adults may benefit from supplemental vitamin D. Home bound individuals, people living in northern latitudes such as in New England and Alaska, women who wear robes and head coverings for religious reasons, and individuals working in occupations that prevent sun exposure are unlikely to obtain much vitamin D from sunlight. It is important for people with limited sun exposure to consume recommended amounts of vitamin D in their diets or consider vitamin D supplementation.[62,63,64] Melanin is the pigment that gives skin its color. Greater amounts of melanin result in darker skin. The high melanin content in darker skin reduces the skin's ability to produce vitamin D from sunlight. It is very important for African Americans and other populations with dark-pigmented skin to consume recommended amounts of vitamin D. Some studies suggest that older adults, especially women, in these groups are at even higher risk of vitamin D deficiency.[51,65] Individuals with darkly pigmented skin who are unable to get adequate sun exposure and/or consume recommended amounts of vitamin D may benefit from a vitamin D supplement.

As a fat soluble vitamin, vitamin D requires some dietary fat for absorption. Individuals who have a reduced ability to absorb dietary fat may require vitamin D supplements.[66]   A deficiency of vitamin D also contributes to osteoporosis by reducing calcium absorption.[68] While rickets and osteomalacia are extreme examples of vitamin D deficiency, osteopororsis is an example of a long-term effect of vitamin D insufficiency.[69] Adequate storage levels of vitamin D help keep bones strong and may help prevent osteoporosis in older adults, in non-ambulatory individuals (those who have difficulty walking and exercising), in post-menopausal women, and in individuals on chronic steroid therapy.[70]

Caffeine may inhibit vitamin D receptors, thus limiting absorption of vitamin D and decreasing bone mineral density. A study found that elderly postmenopausal women who consumed more than 300 milligrams per day of caffeine (which is equivalent to approximately 18 oz of caffeinated coffee) lost more bone in the spine than women who consumed less than 300 milligrams per day.[92]   However, there is also evidence that increasing calcium intake (by, for example, adding milk to coffee) can counteract any potential negative effect that caffeine may have on bone loss. More evidence is needed before health professionals can confidently advise adults to decrease caffeine intake as a means of preventing osteoporosis.

Dietary Reference Intakes[39]

Recommendations for vitamin D are provided in the Dietary Reference Intakes (DRIs) developed by the Institute of Medicine (IOM) of the National Academy of Sciences.[39]   The RDA recommends the average daily intake that is sufficient to meet the nutrient requirements of nearly all (97-98%) healthy individuals in each age and gender group.[39]

The IOM determined there was insufficient scientific information to establish a RDA for vitamin D. Instead, the recommended intake is listed as an Adequate Intake (AI), which represents the daily vitamin D intake that should maintain bone health and normal calcium metabolism in healthy people. AIs meet or exceed the amount needed to maintain a nutritional state of adequacy in nearly all members of a specific age and gender group. The UL, on the other hand, is the maximum daily intake unlikely to result in adverse health effects.[35]   AIs for vitamin D may be listed on food and dietary supplement labels as either micrograms (mcg) or International Units (IU).   The biological activity of 1 mcg vitamin D is equal to 40 IUs.[39]

Adequate Intake for vitamin D for infants, children, and adults[39]

Age	Children(g/day)	Men(g/day)	Women(g/day)	Pregnancy(g/day)
Birth to 13 years	5(=200 IU)			
14 to 18 years	5(=200 IU)	5(=200 IU)	5(=200 IU)	5(=200 IU)
19 to 50 years	5(=200 IU)	5(=200 IU)	5(=200 IU)	5(=200 IU)
51 to 70 years		10(=400 IU)	10(=400 IU)	
71+ years		15(=600 IU)	15(=600 IU)	

Toxicity

Vitamin D toxicity can cause nausea, vomiting, poor appetite, constipation, weakness, and weight loss. It can also raise blood levels of calcium, causing mental status changes such as confusion. High blood levels of calcium also can cause heart rhythm abnormalities. Calcinosis, the deposition of calcium and phosphate in the body's soft tissues such as the kidney, can also be caused by vitamin D toxicity.[39] Sun exposure is unlikely to result in vitamin D toxicity. Diet is also unlikely to cause vitamin D toxicity, unless large amounts of cod liver oil are consumed.   Vitamin D toxicity is much more likely to occur from high intakes of vitamin D in supplements. The Food and Nutrition Board of the Institute of Medicine has set the tolerable upper intake level (UL) for vitamin D at 25 mcg (1,000 IU) for infants up to 12 months of age and 50 mg (2,000 IU) for children, adults, pregnant, and lactating women. Long term intakes above the UL increase the risk of adverse health effects.[39]

Vitamin E

Vitamin E is a fat-soluble vitamin that exists in eight different forms. Each form has its own biological activity, which is the measure of potency or functional use in the body. Alpha-tocopherol is the name of the most active form of vitamin E in humans. It is also a powerful biological antioxidant.[98] Vitamin E in supplements is usually sold as alpha-tocopheryl acetate, a form of alpha-tocopherol that protects its ability to function as an antioxidant. The synthetic form is labeled "D, L" while the natural form is labeled "D". The synthetic form is only half as active as the natural form. Antioxidants such as vitamin E act to protect cells against the effects of free radicals, which are potentially damaging by-products of energy metabolism. Free radicals can damage cells and may contribute to the development of cardiovascular disease and cancer. Studies are underway to determine whether vitamin E, through its ability to limit production of free radicals, might help prevent or delay the development of those chronic diseases. Vitamin E has also been shown to play a role in immune function, in DNA repair, and other metabolic processes.[98,99]

Preliminary research has led to a widely held belief that vitamin E may help prevent or delay coronary heart disease.[101] Researchers have reported that oxidative changes to LDL-cholesterol (sometimes called "bad" cholesterol) promote blockages (atherosclerosis) in coronary arteries that may lead to heart attacks. Vitamin E may help prevent or delay coronary heart disease by limiting the oxidation of LDL-cholesterol.[102] Vitamin E also may help prevent the formation of blood clots, which could lead to a heart attack. Observational studies have associated lower rates of heart disease with higher vitamin E intake. A study of approximately 90,000 nurses suggested that the incidence of heart disease was 30% to 40% lower among nurses with the highest intake of vitamin E from diet and supplements. Researchers found that the apparent benefit was mainly associated with intake of vitamin E from dietary supplements. High vitamin E intake from food was not associated with significant cardiac risk reduction.[103] A 1994 review of 5,133 Finnish men and women aged 30-69 years also suggested that increased dietary intake of vitamin E was associated with decreased mortality (death) from heart disease.[104]

Even though these observations are promising, randomized clinical trials raise questions about the efficacy of vitamin E supplements in the prevention of heart disease. The Heart Outcomes Prevention Evaluation (HOPE) Study followed almost 10,000 patients for 4.5 years who were at high risk for heart attack or stroke.[105] In this intervention study the subjects who received 265 mg (400 IU) of vitamin E daily did not experience significantly fewer cardiovascular events or hospitalizations for heart failure or chest pain when compared to those who received a placebo (sugar pill). The researchers suggested that it is unlikely that the vitamin E supplement provided any protection against cardiovascular disease in the HOPE study. This study is continuing, with the goal of determining whether a longer duration of intervention with vitamin E supplements will provide any protection against cardiovascular disease.

In a study sponsored by the National Heart, Lung, and Blood Institute (NHLBI) of the National Institutes of Health, postmenopausal women with heart disease who took supplements providing 400 IU vitamin E and 500 mg vitamin C twice a day, either alone or in combination with hormones, did not have fewer heart attacks or deaths. There was also no change in progression of their coronary disease. This study, The Women's Angiographic Vitamin and Estrogen (WAVE) trial, studied 423 postmenopausal women at seven clinical centers in the U.S. and Canada. In postmenopausal women with coronary disease enrolled in this trial, neither hormone replacement therapy nor antioxidant vitamin supplements provided cardiovascular benefit.[106]

Antioxidants such as vitamin E are believed to help protect cell membranes against the damaging effects of free radicals, which may contribute to the development of chronic diseases such as cancer.[4] Vitamin E also may block the formation of nitrosamines, which are carcinogens formed in the stomach from nitrites consumed in the diet. It also may protect against the development of cancers by enhancing immune function.[107] Unfortunately, human trials and surveys that have tried to associate vitamin E intake with incidence of cancer have been generally inconclusive.

Some evidence associates higher intake of vitamin E with a decreased incidence of prostate cancer and breast cancer.[108] However, an examination of the effect of dietary factors, including vitamin E, on incidence of postmenopausal breast cancer in over 18,000 women from New York State did not associate a greater vitamin E intake with a reduced risk of developing breast cancer.[109]

A study of women in Iowa provides evidence that an increased dietary intake of vitamin E may decrease the risk of colon cancer, especially in women under 65 years of age.[110] On the other hand, a study of 87,998 females from the Nurses' Health Study and 47,344 males from the Health Professionals Follow-up Study failed to support the theory that an increased dietary intake of vitamin E may decrease the risk of colon cancer.[111]

The American Cancer society recently released the results of a long-term study that evaluated the effect of regular use of vitamin C and vitamin E supplements on bladder cancer mortality in almost 1,000,000 adults in the U.S. The study, conducted between the years 1982 to 1998, found that subjects who regularly consumed a vitamin E supplement for longer than 10 years had a reduced risk of death from bladder cancer. No benefit was seen from vitamin C supplements.[112] At this time researchers cannot confidently recommend vitamin E supplements for the prevention of cancer because the evidence on this issue is inconsistent and limited.

Cataracts are abnormal growths in the lens of the eye. These growths cloud vision. They also increase the risk of disability and blindness in aging adults. Antioxidants are being studied to determine whether they can help prevent or delay cataract growth. Observational studies have found that lens clarity, which is used to diagnose cataracts, was better in regular users of vitamin E supplements and in persons with higher blood levels of vitamin E.[113] A study of middle-aged male smokers, however, did not demonstrate any effect from vitamin E supplements on the incidence of cataract formation.[1164] The effects of smoking, a major risk factor for developing cataracts, may have overridden any potential benefit from the vitamin E, but the conflicting results also indicate a need for further studies before researchers can confidently recommend extra vitamin E for the prevention of cataracts.

Food Sources

Wheat germ oil, sunflower seeds, oils (such as almond, peanut, corn, olive, sesame), whole wheat flour, fish oils, green leafy vegetables and fortified cereals

Deficiency

Vitamin E deficiency is rare in humans. There are three specific situations when a vitamin E deficiency is likely to occur.   Persons who cannot absorb dietary fat due to an inability to secrete bile or with rare disorders of fat metabolism are at risk of vitamin E deficiency; individuals with rare genetic abnormalities in the alpha-tocopherol transfer protein are at risk of vitamin E deficiency; and premature, very low birth weight infants (birth weights less than 1500 grams, or 3 pounds, 4 ounces) are at risk of vitamin E deficiency.[98]

Individuals who cannot absorb fat require a vitamin E supplement because some dietary fat is needed for the absorption of vitamin E from the gastrointestinal tract. Intestinal disorders that often result in malabsorption of vitamin E and may require vitamin E supplementation include:[99]
> · Crohn's Disease is an inflammatory bowel disease that affects the small intestines. People with Crohn's disease often experience diarrhea and nutrient malabsorption.
> · Cystic Fibrosis is an inherited disease that affects the lungs, gastrointestinal tract, pancreas, and liver. Cystic fibrosis can interfere with normal digestion and absorption of nutrients, especially of fat soluble vitamins including vitamin E. People who cannot absorb fat often pass greasy stools or have chronic diarrhea. People with an inability to secrete bile, a substance that helps fat digestion, may need a special water-soluble form of vitamin E.

Dietary Reference Intakes[115]

Recommendations for vitamin E are provided in the Dietary Reference Intakes developed by the Institute of Medicine.[115] *Dietary Reference Intakes* (DRIs) is the general term for a set of reference values used for planning and assessing nutrient intake for healthy people. Three important types of reference values included in the DRIs are *Recommended Dietary Allowances* (RDA), *Adequate Intakes* (AI), and *Tolerable Upper Intake Levels* (UL). The RDA recommends the average daily dietary intake level that is sufficient to meet the nutrient requirements of nearly all (97-98%) healthy individuals in each age and gender group .[117] An AI is set when there is insufficient scientific data available to establish a RDA. AIs meet or exceed the amount needed to maintain a nutritional state of adequacy in nearly all members of a specific age and gender group. The UL, on the other hand, is the maximum daily intake unlikely to result in adverse health effects.[115]

RDAs for vitamin E are based only on the alpha-tocopherol form of vitamin E.

Recommended Dietary Allowances for Vitamin E for Children and Adults[115]			
Age(years) Children(mg/day)	Men(mg/day)	Women(mg/day)	Pregnancy(mg/day)
1-3 6 mg(=9 IU)			
4-8 7 mg(=10.5 IU)			
9-13	11 mg(=16.5 IU)	11 mg(=16.5 IU)	15 mg(=22.5 IU)
14 +	15 mg(=22.5 IU)	15 mg(=22.5 IU)	15 mg(=22.5 IU)

There is insufficient scientific data on vitamin E to establish an RDA for infants. An Adequate Intake (AI) has been established that is based on the amount of vitamin E consumed by healthy infants who are fed breast milk.

Most studies of the safety of vitamin E supplementation have lasted for several months or less, so there is little evidence for the long-term safety of vitamin E supplementation.

Toxicity

The Food and Nutrition Board of the Institute of Medicine has set an upper tolerable intake level (UL) for vitamin E at 1,000 mg (1,500 IU) for any form of supplementary alpha-tocopherol per day. Based for the most part on the result of animal studies, the Board decided that because vitamin E can act as an anticoagulant and may increase the risk of bleeding problems this UL is the highest dose unlikely to result in bleeding problems.[115]

Many people are concerned about their fat intake today. Your overall diet should be moderate in fat, but it is important to include some healthful sources of fat, including those oils and nuts that provide vitamin E. Including these foods in your diet will help you meet your daily need for vitamin E. Meats, grain products, dairy products, and most fruits and vegetables are generally not good sources of vitamin E. According to the 2005 *Dietary Guidelines for Americans*, "Nutrient needs should be met primarily through consuming foods. Foods provide an array of nutrients and other compounds that may have beneficial effects on health. In certain cases, fortified foods and dietary supplements may be useful sources of one or more nutrients that otherwise might be consumed in less than recommended amounts. However, dietary supplements, while recommended in some cases, cannot replace a healthful diet."

Reference Notes

All cells use oxygen to produce energy. Oxygen is a potent producer of radicals during normal metabolism. These radicals attack the unsaturated fatty acids in cell membranes—lipid peroxidation. If left uncontrolled cell membranes would be destroyed thus compromising cellular function. Vitamin E is the first line of defense against these radicals. An important area where vitamin E exerts its antioxidant effects is in the lungs where exposure to oxygen is the greatest.

Vitamin K

Worldwide, only a handful of researchers study vitamin K—long known for its critical role in blood clotting. But with the aging of the U.S. population, this vitamin may command a bigger following as its importance to the integrity of bones becomes increasingly clear. It activates at least three proteins involved in bone health, says Sarah Booth at the Jean Mayer USDA Human Nutrition Research Center on Aging at Tufts University in Boston.[118]

"Not too long ago," Booth says, "it looked like Americans consumed several times the recommended dietary allowance for vitamin K. But improved analytical methods show that the vitamin isn't as abundant in the diet as once thought." Booth and colleagues estimated vitamin K intake from 14-day food intake diaries of a nationwide sample of about 2,000 households.[118]

Phylloquinone, the most common form of vitamin K, was the researchers' benchmark for vitamin K intake. "People over age 65 consumed more phylloquinone than those in the 20 to 40 age bracket," she says. Only half the females age 13 and over and less than half the males got the RDA, she notes. "This confirms there are very low intakes nationwide."[118]

Booth says recent evidence suggests the current RDA may not be sufficient for maximizing vitamin K's function in bones. The vitamin adds chemical entities called carboxyl groups to osteocalcin and other proteins that build and maintain bone. Exactly how much vitamin K is needed to optimize this function is still being established.[118]

Most of the survey respondents also consumed another form of vitamin K—dihydrophylloquinone—produced during the hydrogenation of oils. About half of U.S. soybean oil is hydrogenated, according to the Institute of Shortening and Edible Oils in Washington, D.C. The degree of hydrogenation ranges from light, for margarines, spreads, and cooking oils used in restaurants, to heavy, for deep frying and bakery products. Booth says that as much as 30 percent of total vitamin K intake may come in the form of dihydrophylloquinone, but it is less biologically active than phylloquinone. In fact, it was half as active with a clot-forming protein and was completely inactive with a bone-forming protein. "So hydrogenated oils shouldn't be considered an important source of vitamin K," she emphasizes.[118]

Booth says scientists are now using different measures of vitamin K status because the traditional yardstick—blood coagulation time—is not sensitive enough to detect changes in status. So the researchers relied on changes in plasma phylloquinone levels and two functional markers.[118]

One functional marker is the bone-building protein osteocalcin. To be fully active, it must be saturated with carboxyl groups, and that's vitamin K's job. So the researchers looked for changes in saturation in the osteocalcin. After 5 days of eating broccoli or oil fortified with vitamin K, says Booth, more osteocalcin was saturated with carboxyl groups.[118]

The second functional marker—urinary Gla—didn't change. Short for gamma carboxyglutamic acid, Gla indicates overall vitamin K activity in the body. Its lack of change was expected, says Booth, because the supplementation period was short. She has since found that it takes 10 days on the same diet to cause a change in urinary Gla. But they are not good markers of long-term vitamin K status because they fluctuate according to the diet.[118]

"Older people tend to have higher blood levels of phylloquinone," explains Booth. Our study showed that older people can get just as much benefit from increasing vitamin K intake." And that's good news because there is some evidence that hip fractures may be associated with lower saturation of osteocalcin.[118]

Food Sources

Phylloquinone is found in some oils, especially soybean oil, and in dark-green vegetables such as spinach and broccoli. For instance, one serving of spinach or two servings of broccoli provide four to five times the RDA of phylloquinone.

Deficiency

Deficiency of this vitamin causes hemorrhaging. If the vitamin is unavailable, persons will bleed to death. Newborns are born with a sterile digestive tract. To prevent hemorrhaging, newborns are given a single dose of vitamin K at birth. Certain drugs given to "thin" the blood of those at risk for blood clots destroy the vitamin K cycle.

Dietary Reference Intakes[6]

The RDA is 65 micrograms per day for adult females and 80 micrograms per day for adult males.[118]

Toxicity

Toxicity is not common but can result when water-soluble substances for vitamin K are prescribed, especially in infants and pregnant women. Toxicity symptoms include red cell hemolysis, brain damage, and jaundice.

SUMMARY

Vitamins are a group of organic compounds that are required in small amounts for specific functions of growth, maintenance, reproduction and repair of tissue. Vitamins differ from the energy nutrients in that they are needed in smaller amounts, do not provide energy, act singly, not as macromolecules, require no digestion and are absorbed intact into the blood stream. Two major categories of vitamins are the water soluble vitamins and fat soluble vitamins.

Determining adequate intake of each micronutrient individually can be an "arduous task". Computerized software can make the task manageable. However, individuals can be assured of obtaining all the micro nutrients in adequate amounts if their diets include 7 to 9 servings of fruits and vegetables, whole grain, all natural products, and calcium through dairy products or supplements.

The latest research shows that supplements are not equivalent to eating fruits and vegetables. Studies have shown that subjects taking pills did not have decreased risk for chronic disease, only those who ate the real thing—fruit and vegetables—did; these foods contain over 200 phytochemicals that have antioxidant properties. Bottom line: Persons should not be fooled into thinking that they can take a pill every day, and never have to eat a fruit or vegetable again in order to be healthy. See section on nutrition and disease.

CHAPTER 7 - SAMPLE TEST

1. List the major roles for each of the following water soluble vitamins: folate, B6, and vitamin C.

2. List the major roles for each of the following: Vitamin A, Vitamin D, Vitamin E, and Vitamin K.

3. List two sources for the vitamins listed in question #1.

4. List two sources for the vitamins listed in question #2.

5. Why would it be unwise to take three times the DRI of vitamin D?

6. What are the number of servings of fruits and vegetables in your diet? What are the recommended number of servings of fruits and vegetables? Keep a food log and determine the number of servings of fruits and vegetables in your diet.

7. What advice would you give to a client who tells you that he or she is taking three grams (3000 mg) of vitamin C per day?

REFERENCES

1. Guyton, A, *Textbook of Medical Physiology,* 8th ed. Phil: W.B. Saunders Co., 1991.

2. Shils, M, V Young. *Modern Nutrition in Health & Disease*, 7th ed. Philadelphia PA: Lea & Febiger, 1987.

3. Russell, R. How Much Is Too Much? - National Academy of Science issues tolerable upper intake levels for nutritional supplements - Interview. Nutrition Action Healthletter, June, 2001.

4. Whitney, E, S Rolfes. *Understanding Nutrition,* 6th ed. NY: West Publishing Co., 1993.

5. Evans, W, I H Rosenberg. *Biomarkers.* NY: Simon & Schuster, 1991.

6. Tucker, K. Plasma vitamin B12 concentrations relate to intake source in the Framingham offspring Study. *Am J of Clin Nutr,* 71(2),514,2000.

7. Recommended Dietary Allowances, 10th ed. Subcommittee on the tenth edition of the RDAs, Food and Nutrition Board Commission on Life Sciences, National Research Council. Washington, DC: National Academy Press, 1989.

8. Liebman, B. Calcium: after the craze. Nutrition Action Healthletter. 21:5, p. 1. 1994.

9. Institute of Medicine, Food and Nutrition Board. Dietary Reference Intakes for Vitamin C, Vitamin E, Selenium and Carotenoids. A report of the Panel on dietary Antioxidants and Related Compounds, Subcommittees on Upper Reference Levels of Nutrients and Interpretation and Uses of Dietary Reference Intakes, and the Standing Committee on the Scientific Evaluation of Dietary Reference Intakes. Washington, D.C, National Academy Press, 2000.

10. Institute of Medicine, Food and Nutrition Board. Dietary Reference Intakes for Thiamin, Riboflavin, Niacin, Vitamin B6, Folate, Vitamin B12, Pantothenic Acid, Biotin, and Choline. A Report of the Standing Committee on the Scientific Evaluation of Dietary Reference Intakes and its Panel on Folate, other B vitamins and Choline and Subcommittee on Upper Reference Levels of Nutrients. Washington, D.C, National Academy Press, 2000.

11. Wikipedia, The Free Encyclopedia, *Vitamin C.* Retrieved Jan, 2008.

12. Vitamin C (Ascorbic acid). *MedLine Plus.* National Institute of Health (2006-08-01). Retrieved on 2007-08-03.

13. http://www.nlm.nih.gov/medlineplus/ency/article/002404.htm. Retrieved Jan, 2008.

14. Gerster H. Vitamin A-functions, dietary requirements and safety in humans. Int J Vitam Nutr Res 1997;67:71-90. [PubMed abstract]

15. Ross DA. Vitamin A and public health: Challenges for the next decade. Proc Nutr Soc 1998;57:159-65. [PubMed abstract]

16. Harbige LS. Nutrition and immunity with emphasis on infection and autoimmune disease. Nutr Health 1996;10:285-312. [PubMed abstract]

17. Semba RD. The role of vitamin A and related retinoids in immune function. Nutr Rev 1998;56:S38-48. [PubMed abstract].

18. de Pee S, West CE. Dietary carotenoids and their role in combating vitamin A deficiency: A review of the literature. Eur J Clin Nutr 1996;50 Suppl 3:S38-53. [PubMed abstract].

19. Olson JA, Kobayashi S. Antioxidants in health and disease: Overview. Proc Soc Exp Biol Med 1992;200:245-7. [PubMed abstract].

20. Olson JA. Benefits and liabilities of vitamin A and carotenoids. J Nutr 1996;126:1208S-12S. [PubMed abstract]

21. Pavia SA, Russell RM. Beta-carotene and other carotenoids as antioxidants. J Am Coll Nutr

1999;18:426-33. [PubMed abstract].

22. Bendich A, Olson JA. Biological actions of carotenoids. FASEB J 1989:3;1927-32 [PubMed abstract]

23. Fontham ETH. Protective dietary factors and lung cancer. Int J Epidemiol 1990;19:S32-S42. [PubMed abstract].

24. Rock CL, Jacob RA, Bowen PE. Update on the biological characteristics of the antioxidant micronutrients: Vitamin C, vitamin E, and the carotenoids. J Am Diet Assoc 1996;96:693-702. [PubMed abstract].

25. Albanes D, Heinonen OP, Taylor PR, Virtamo J, Edwards BK, Rautalahti M, Hartman AM, Palmgren J, Freedman LS, Haapakoski J, Barrett MJ, Pietinen P, Malila N, Tala E, Lippo K, Salomaa ER, Tangrea JA, Teppo L, Askin FB, Taskinen E, Erozan Y, Greenwald P, Huttunen JK. Alpha-tocopherol and beta-carotene supplement and lung cancer incidence in the alpha-tocopherol, beta-carotene cancer prevention study: Effects of base-line characteristics and study compliance. J Natl Cancer Inst 1996;88:1560-70. [PubMed abstract].

26. Redlich CA, Blaner WS, Van Bennekum AM, Chung JS, Clever SL, Holm CT, Cullen MR. Effect of supplementation with beta-carotene and vitamin A on lung nutrient levels. Cancer Epidemiol Biomarkers Prev 1998;7:211-14. [PubMed abstract].

27. Pryor WA, Stahl W, Rock CL. Beta carotene: from biochemistry to clinical trials. Nutr Rev 2000;58:39-53.

28. National Institutes of Health. Osteoporosis prevention, diagnosis, and therapy. NIH Consensus Statement Online, 2000 March 27-29, 2000:1-36.

29. National Osteoporosis Foundation. NOF osteoporosis prevention-risk factors for osteoporosis. 2003. http://www.nof.org/prevention/risk.htm.

30. Binkley N, Krueger D. Hypervitaminosis A and bone. Nutr Rev 2000;58:138-44. [PubMed abstract]

31. Forsyth KS, Watson RR, Gensler HL. Osteotoxicity after chronic dietary administration of 13-cis-retinoic acid, retinyl palmitate or selenium in mice exposed to tumor initiation and promotion. Life Sci 1989;45:2149-56. [PubMed abstract].

32. Whiting SJ, Lemke B. Excess retinol intake may explain the high incidence of osteoporosis in northern Europe. Nutr Rev 1999;57:249-50. [PubMed abstract].

33. Harrison EH. Mechanisms of digestion and absorption of dietary vitamin A. Annu Rev Nutr 2005;25:5.1-5.18.

34. Rodrigues MI, Dohlman CH. Blindness in an American boy caused by unrecognized vitamin A deficiency. Arch Ophthalmol 2004;122:1228-9.

35. http://dietary-supplements.info.nih.gov/factsheets/vitamind.asp.

36. DeLuca HF and Zierold C. Mechanisms and functions of vitamin D. Nutr Rev 1998;56:S4-10. [PubMed abstract].

37. Reichel H, Koeffler H, Norman AW. The role of vitamin D endocrine system in health and disease. N Engl J Med 1989;320:980-91. [PubMed abstract].

38. van den Berg H. Bioavailability of vitamin D. Eur J Clin Nutr 1997;51 Suppl 1:S76-9. [PubMed abstract] 39. Institute of Medicine, Food and Nutrition Board. Dietary Reference Intakes: Calcium, Phosphorus, Magnesium, Vitamin D and Fluoride. National Academy Press, Washington, DC, 1999.

40. Goldring SR, Krane S, Avioli LV. Disorders of calcification: Osteomalacia and rickets. In: LJ D, ed. Endocrinology. 3rd ed. Philadelphia: WB Saunders, 1995:1204-27.

41. Favus MJ and Christakos S. Primer on the Metabolic Bone Diseases and Disorders of Mineral

Metabolism. 3rd ed. Philadelphia, PA: Lippincott-Raven, 1996.

42. Holick MF. Evolution and function of vitamin D. Recent Results Cancer Res 2003;164:3-28.

43. Hayes CE, Hashold FE, Spach KM, Pederson LB. The immunological functions of the vitamin D endocrine system. Cell Mol Biol 2003;49:277-300.

44. Holick MF. Vitamin D. In: Shils M, Olson J, Shike M, Ross AC, ed. Modern Nutrition in Health and Disease, 9th ed. Baltimore: Williams and Wilkins, 1999.

45. J P. Bowes and Church's Food Values of Portions Commonly Used. 17th ed. Philadelphia: Lippincot-Raven, 1998.

46. Nutrition Coordinating Center. Nutrition Data System for Research (NDS-R). Version 4.06/34 Minnesota: University of Minnesota, 2003.

47. U.S. Department of Agriculture, Agricultural Research Service. 2003. USDA Nutrient Database for Standard Reference, Release 16. Nutrient Data Laboratory Home Page, http:// www.nal.usda.gov/fnic/foodcomp online.

48. Holick MF. McCollum Award Lecture, 1994: Vitamin D: new horizons for the 21st century. Am J Clin Nutr 1994;60:619-30. [PubMed abstract.]

49. Holick MF. Vitamin D: the underappreciated D-lightful hormone that is important for skeletal and cellular health. Curr Opin Endocrinol Diabetes 2002;9:87-98.

50. Wharton B and Bishop N. Rickets. The Lancet 2003;362:1389-1400.

51. Nesby-O'Dell S, Scanlon KS, Cogswell ME, Gillespie C, Hollis BW, Looker AC, Allen C, Doughertly C, Gunter EW, Bowman BA. Hypovitaminosis D prevalence and determinants among African-American and white women of reproductive age: third National Health and Nutrition Examination Survey, 1988-1994. Am J Clin Nutr 2002;76:187-92.

52. Biser-Rohrbaugh A, Hadley-Miller N. Vitamin D deficiency in breast-fed toddlers. J of Pediatr Orthaped 2001;21:508-11.

53. Chesney R. Rickets: An old form for a new century. Pediatrics International 2003;45:509-11.

54. Picciano MF. Nutrient composition of human milk. Pediatr Clin North Am 2001;48:53-67.

55. Gartner LM, Greer FR, American Academy of Pediatrics Committee on Nutrition. Prevention of rickets and vitamin D deficiency: new guidelines for vitamin D Intake. Pediatrics 2003:111:908-10.

56. American Academy of Pediatrics committee on Environmental Health. Ultraviolet light: a hazard to children. Pediatrics 1999;104:328-33.

57. Fomom SJ. Reflections on infant feeding in the 1970s and 1980s. Am J Clin Nutr 198;46:171-82.

58. Lips P. Vitamin D deficiency and secondary hyperparathyriodism in the elderly: consequences for bone loss and fractures and therapeutic implications. Endocrine Rev 2001;22:477-501.

59. MacLaughlin J and Holick MF. Aging decreases the capacity of human skin to produce vitamin D3. J Clin Invest 1985;76:1536-38. [PubMed abstract].

60. Holick MF, Matsuoka LY, Wortsman J. Age, vitamin D, and solar ultraviolet. Lancet 1989;2:1104-5. [PubMed abstract].

61. Need AG, MorrisHA, Horowitz M, Nordin C. Effects of skin thickness, age, body fat, and sunlight on serum 25-hydroxyvitamin D. Am J Clin Nutr 1993;58:882-5. [PubMed abstract].

62. Webb AR, Kline L, Holick MF. Influence of season and latitude on the cutaneous synthesis of vitamin D3: Exposure to winter sunlight in Boston and Edmonton will not promote vitamin D3 synthesis in human skin. J Clin Endocrinol Metab 1988;67:373-78. [PubMed abstract].

63. Webb AR, Pilbeam C, Hanafin N, Holick MF. An evaluation of the relative contributions of exposure to sunlight and of diet to the circulating concentrations of 25-hydroxyvitamin D in an elderly nursing home population in Boston. Am J Clin Nutr 1990;51:1075-81. [PubMed abstract].

64. Fairfield KM, and Fletcher RH. Vitamins for chronic disease prevention in adults. J Am Med Assoc 2002;287:3116-26.

65. Harris SS, Soteriades E, Coolidge JAS, Mudgal S, Dawson-Hughes B. Vitamin D insufficiency and hyperparathyroidism in a low income, multiracial, elderly population. J Clin Endocrinol Metab 2000;85:4125-30.

66. Lo CW, Paris PW, Clemens TL, Nolan J, Holick MF. Vitamin D absorption in healthy subjects and in patients with intestinal malabsorption syndromes. Am J Clin Nutr 1985;42:644-49. [PubMed abstract]

67. Reid IR. The roles of calcium and vitamin D in the prevention of osteoporosis. Endocrinol Metab Clin North Am 1998;27:389-98. [PubMed abstract] .

68 Heaney RP. Long-latency deficiency disease: insights from calcium and vitamin D. Am J Clin Nutr 2003;78:912-9.

69. Parfitt AM. Osteomalacia and related disorders. In: Avioli LV, Krane SM, etc. Metabolic bone disease and clinically related disorders. 2nd ed. Philadelphia: WB Saunders. 1990:329-96.

70. LeBoff MS, Kohlmeier L, Hurwitz S, Franklin J, Wright J, Glowacki J. Occult vitamin D deficiency in postmenopausal US women with acute hip fracture. J Am Med Assoc 1999;251:1505-11. [PubMed abstract].

71. Menopausal Hormone Therapy: Summary of a Scientific Workshop. Annals of Internal Medicine 2003;138:361-4.

72. ACOG, Questions and Answers on Hormone Therapy, in American College of Obstetricians and Gynecologists Web site response to the WHI Study Results on Estrogen and Progestin Hormone Therapy 2002. p. 1-8. Position Statement: Role of progestrogen in hormone therapy for postmenopausal women: position statement of The North American Menopause Society. Menopause: The Journal of the North American Menopause Society 2003;10:113-32. Chapuy MC Arlot ME, Duboeuf F, Brun J, Crouzet B, Arnaud S, Delmas PD, Meunier PJ. Vitamin D3 and calcium to prevent hip fractures in elderly women. N Engl J Med 1992;327:1637-42. [PubMed abstract].

75. Dawson-Hughes B, Harris SS, Krall EA, Dallal GE, Falconer G, Green CL. Rates of bone loss in postmenopausal women randomly assigned to one of two dosages of vitamin D. Am J Clin Nutr 1995;61:1140-45. [PubMed abstract].

76. Rodriguez-Martinez MA and Garcia-Cohen EC. Role of Ca2+and vitamin D in the prevention and treatment of osteoporosis. Pharmacology & Therapeutics 2002;93:37-49. Reid IR. Therapy of osteoporosis: Calcium, vitamin D, and exercise. Am J Med Sci 1996;312:278-86. [PubMed abstract].

77. Chapuy MC, Pamphile R, Paris E, Kempf C, Schlichting M, Arnaud S, Garnere P, Meunier PJ. Combined calcium and vitamin D3 supplementation in elderly women: confirmation of reversal of secondary hyperparathyroidism and hip fracture risk: the Decalyos II study. Osteoporosis Int 2002;13:257-64.

78. Posner G. Low-Calcemic Vitamin D Analogs (Deltanoids) for Human Cancer Prevention. J. Nutr 2002;132:3802S-3S.

79. Martinez ME and Willett W C. Calcium, vitamin D, and colorectal cancer: a review of the epidemiologic evidence. Cancer Epidemiol. Biomark. Prev 1998;7:163-68.

80. Garland C, Shekelle R B, Barrett-Connor E, Criqui MH, Rossof A H and Paul O. Dietary vitamin D and calcium and risk of colorectal cancer: a 19-year prospective study in men. Lancet 1985;1:307-9.

81. Holt PR. Studies of calcium in food supplements in humans. Ann N Y Acad Sci 1999;889:128-

37. [PubMed abstract].

82. Langman M and Boyle P. Chemoprevention of colorectal cancer. Gut 1998;43:578-85.

83. Glinghammar B, Venturi M, Rowland IR, Rafter JJ. Shift from a dairy product-rich to a dairy product-free diet: Influence on cytotoxicity and genotoxicity of fecal water—potential risk factors for colon cancer. Am J Clin Nutr 1997;66:1277-82. [PubMed abstract].

84. La Vecchia C, Braga C, Negri E, Franceschi S, Russo A, Conti E, Falcini F, Giacosa A, Montella M, Decarli A. Intake of selected micronutrients and risk of colorectal cancer. Int J Cancer 1997;73:525-30. [PubMed abstract].

85. ieth R. Vitamin D supplementation, 25-hydroxyvitamin D concentrations, and safety. Am J Clin Nutr 1999 69 :842-56. [PubMed abstract].

86. Lieberman DA, Prindiville S, Weiss DG, Willett W. Risk factors for advanced colonic neoplasia and hyperplastic polyps in asymptomatic individuals. J Am Med Assoc 2003;290:2959-67.

87. Buckley LM, Leib ES, Cartularo KS, Vacek PM, Cooper SM. Calcium and vitamin D3 supplementation prevents bone loss in the spine secondary to low-dose corticosteroids in patients with rheumatoid arthritis. A randomized, double-blind, placebo-controlled trial. Ann Intern Med 1996;125:961-8. [PubMed abstract].

88. Lukert BP and Raisz LG. Gucocorticoid-induced osteoporosis: Pathogenesis and management. Annals of Internal Medicine 1990;112:352-64. [PubMed abstract].

89. de Sevaux RGL, Hoitsma AJ, Corstens FHM, Wetzels JFM. Treatment with vitamin D and calcium reduces bone loss after renal transplantation: A randomized study. J Am Soc Nephrol 2002;13:1608-14.

90. Buchner DM and Larson EB. Falls and fractures in patients with Alzheimer-type dementia. J Am Med Assoc 1987;20:1492-5. [PubMed abstract].

91. Sato Y, Asoh T, Oizumi K. High prevalence of vitamin D deficiency and reduced bone mass in elderly women with Alzheimer's disease. Bone 1998;23:555-7. [PubMed abstract].

92. Rapuri PB, Gallagher JC, Kinyamu HK, Ryschon KL. Caffeine intake increases rate of bone loss in elderly women and interacts with vitamin D receptor genotypes. Am J Clin Nutr 2001;74:694-700.

93. Chesney RW. Vitamin D: Can an upper limit be defined? J Nutr 1989;119 (12 Suppl):1825-8. [PubMed abstract].

94. Vieth R, Chan PR, MacFarlane GD. Efficacy and safety of vitamin D3 intake exceeding the lowest observed adverse effect level. Am J Clin Nutr 2001;73(2):288-94.

95. U.S. Department of Agriculture (USDA) and U.S. Department of Health and Human Services. Nutrition and Your Health: Dietary Guidelines for Americans. 5th ed. USDA Home and Garden Bulleting No. 232, Washington, DC: USDA, 2000. http://www.cnpp.usda.gov/DietGd.pdf.

96. Center for Nutrition Policy and Promotion. United States Department of Agriculture. Food Guide Pyramid, 1992 (slightly revised 1996). http://www.nal.usda.gov/fnic/Fpyr/pyramid.html.

97. http://dietary-supplements.info.nih.gov/factsheets/vitamine.asp. NIH Clinical Center Fact Sheets in conjunction with ODS.

98. Traber MG. Vitamin E. In: Shils ME, Olson JA, Shike M, Ross AC, ed. Modern Nutrition in Health and Disease. 10th ed. Baltimore: Williams & Wilkins, 1999:347-62.

99. Farrell P and Roberts R. Vitamin E. In: Shils M, Olson JA, and Shike M, ed. Modern Nutrition in Health and Disease. 8th ed. Philadelphia, PA: Lea and Febiger, 1994:326-41.

100. U.S. Department of Agriculture, Agricultural Research Service. 2004. USDA National Nutrient Database for Standard Reference, Release 16-1. Nutrient Data Laboratory Home Page, http://www.ars.usda.gov/ba/bhnrc/ndl.

101. Lonn EM and Yusuf S. Is there a role for antioxidant vitamins in the prevention of cardiovascular diseases? An update on epidemiological and clinical trials data. Can J Cardiol 1997;13:957-65. [PubMed abstract].

102. Jialal I and Fuller CJ. Effect of vitamin E, vitamin C and beta-carotene on LDL oxidation and atherosclerosis. Can J Cardiol 1995;11 Suppl G:97G-103G. [PubMed abstract].

103. Stampfer MJ, Hennekens CH, Manson JE, Colditz GA, Rosner B, Willett WC. Vitamin E consumption and the risk of coronary disease in women. N Engl J Med 1993;328:1444-9 [PubMed abstract].

104. Knekt P, Reunanen A, Jarvinen R, Seppanen R, Heliovaara M, Aromaa A. Antioxidant vitamin intake and coronary mortality in a longitudinal population study. Am J Epidemiol 1994;139:1180-9. [PubMed abstract].

105. The Heart Outcomes Prevention Evaluation Study Investigators. Vitamin E supplementation and cardiovascular events in high-risk patients. N Engl J Med 2000;342:154-60. [PubMed abstract]

106. Waters DD, Alderman EL, Hsia J, Howard BV, Cobb FR, Rogers WJ, Ouyang P, Thompson P, Tardif JC, Higginson L, Bittner V, Steffes M, Gordon DJ, Proschan M, Younes N, Verter JI. Effects of hormone replacement therapy and antioxidant vitamin supplements on coronary atherosclerosis in postmenopausal women: a randomized controlled trial. J Am Med Assoc 2002;288:2432-40.

107. Weitberg AB and Corvese D. Effect of vitamin E and beta-carotene on DNA strand breakage induced by tobacco-specific nitrosamines and stimulated human phagocytes. J Exp Clin Cancer Res 1997;16:11-4. [PubMed abstract].

108. Chan JM, Stampfer MJ, Giovannucci EL. What causes prostate cancer? A brief summary of the epidemiology. Semin Cancer Biol 1998;8:263-73. [PubMed abstract].

109. Graham S, Sielezny M, Marshall J, Priore R, Freudenheim J, Brasure J, Haughey B, Nasca P, Zdeb M. Diet in the epidemiology of Postmenopausal Breast Cancer in the New York State Cohort. Am J Epidemiol 1992;136:3127-37. [PubMed abstract].

110. Bostick RM, Potter JD, McKenzie DR, Sellers TA, Kushi LH, Steinmetz KA, Folsom AR. Reduced risk of colon cancer with high intakes of vitamin E: The Iowa Women's Health Study. Cancer Res 1993;15:4230-17. [PubMed abstract].

111. Wu K, Willett WC, Chan JM, Fuchs CS, Colditz GA, Rimm EB, Giovannucci EL. A prospective study on supplemental vitamin E intake and risk of colon cancer in women and men. Cancer Epidemiol Biomarkers Prev 2002;11:1298-304.

112. Jacobs EJ, Henion AK, Briggs PJ, Connell CJ, McCullough ML, Jonas CR, Rodriguez C, Calle EE, Thun MJ. Vitamin C and vitamin E supplement use and bladder cancer mortality in a large cohort of US men and women. American Journal of Epidemiology 2002;156: 1002-10.

113. Leske MC, Chylack LT Jr., He Q, Wu SY, Schoenfeld E, Friend J, Wolfe J. Antioxidant vitamins and nuclear opacities: The longitudinal study of cataract. Ophthalmology 1998;105:831-6. [PubMed abstract].

114. Teikari JM, Virtamo J, Rautalahti M, Palmgren J, Liesto K, Heinonen OP. Long-term supplementation with alpha-tocopherol.

115. Institute of Medicine, Food and Nutrition board. Dietary Reference Intakes: Vitamin C, Vitamin E, Selenium, and Carotenoids. National Academy Press, Washington, DC, 2000. I and beta-carotene and age-related cataract. Acta Ophthalmol Scand 1997;75:634-40. [PubMed abstract].

116. Booth, S. http://www.ars.usda.gov/is/AR/archive/jan00/green0100.htm. Vitamin K - Another good Reason to Eat your Greens. Jan, 2008. "Vitamin K: Another Reason To Eat Your Greens" was published in the January 2000 issue of *Agricultural Research* magazine.

Chapter 8
Micronutrients - Minerals

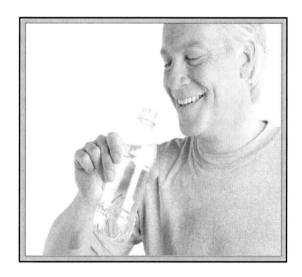

In this chapter we will take a more in depth look at minerals. Minerals are involved in all aspects of metabolism, whether catabolic or anabolic.

Please do not feel that you must memorize all the information in this chapter. Some of the information presented here is meant to be a resource for future reference. The goal of this textbook is to have you become familiar with the major roles of each micronutrient and with foods containing substantial amounts of each nutrient.

Objectives

After reading and studying this chapter you should:

1. Be able to discuss the major minerals, and be able to discuss the roles, food sources, Dietary Reference Intakes, toxicities, and anti-minerals.

2. Be able to discuss the trace minerals: roles, food sources, Dietary Reference Intakes, toxicities, and anti-nutrients.

INTRODUCTION

Minerals are inorganic elements essential to life that act as control agents in body reactions and cooperative factors in energy production, body building and maintenance of tissues. They retain their identity (they cannot be changed into anything else), and they cannot be destroyed by heat, air, acid, or mixing (can be lost in cooking water).

Minerals require no digestion and are absorbed intact from the small intestines. They can become charged particles and can form compounds. Sodium and chloride are a familiar example of a compound i.e., sodium chloride (table salt).[1]

Like the water soluble vitamins, some minerals are readily absorbed into the blood, transported freely, and readily excreted by the kidneys. Some minerals must have carriers to be absorbed and transported just like the fat soluble vitamins.[1]

Minerals are divided into two categories - the major minerals and the trace minerals. The trace minerals are found in smaller amounts in the body, while the major minerals are found in larger amounts. The major minerals are calcium, sodium, chloride, potassium, sulfur, phosphorous and magnesium. The trace minerals are iron, zinc, iodine, copper, manganese, fluoride, chromium, selenium and others.[1]

As with all the other essential nutrients, minerals are vital to life.

MAJOR MINERALS

Calcium

Calcium, the most abundant mineral in the human body, has several important functions. More than 99% of total body calcium is stored in the bones and teeth where it functions to support their structure.[1] The remaining 1% is found throughout the body in blood, muscle, and the fluid between cells. Calcium is needed for muscle contraction, blood vessel contraction and expansion, the secretion of hormones and enzymes, and sending messages through the nervous system.[1] A constant level of calcium is maintained in body fluid and tissues so that these vital body processes function efficiently.

Bone undergoes continuous remodeling, with constant resorption (breakdown of bone) and deposition of calcium into newly deposited bone (bone formation).[2] The balance between bone resorption and deposition changes as people age. During childhood there is a higher amount of bone formation and less breakdown. In early and middle adulthood, these processes are relatively equal. In aging adults, particularly among postmenopausal women, bone breakdown exceeds its formation, resulting in bone loss, which increases the risk for osteoporosis (a disorder characterized by porous, weak bones).[2]

Bones are living tissues and continue to change throughout life. During childhood and adolescence, bones increase in size and mass. Bones continue to add more mass until around age 30, when peak bone mass is reached. Peak bone mass is the point when the maximum amount of bone is achieved. Because bone loss, like bone growth, is a gradual process, the stronger your bones are at age 30, the more your bone loss will be delayed as you age. Therefore, it is particularly important to consume adequate calcium and vitamin D throughout infancy, childhood, and adolescence. It is also important to engage in weight-bearing exercise to maximize bone strength and bone density (amount of bone tissue in a certain volume of bone) to help prevent osteoporosis later in life. Weight bearing exercise is the type of exercise that causes your bones and muscles to work against gravity while they bear your weight. Resistance exercises such as weight training are also important because they help to improve muscle mass and bone strength.

Calcium control or homeostasis is regulated through bone and the regulating agents are a system of hormones and vitamin D. Food calcium never directly affects blood calcium. If calcium intake is too low, the body will take calcium from bone in order to maintain blood levels. Bone is continually being destroyed and rebuilt to adapt to mechanical strain. About 1/5 of bone is replaced every year. But remodeling is not always a zero sum game. During the first few decades of life, each rebuilding makes the bones denser. They peak somewhere between twenty-five and thirty-five. At menopause women's bodies begin to dissolve old bone at an accelerated rate, and new bone is not formed. Women who stock up on bone when they're young have enough left over after these losses to avoid fractures. Women who do not stock up on bone in youth are at increased risk for osteoporosis.

Food Sources

In the United States (U.S.), milk, yogurt and cheese are the major contributors of calcium in the typical diet.[3] The inadequate intake of dairy foods may explain why some Americans are deficient in calcium since dairy foods are the major source of calcium in the diet.[3] The U.S. Department of Agriculture's Food Guide Pyramid recommends that individuals two years and older eat 2-3 servings of dairy products per day. A serving is equal to: 1 cup (8 fl oz) of milk; 8 oz of yogurt; 1.5 oz of natural cheese (such as Cheddar); 2.0 oz of processed cheese (such as American). A variety of non-fat and reduced fat dairy products that contain the same amount of calcium as regular dairy products are available in the U.S. today for individuals concerned about saturated fat content from regular dairy products.

Although dairy products are the main source of calcium in the U.S. diet, other foods also contribute to overall calcium intake. Individuals with lactose intolerance (those who experience symptoms such as bloating and diarrhea because they cannot completely digest the milk sugar lactose) and those who are vegan (people who consume no animal products) tend to avoid or completely eliminate dairy products from their diets.[2] Thus, it is important for these individuals to meet their calcium needs with alternative calcium sources if they choose to avoid or eliminate dairy products from their diet. Foods such as Chinese cabbage, kale and broccoli are other alternative calcium sources.[2] Although most grains are not high in calcium (unless fortified), they do contribute calcium to the diet because they are consumed frequently.[2] Additionally, there are several calcium-fortified food sources presently available, including fruit juices, fruit drinks, tofu and cereals. Certain plant-based foods such as some vegetables contain substances which can reduce calcium absorption. Thus, you may have to eat several servings of certain foods such as spinach to obtain the same amount of calcium in one cup of milk, which is not only calcium-rich but also contains calcium in an easily absorbable form.

Deficiency

When calcium intake is low or calcium is poorly absorbed, bone breakdown occurs because the body must use the calcium stored in bones to maintain normal biological functions such as nerve and muscle function. Bone loss also occurs as a part of the aging process. A prime example is the loss of bone mass observed in post-menopausal women because of decreased amounts of the hormone estrogen. Researchers have identified many factors that increase the risk for developing osteoporosis. These factors include being female, thin, inactive, of advanced age, cigarette smoking, excessive intake of alcohol, and having a family history of osteoporosis.[4]

Inadequate calcium intake, decreased calcium absorption, and increased calcium loss in urine can decrease total calcium in the body, with the potential of producing osteoporosis and the other consequences of chronically low calcium intake. If an individual does not consume enough dietary calcium or experiences rapid losses of calcium from the body, calcium is withdrawn from their bones in order to maintain calcium levels in the blood.

Because circulating blood calcium levels are tightly regulated in the bloodstream, hypocalcemia (low blood calcium) does not usually occur due to low calcium intake, but rather results from a medical problem or treatment such as renal failure, surgical removal of the stomach (which significantly decreases calcium absorption), and use of certain types of diuretics (which result in increased loss of calcium and fluid through urine). Simple dietary calcium deficiency produces no signs at all. Hypocalcemia can cause numbness and tingling in fingers, muscle cramps, convulsions, lethargy, poor appetite, and mental confusion.[1] It can also result in abnormal heart rhythms and even death.

Individuals with medical problems that result in hypocalcemia should be under a medical doctor's care and receive specific treatment aimed at normalizing calcium levels in the blood. It is important to consult a health professional if you experience any of these symptoms.

Menopause often leads to increases in bone loss with the most rapid rates of bone loss occurring during the first five years after menopause. Drops in estrogen production after menopause result in increased bone resorption, and decreased calcium absorption. Annual decreases in bone mass of 3-5% per year are often seen during the years immediately following menopause, with decreases less than 1% per year seen after age 65. Two studies are in agreement that increased calcium intakes during menopause will not completely offset menopause bone loss.[5,6] Hormone therapy (HT), previously known as hormone replacement therapy (HRT), with sex hormones such as estrogen and progesterone, helps to prevent osteoporosis and fractures. However, some medical groups and professional societies such as the American College of Obstetricians and Gynecologists, The North American Menopause Society and The American Society for Bone and Mineral Research recommend that postmenopausal women consider using other agents such as bisphosphonates (medication used to slow or stop bone-resorption) because of potential health risks of HT if combination HT (estrogen and progestin) is solely being administered to prevent or treat osteoporosis.[7,8] Postmenopausal women using combination HT to reduce bone loss should consult with their physician about the risks and benefits of estrogen therapy for their health.

Estrogen therapy works to restore postmenopausal bone remodeling levels back to those of pre-menopause, leading to a lower rate of bone loss. Estrogen appears to interact with supplemental calcium by increasing calcium absorption in the gut. However, including adequate amounts of calcium in the diet may help slow the rate of bone loss for all women. Amenorrhea is the condition when menstrual periods stop or fail to initiate in women who are of childbearing age. Secondary amenorrhea is the absence of three or more consecutive menstrual cycles after menarche occurs (first menstrual period). The secondary type of amenorrhea can be induced by exercise in athletes and is referred to as "athletic amenorrhea". Potential causes of athletic amenorrhea include low body weight and low percent body fat, rapid weight loss, sudden onset of vigorous exercise, disordered eating and stress. Amenorrhea results from decreases in circulating estrogen, which then negatively affect calcium balance.[2]   Studies comparing healthy women with normal menstrual cycles to amenorrheic women with anorexia nervosa (a type of disordered eating) found decreased levels of calcium absorption, a higher urinary calcium excretion, and a lower rate of bone formation in women with anorexia.

The condition "female athlete triad" refers to the combination of disordered eating, amenorrhea, and osteoporosis. Exercise-induced amenorrhea has been shown to result in decreases in bone mass [86,87]. In female athletes, low bone mineral density, menstrual irregularities, dietary factors, and a history of prior stress fractures are associated with an increased risk of future stress fractures [88]. Stress fractures can severely impact health and cause financial burden, especially in physically active females such women in the military.[9] Thus, it is important for amenorrheic women to maintain the recommended Adequate Intake for calcium.

Lactose maldigestion (or "lactase non-persistence") describes the inability of an individual to completely digest lactose, the naturally occurring sugar in milk. Lactose intolerance refers to the symptoms that occur when the amount of lactose exceeds the ability of an individual's digestive tract to break down lactose. In the US, approximately 25% of all adults have a limited ability to digest lactose. Lactose maldigestion varies by ethnicity, with a prevalence of 85% in Asians, 50% in African Americans, and 10% in Caucasians.[9,10] Symptoms of lactose intolerance include bloating, flatulence, and diarrhea after consuming large amounts of lactose (such as the amount in 1 quart of milk).[11] Lactose maldigesters may be at risk for calcium deficiency, not due to an inability to absorb calcium, but rather from the avoidance of dairy products. Although some lactose maldigesters avoid dairy products, others are able to consume moderate amounts of lactose, such as the amount in an 8-oz glass of milk. Some individuals may be able to consume two 8-oz glasses of milk a day if they do so at different meals.

Symptoms of lactose intolerance vary from individual to individual depending on the amount of lactose consumed, history of previous consumption of foods with lactose and the type of meal with which the lactose is consumed. Drinking milk with a meal helps reduce symptoms of lactose intolerance substantially. In addition, regularly eating foods (e.g. daily for 2-3 weeks) with lactose (such as milk) can help the body adapt to the lactose and thus reduce symptoms of lactose intolerance.[12] Other dietary options for lactose maldigesters include choosing aged cheeses (such as Cheddar and Swiss) which contain little lactose, yogurt which contains live active cultures that aid in lactose digestion, or lactose reduced and lactose free milk. If an individual is a lactose maldigester and chooses to avoid dairy products, it is important for them to include non-dairy sources of calcium in their daily diet or consider taking a calcium supplement to help meet their recommended calcium needs.

There are several types of vegetarian eating practices. Individuals may choose to include some animal products (ovo-vegetarian, lacto-vegetarian, lacto-ovo vegetarian, pesco-vegetarian) or no animal products (vegan) in their diet. Calcium intakes between lacto-ovo-vegetarians (those who consume eggs and dairy products) and non-vegetarians have been shown to be similar.[13,14] Calcium absorption may be reduced in vegetarians because they eat more plant foods containing oxalic and phytic acids, compounds which interfere with calcium absorption.[2] However, vegetarian diets that contain less protein may reduce calcium excretion.[1] Yet, vegans may be at increased risk for inadequate intake of calcium because of their lack of consumption of dairy products.[15] Therefore, it is important for vegans to include adequate amounts of non-dairy sources of calcium in their daily diet or consider taking a calcium supplement to meet their recommended calcium intake.[16]

Osteoporosis is a disorder characterized by porous, fragile bones. It is a serious public health problem for more than 10 million Americans, 80% of whom are women. Another 34 million Americans have osteopenia, or low bone mass, which precedes osteoporosis. Osteoporosis is a concern because of its association with fractures of the hip, vertebrae, wrist, pelvis, ribs, and other bones. Each year, Americans suffer from 1.5 million fractures because of osteoporosis. Osteoporosis and osteopenia can result from dietary factors such as: chronically low calcium intake; low vitamin D intake; poor calcium absorption; excess calcium excretion.

Dietary Reference Intakes

Recommendations for calcium are provided in the Dietary Reference Intakes (DRIs) developed by the Institute of Medicine (IOM) of the National Academy of Sciences. *Dietary Reference Intake* (DRI) is the general term for a set of reference values used for planning and assessing nutrient intakes of healthy people. Three important types of reference values included in the DRIs are *Recommended*

Dietary Allowances (RDA), *Adequate Intakes* (AI), and *Tolerable Upper Intake Levels* (UL). The RDA recommends the average daily intake that is sufficient to meet the nutrient requirements of nearly all (97-98%) healthy individuals in each age and gender group. An AI is set when there is insufficient scientific data available to establish a RDA. AIs meet or exceed the amount needed to maintain a nutritional state of adequacy in nearly all members of a specific age and gender group. The UL, on the other hand, is the maximum daily intake unlikely to result in adverse effects.

For calcium, the recommended intake is listed as an Adequate Intake (AI), which is a recommended average intake level based on observed or experimentally determined levels. Current calcium recommendations for nonpregnant women are also sufficient for pregnant women because intestinal calcium absorption increases during pregnancy.[2] For this reason, the calcium recommendations established for pregnant women are not different than the recommendations for women who are not pregnant.

Male and Female Age	Calcium (mg/day)	Pregnancy & Lactation
0 to 6 months	210	N/A
7 to 12 months	270	N/A
1 to 3 years	500	N/A
4 to 8 years	800	N/A
9 to 13 years	1300	N/A
14 to 18 years	1300	1300
19 to 50 years	1000	1000
51+ years	1200	N/A

The Tolerable Upper Limit (UL) is the highest level of daily intake of calcium from food, water and supplements that is likely to pose no risks of adverse health effects to almost all individuals in the general population.[2] The UL for children and adults ages 1 year and older (including pregnant and lactating women) is 2500 mg/day. It was not possible to establish a UL for infants under the age of 1 year.

Toxicity

While low intakes of calcium can result in deficiency and undesirable health conditions, excessively high intakes of calcium can also have adverse effects. Adverse conditions associated with high calcium intakes are hypercalcemia (elevated levels of calcium in the blood), impaired kidney function and decreased absorption of other minerals.[2] Hypercalcemia can also result from excess intake of vitamin D, such as from supplement overuse at levels of 50,000 IU or higher.[1] However, hypercalcemia from diet and supplements is very rare. Most cases of hypercalcemia occur as a result of malignancy - especially in the advanced stages.

Another concern with high calcium intakes is the potential for calcium to interfere with the absorption of other minerals, iron, zinc, magnesium, and phosphorus.[17]

Most Americans should consider their intake of calcium from all foods including fortified ones before adding supplements to their diet to help avoid the risk of reaching levels at or near the UL for calcium (2500 mg). If you need additional assistance regarding your calcium needs, consider checking with a physician or registered dietitian. The 2000 Dietary Guidelines for Americans recommend that individuals consume a variety of foods to meet their nutrient needs since no single food can supply all the nutrients in the amounts needed by an individual.[18]   However, for some people it may be necessary to take supplements in order to meet the recommended intakes for calcium. In 2002, calcium supplements were the number one selling mineral supplement and the 3rd highest selling supplement overall in the U.S. nutrition industry totaling approximately $877 million in sales.[219]

The two main forms of calcium found in supplements are carbonate and citrate. Calcium carbonate is the most common because it is inexpensive and convenient. The absorption of calcium citrate is similar to calcium carbonate. For instance, a calcium carbonate supplement contains 40% calcium while a calcium citrate supplement only contains 21% calcium. However, you have to take more pills of calcium citrate to get the same amount of calcium as you would get from a calcium carbonate pill since citrate is a larger molecule than carbonate. One advantage of calcium citrate over calcium carbonate is better absorption in those individuals who have decreased stomach acid. Calcium citrate malate is a form of calcium used in the fortification of certain juices and is also well absorbed.[20] Other forms of calcium in supplements or fortified foods include calcium gluconate, lactate, and phosphate.

The amount of calcium your body obtains from various supplements depends on the amount of elemental calcium in the tablet. The amount of elemental calcium is the amount of calcium that actually is in the supplement. Calcium absorption also depends on the total amount of calcium consumed at one time and whether the calcium is taken with food or on an empty stomach. Absorption from supplements is best in doses 500 mg or less because the percent of calcium absorbed decreases as the amount of calcium in the supplement increases. Therefore, someone taking 1000 mg of calcium in a supplement should take 500 mg twice a day instead of 1000 mg calcium at one time.

Some common complaints of calcium supplement use are gas, bloating and constipation. If you have such symptoms, you may want to spread the calcium dose out throughout the day, change supplement brands, take the supplement with meals and/or check with your pharmacist or health care provider.

Reference Notes[23]

Calcium absorption refers to the amount of calcium that is absorbed from the digestive tract into our body's circulation. Calcium absorption can be affected by the calcium status of the body, vitamin D status, age, pregnancy and plant substances in the diet. The amount of calcium consumed at one time such as in a meal can also affect absorption. For example, the efficiency of calcium absorption decreases as the amount of calcium consumed at a meal increases. Net calcium absorption can be as high as 60% in infants and young children, when the body needs calcium to build strong bones. Absorption slowly decreases to 15-20% in adulthood and even more as one ages. Because calcium absorption declines with age, recommendations for dietary intake of calcium are higher for adults ages 51 and over. Vitamin D helps improve calcium absorption. Your body can obtain vitamin D from food and it can also make vitamin D when your skin is exposed to sunlight. Thus, adequate vitamin D intake from food and sun exposure is essential to bone health. The Office of Dietary Supplement's vitamin D fact sheet provides more information: http://ods.od.nih.gov/factsheets/vitamind.asp.

Phytic acid and oxalic acid, which are found naturally in some plants, may bind to calcium and prevent it from being absorbed optimally. These substances affect the absorption of calcium from the plant itself not the calcium found in other calcium-containing foods eaten at the same time. Examples of foods high in oxalic acid are spinach, collard greens, sweet potatoes, rhubarb, and beans. Foods high in phytic acid include whole grain bread, beans, seeds, nuts, grains, and soy isolates.[2] Although soybeans are high in phytic acid, the calcium present in soybeans is still partially absorbed. Fiber, particularly from wheat bran, could also prevent calcium absorption because of its content of phytate. However, the effect of fiber on calcium absorption is more of a concern for individuals with low calcium intakes. The average American tends to consume much less fiber per day than the level that would be needed to affect calcium absorption.

Calcium excretion refers to the amount of calcium eliminated from the body in urine, feces and sweat. Calcium excretion can be affected by many factors including dietary sodium, protein, caffeine and potassium. Typically, dietary sodium and protein increase calcium excretion as the amount of their intake is increased. However, if a high protein, high sodium food also contains calcium, this may help counteract the loss of calcium.

Increasing dietary potassium intake (such as from 7-8 servings of fruits and vegetables per day) in the presence of a high sodium diet (>5100 mg/day, which is more than twice the Tolerable Upper Intake Level of 2300 mg for sodium per day) may help decrease calcium excretion particularly in postmenopausal women.

Caffeine has a small effect on calcium absorption. It can temporarily increase calcium excretion and may modestly decrease calcium absorption, an effect easily offset by increasing calcium consumption in the diet. One cup of regular brewed coffee causes a loss of only 2-3 mg of calcium easily offset by adding a tablespoon of milk [14]. Moderate caffeine consumption, (1 cup of coffee or 2 cups of tea per day), in young women who have adequate calcium intakes has little to no negative effects on their bones.

Other factors

Phosphorus: The effect of dietary phosphorus on calcium is minimal. Some researchers speculate that the detrimental effects of consuming foods high in phosphate such as carbonated soft drinks is due to the replacement of milk with soda rather than the phosphate level itself.

Alcohol: Alcohol can affect calcium status by reducing the intestinal absorption of calcium. It can also inhibit enzymes in the liver that help convert vitamin D to its active form which in turn reduces calcium absorption. However, the amount of alcohol required to affect calcium absorption is unknown. Evidence is currently conflicting whether moderate alcohol consumption is helpful or harmful to bone.

In summary, a variety of factors that may cause a decrease in calcium absorption and/or increase in calcium excretion may negatively affect bone health.

Sodium, Potassium, Chloride

Electrolyte is a "medical/scientific" term for salts, specifically ions. The term electrolyte means that this ion is electrically-charged and moves to either a negative (cathode) or positive (anode) electrode:

- ions that move to the cathode (cations) are positively charged
- ions that move to the anode (anions) are negatively charged

Electrolytes are important because they are what your cells (especially nerve, heart, muscle) use to maintain voltages across their cell membranes and to carry electrical impulses (nerve impulses, muscle contractions) across themselves and to other cells. Kidneys work to keep the electrolyte concentrations in your blood constant despite changes in your body. For example, when you exercise heavily, you lose electrolytes in sweat, particularly sodium and potassium. Without the presence of these electrolytes water would move freely across cell membranes, thus destroying cellular integrity. Electrolytes, through their charge, control water flow into and out of cells.

Food sources[1]

Diets rarely lack sodium. Table salt is sodium chloride which contains about 40% sodium. Chloride is never naturally lacking in the diet. It abounds in foods as part of sodium chloride and other salts. Potassium is found in both plant and animal foods.

Deficiency

Deficiency of these nutrients is rare. Deficiency of sodium can occur in dehydration situations such as vomiting, diarrhea, or heavy sweating. In normal sweating during exercise, salt losses can safely be replaced later in the day with plain foods. Deficiency of chloride has never been seen. Deficiency of potassium is unlikely, but diets low in fresh fruits and vegetables make it a possibility.

Toxicity: Toxicity of sodium produces edema and hypertension, but this is not a problem as long as water needs are met. In sensitive persons, prolonged excess can lead to hypertension. Toxicity of chloride can only result from dehydration due to water deficiency. Toxicity of potassium does not occur from overeating foods high in potassium.

Dietary Reference Intakes[s4]

In 2004, The Food and Nutrition Board released the sixth in a series of reports presenting dietary reference values for the intake of nutrients by Americans and Canadians. This new report establishes nutrient recommendations on water, salt and potassium to maintain health and reduce chronic disease risk. There is no DRI set for these three nutrients; rather, an estimated minimum requirement has been recommended. The minimum requirement for sodium is 500 milligrams. The American Heart Association recommends limiting sodium intake to 3000 milligrams per day. The estimated minimum requirement for chloride is 750 milligrams per day; and the estimated minimum requirement for potassium is 2000 milligrams per day.

The vast majority of healthy people adequately meet their daily hydration needs by letting thirst be their guide. The report did not specify exact requirements for water, but set general recommendations for women at approximately 2.7 liters (91 ounces) of total water — from all beverages and foods — each day, and men an average of approximately 3.7 liters (125 ounces daily) of total water. The panel did not set an upper level for water.

About 80 percent of people's total water intake comes from drinking water and beverages — including caffeinated beverages — and the other 20 percent is derived from food. Prolonged physical activity and heat exposure will increase water losses and therefore may raise daily fluid needs, although it is important to note that excessive amounts can be life-threatening. Healthy 19- to 50-year-old adults should consume 1.5 grams of sodium and 2.3 grams of chloride each day — or 3.8 grams of salt — to replace the amount lost daily on average through sweat and to achieve a diet that provides sufficient amounts of other essential nutrients. Visit http://www.iom.edu/Object.File/Master/20/004/0.pdf for a complete list of recommendations.

Toxicity

The tolerable upper intake level (UL) for salt is set at 5.8 grams per day. More than 95 percent of American men and 90 percent of Canadian men ages 31 to 50, and 75 percent of American women and 50 percent of Canadian women in this age range regularly consume salt in excess of the UL.

Older individuals, African Americans, and people with chronic diseases including hypertension, diabetes, and kidney disease are especially sensitive to the blood pressure-raising effects of salt and should consume less than the UL. Adults should consume at least 4.7 grams of potassium per day to lower blood pressure, blunt the effects of salt, and reduce the risk of kidney stones and bone loss. However, most American women 31 to 50 years old consume no more than half of the recommended amount of potassium, and men's intake is only moderately higher. There was no evidence of chronic excess intakes of potassium in apparently health individuals and thus no UL was established.

Sulfur

The body does not use sulfur as a nutrient. Sulfur occurs in essential nutrients. Two amino acids are sulfur containing amino acids—methionine and cysteine. Sulfur forms bridges in proteins and is crucial to the contour of protein molecules. There is no recommended intake for sulfur and no deficiencies are known.

Phosphorus

Phosphorus is the second most abundant mineral in the body. Phosphorous is a component of bone, teeth, nucleic acids, phospholipids, ATP, and a number of enzymes and coenzymes. Phosphorylation of glucose is a requirement for its metabolism. Phosphorylation/dephosphorylation of cellular compounds is a mechanism for regulating enzyme activity and for transport and storage of cell compounds. Approximately 85% of the total body phosphate pool is found in bone as hydroxyapatite. The remaining amount of phosphate is distributed in blood and soft tissues. In the blood, phosphate is part of the monobasic-dibasic buffer system.[25]

Phosphorus is part of DNA and RNA. Phosphorus is also involved in the energy cycle. Many enzymes and the B vitamins become active when a phosphate group is added. Phosphate is also part of lipids—phospholipids.[25]

Phosphorus is well absorbed by the intestines and does not change with changing needs. The total body phosphorus pool is regulated by renal excretion.

Food sources[25]

Beans, peas, cereals and nuts contain phytate or inositol phosphate which is resistant to digestion. However, phytase from yeast added during leavening of breads, can release some phosphate from phytate. Intestinal microflora can also release phosphate from phytic acid in the colon. Phytase activity from endogenous and exogenous sources can increase the bioavailability of phosphate from plant sources by approximately 50%. Good Dietary Sources of phosphorous are typically also rich in protein. These foods are mainly milk, meat, nuts, legumes, and grains. Additional Dietary Sources of phosphorous are listed in the table below.

Deficiency[25]

Phosphorus Deficiency caused by inadequate dietary intake does not occur. However, chronic and excessive use of anticonvulsants, calcium carbonate supplements, or aluminum hydroxide-containing antacids can decrease phosphate absorption. Hypophosphatemia can also develop in individuals with gastrointestinal malabsorption, diabetes mellitus, hyperparathyroidism, renal dysfunction, or alcoholism whether or not it is accompanied by decompensated liver disease. Hypophosphatemia results in bone loss, weakness, and poor appetite. Imbalances in phosphate intake may contribute to negative calcium balance when inadequate calcium intake is accompanied by excessive intake of phosphorous. Elevations in serum phosphate following a meal will inhibit activation of vitamin D which is necessary for stimulation of intestinal calcium absorption. In response to diminished levels of calcitriol, additional amounts of parathyroid hormone are secreted to compensate for interference with vitamin D activation by elevated serum phosphate. This condition is described as a nutritional secondary hyperparathyroidism which contributes to increased rates of bone turnover and eventually to a reduction of bone mass and density. Elevated blood phosphorous levels are usually secondary to inadequate renal filtration due to acute or chronic renal failure.

Dietary Reference Intakes[2]

Age	Phosphorus(mg)
Infants	
0-6 months	100
7-12 months	275
Children	
1-3 years	460
4-8 years	500
Males	
9-13 years	1250
14-18 years	1250
19-30 years	700
31-50 years	700
51-70 years	700
>70 years	700

Toxicity

The upper limit of safety for phosphorus established by the Food and Nutrition Board of the Institute of Medicine is 3 to grams daily for adults.

Magnesium

Magnesium is the fourth most abundant mineral in the body and is essential to good health. Approximately 50% of total body magnesium is found in bone. The other half is found predominantly inside cells of body tissues and organs. Only 1% of magnesium is found in blood, but the body works very hard to keep blood levels of magnesium constant.[27]

Magnesium is needed for more than 300 biochemical reactions in the body. It helps maintain normal muscle and nerve function, keeps heart rhythm steady, supports a healthy immune system, and keeps bones strong. Magnesium also helps regulate blood sugar levels, promotes normal blood pressure, and is known to be involved in energy metabolism and protein synthesis.[28,29] There is an increased interest in the role of magnesium in preventing and managing disorders such as hypertension, cardiovascular disease, and diabetes. Dietary magnesium is absorbed in the small intestines. Magnesium is excreted through the kidneys.[27,29,30]

Food sources

Green vegetables such as spinach are good sources of magnesium because the center of the chlorophyll molecule (which gives green vegetables their color) contains magnesium. Some legumes (beans and peas), nuts and seeds, and whole, unrefined grains are also good sources of magnesium.[31] Refined grains are generally low in magnesium.[30,31] When white flour is refined and processed, the magnesium-rich germ and bran are removed. Bread made from whole grain wheat flour provides more magnesium than bread made from white refined flour. Tap water can be a source of magnesium, but the amount varies according to the water supply. Water that naturally contains more minerals is described as "hard". "Hard" water contains more magnesium than "soft" water.

Deficiency

Even though dietary surveys suggest that many Americans do not consume recommended amounts of magnesium, symptoms of magnesium deficiency are rarely seen in the US. However, there is concern about the prevalence of sub-optimal magnesium stores in the body. For many people, dietary intake may not be high enough to promote an optimal magnesium status, which may be protective against disorders such as cardiovascular disease and immune dysfunction.[32,33]

Early signs of magnesium deficiency include loss of appetite, nausea, vomiting, fatigue, and weakness. As magnesium deficiency worsens, numbness, tingling, muscle contractions and cramps, seizures, personality changes, abnormal heart rhythms, and coronary spasms can occur.[27,29,30] Severe magnesium deficiency can result in low levels of calcium in the blood (hypocalcemia). Magnesium deficiency is also associated with low levels of potassium in the blood (hypokalemia).[27]

Many of these symptoms are general and can result from a variety of medical conditions other than magnesium deficiency. It is important to have a physician evaluate health complaints and problems so that appropriate care can be given.

Deficiency does not occur under normal circumstances, even when intake is half of the RDA. Magnesium deficiency occurs in alcohol abuse, protein malnutrition, or diseases that cause prolonged vomiting or diarrhea.[35] The UL has been set at 350 mg from non food sources which has been shown to be toxic.

Dietary Reference Intakes[30]

Recommended Dietary Allowances for magnesium[30]		
Age (years)	Male(mg/day)	Female(mg/day)
1-3	80	80
4-8	130	130
9-13	240	240
14-18	410	360
19-30	400	310
31+	420	320

There is insufficient information on magnesium to establish a RDA for infants. For infants 0 to 12 months, the DRI is in the form of an Adequate Intake (AI), which is the mean intake of magnesium in healthy, breast-fed infants.

Toxicity

Magnesium toxicity is very rare except in certain instances where renal failure prevents urinary excretion (i.e., in the situation where magnesium-containing drugs are given to a patient with renal inabilities). Symptoms include central nervous system depression, skeletal muscle paralysis, and in extreme cases, coma and death. Calcium infusion tends to counteract magnesium toxicity.

Healthy kidney function excretes magnesium rapidly and efficiently, with little possibility for toxic buildup. Levels up to 1600 mg daily have proven to be no problem as long as there as a balance of at least 50% calcium intake at the same time.

TRACE MINERALS

The trace minerals are iron, zinc, iodine, selenium, copper, manganese, chromium, and molybdenum. The purpose of this discussion is to familiarize you with the roles of these nutrients.

Iron

Most of the body's iron is in the proteins hemoglobin in the red blood cells and myoglobin in muscle cells. Hemoglobin is the molecule responsible for carrying oxygen to all our cells, while myoglobin accepts, stores, and releases oxygen in the muscles.[36] About 65 to 75 percent of the body's iron is in the blood in the form of hemoglobin. Iron is also required for the making of amino acids, hormones, and neurotransmitters. The body conserves iron zealously; iron is recycled when hemoglobin and myoglobin are degraded. Iron has many different roles in the body. In addition, iron is involved in reactions within the body that produce energy. Any excess iron is stored in the body as a reserve.[36] A lack of iron in the diet may result in the development of iron deficiency anemia. The greatest need for iron is during growth or periods of blood loss.[36]

There are two forms of iron - heme and non-heme. The iron in meat is about 40 percent heme and 60 percent non-heme. Much of the iron in the diet, however, is in the non-heme form. This is the form found in plant sources such as fruits, vegetables and grain products. About 25 percent to 35 percent of heme iron is absorbed, yet this percentage drops to 3 percent for non-heme iron. This difference is important because heme iron is found only in animal flesh.[36]

Vegetarians in particular need to be aware of the low absorption of non-heme iron. There are, however, a number of methods to improve iron absorption. One of these methods is to include foods rich in vitamin C in the diet. Good sources of vitamin C include citrus fruits and juices, tomatoes, strawberries, melons, dark green leafy vegetables and potatoes. To have an effect, these foods must be eaten at the same meal as the iron source. Another method to improve non-heme iron absorption is to include a source of heme iron (meat) with the meal. Not only will more total iron be eaten, but the percentage of non-heme iron that is absorbed will be greater.[36]

Other factors may decrease the availability of iron. Coffee and tea consumption at the time of a meal can significantly decrease iron absorption. Tea can cause iron absorption to drop by 60 percent and coffee can cause a 50 percent decrease in iron uptake. The tannins in both tea and coffee adversely affect iron availability. Phytates in some grains, phosphates in cola drinks, and possibly fiber may interfere with iron absorption. These may be important factors if the diet already is low in iron.[36]

Food Sources[36]

To meet the recommendations for dietary iron, eat a variety of foods. Iron is not concentrated in many foods except organ meats such as liver and heart. Other foods with lower, yet substantial amounts of iron include most meats (especially red meats), dried beans and peas, green leafy vegetables and dried fruit. Whole-grain, enriched, and iron-fortified bread and cereal products also are good sources. To ensure a diet adequate in iron: Eat a variety of iron-rich foods, eat foods high in vitamin C, and combine plant sources of iron with meat, fish and poultry.

Deficiency[36]

If iron is lacking in the diet, iron reserves in the body are used. Once this supply is depleted the formation of hemoglobin is affected. This means the red blood cells cannot carry oxygen needed by the cells. When this happens, iron deficiency occurs and anemia results.

The greatest need for iron is during growth or periods of blood loss. Young children, adolescents and pregnant women have increased needs because of the growth taking place during these periods. The demands during pregnancy are so large that an iron supplement is recommended for pregnant women. All women of child-bearing age have increased requirements because of the losses from menstruation.[36]

An active female athlete involved in a rigorous training program has an increased risk for iron deficiency anemia. Iron deficiency is common with or without anemia, decreases performance for the athlete, and often is not detected on a standard hematocrit reading. The capacity to transport oxygen to the cells of the muscle via myoglobin is impaired (energy production is limited), which is vital for competition. To ensure optimum iron stores, a female athlete should eat meals or snacks that contain adequate quantities of iron-rich foods and, in some cases, see a physician for a recommended iron supplement.[36]

The elderly are another group at risk for iron deficiency. Seniors should consume adequate quantities of iron-rich foods and be particularly careful to incorporate vitamin C sources with their meals; for example, juice with their toast or cereal or fruit on their morning breakfast food. By eating foods in combination, the absorption of iron can be increased.[36]

Iron deficiency and anemia are not the same. Iron deficiency refers to depleted body iron stores without regard to the degree of depletion or to the presence of anemia. Anemia refers to the severe depletion of iron stores that results in a low hemoglobin concentration. Persons with iron deficiency anemia have red blood cells that can't carry enough oxygen from the lungs to the tissues, so energy release is compromised. These persons feel fatigue, weakness, headaches, and apathy. Populations at increased risk for iron deficiency are persons who have had bleeding episodes; because so much of the body's iron is in blood, iron losses are greatest whenever blood is lost. Bleeding from ulcers, regular blood donations, and menstrual losses can produce iron deficiency. The classic symptoms of iron deficiency are fatigue, weakness, headaches, apathy, pallor, and poor tolerance to cold.[36]

Dietary Reference Intakes[36]

Age	mg iron
Infants and Children	
0-6 months	0.27
7-12 months	11
1-3 years	7
4-8 years	10
Males	
9-13 years	8
14-18 years	11
19+ years	8
Females	
9-13 years	8
14-18 years	15
19-50 years	18
51+ years	8
Pregnancy	
≤18 years	27
18+ years	27
Lactation	
≤18 years	10
18+ years	9

Toxicity

The body normally absorbs less iron if its stores are full. Toxicity, once rare, is emerging among men in the US. Hemochromatosis is caused by a hereditary defect that allows the small intestine to helplessly absorb excess iron.

Notes

Heart disease risk seems to be greater in societies that eat high amounts of red meat versus those that eat minimal amounts. The amount of iron stored in the body can influence a person's potential to develop heart disease. Excess iron is associated with the formation of free radicals, unstable molecules in the body that may injure vessels supplying blood to the heart. It has also been suggested that the incidence of heart disease rises dramatically in women once menstruation stops due to increased amounts of iron in the blood. There is no conclusive evidence that excess iron increases coronary heart disease. It is not recommended to eliminate red meat or other iron rich foods from the diet. Using the Food Guide Pyramid as a guide for daily food choices, red meat is a good source of iron, protein and other important nutrients.

Iron absorption is affected by the iron status of the individual, the type of food eaten and vitamin C intake. Iron has many different roles in the body. About 65 to 75 percent of the body's iron is in the blood in the form of hemoglobin. Myoglobin, the compound that carries oxygen to the muscle cells, also requires iron. In addition, iron is involved in reactions within the body that produce energy. Any excess iron is stored in the body as a reserve.

Zinc

Zinc is an essential mineral that is found in almost every cell. It stimulates the activity of approximately 100 enzymes, which are substances that promote biochemical reactions in your body. Zinc supports a healthy immune system, is needed for wound healing, helps maintain your sense of taste and smell, and is needed for DNA synthesis. Zinc also supports normal growth and development during pregnancy, childhood, and adolescence. Muscle contains the highest proportion of total body zinc. Zinc associates with insulin in the pancreas; zinc interacts with platelets in blood clotting, affects thyroid hormone function, and affects behavior and learning performance.[37]

Food sources[37]

Zinc is found in a wide variety of foods. Oysters contain more zinc per serving than any other food, but red meat and poultry provide the majority of zinc in the American diet. Other good food sources include beans, nuts, certain seafood, whole grains, fortified breakfast cereals, and dairy products. Zinc absorption is greater from a diet high in animal protein than a diet rich in plant proteins. Phytates, which are found in whole grain breads, cereals, legumes and other products, can decrease zinc absorption.

Deficiency[37]

Zinc deficiency most often occurs when zinc intake is inadequate or poorly absorbed, when there are increased losses of zinc from the body, or when the body's requirement for zinc increase. *Signs of zinc deficiency* include growth retardation, hair loss, diarrhea, delayed sexual maturation and impotence, eye and skin lesions, and loss of appetite. There is also evidence that weight loss, delayed healing of wounds, taste abnormalities, and mental lethargy can occur. Since many of these symptoms are general and are associated with other medical conditions, do not assume they are due to a zinc deficiency. It is important to consult with a medical doctor about medical symptoms so that appropriate care can be given.

There is no single laboratory test that adequately measures zinc nutritional status. Medical doctors who suspect a zinc deficiency will consider risk factors such as inadequate caloric intake, alcoholism, digestive diseases, and symptoms such as impaired growth in infants and children when determining a need for zinc supplementation. Vegetarians may need as much as 50% more zinc than non-vegetarians because of the lower absorption of zinc from plant foods, so it is very important for vegetarians to include good sources of zinc in their diet.

Maternal zinc deficiency can slow fetal growth. Zinc supplementation has improved growth rate in some children who demonstrate mild to moderate growth failure and who also have a zinc deficiency (22). Human milk does not provide recommended amounts of zinc for older infants between the ages of 7 months and 12 months, so breast-fed infants of this age should also consume age-appropriate foods containing zinc or be given formula containing zinc. Alternately, pediatricians may recommend supplemental zinc in this situation. Breast-feeding also may deplete maternal zinc stores because of the greater need for zinc during lactation. It is important for mothers who breast-feed to include good sources of zinc in their daily diet and for pregnant women to follow their doctor's advice about taking vitamin and mineral supplements.

Low zinc status has been observed in 30% to 50% of alcoholics. Alcohol decreases the absorption of zinc and increases loss of zinc in urine. In addition, many alcoholics do not eat an acceptable variety or amount of food, so their dietary intake of zinc may be inadequate.

Diarrhea results in a loss of zinc. Individuals who have had gastrointestinal surgery or who have digestive disorders that result in malabsorption, including sprue, Crohn's disease and short bowel syndrome, are at greater risk of a zinc deficiency. Individuals who experience chronic diarrhea should make sure they include sources of zinc in their daily diet (see selected table of food sources of zinc) and may benefit from zinc supplementation. A medical doctor can evaluate the need for a zinc supplement if diet alone fails to maintain normal zinc levels in these circumstances.

Dietary Reference Intakes[37]

The latest recommendations for zinc intake are given in the new Dietary Reference Intakes developed by the Institute of Medicine. Dietary Reference Intakes (DRIs) is the umbrella term for a group of reference values used for planning and assessing nutrient intake for healthy people. The Recommended Dietary Allowance (RDA), one of the DRIs, is the average daily dietary intake level that is sufficient to meet the nutrient requirements of nearly all (97-98%) healthy individuals. For infants 0 to 6 months, the DRI is in the form of an Adequate Intake (AI), which is the mean intake of zinc in healthy, breast-fed infants. The AI for zinc for infants from 0 through 6 months is 2.0 milligrams (mg) per day. The 2001 RDAs for zinc for infants 7 through 12 months, children and adults in mg per day are:

Recommended Dietary Allowances - Zinc			
Age	Infants and Children	Males	Females
7 months to 3 years	3 mg		
4 to 8 years	5 mg		
9 to 13 years	8 mg		
14 to 18 years	11 mg	9 mg	13 mg
19+	11 mg	8 mg	11 mg

Results of two national surveys, the National Health and Nutrition Examination Survey (NHANES III 1988-91) and the Continuing Survey of Food Intakes of Individuals (1994 CSFII) (13) indicated that most infants, children, and adults consume recommended amounts of zinc.

Toxicity

Zinc toxicity has been seen in both acute and chronic forms. Intakes of 150 to 450 mg of zinc per day have been associated with low copper status, altered iron function, reduced immune function, and reduced levels of high-density lipoproteins (the good cholesterol). One case report cited severe nausea and vomiting within 30 minutes after the person ingested four grams of zinc gluconate (570 mg elemental zinc) (35). In 2001 the National Academy of Sciences established tolerable upper levels (UL), the highest intake associated with no adverse health effects, for zinc for infants, children, and adults. The ULs do not apply to individuals who are receiving zinc for medical treatment, but it is important for such individuals to be under the care of a medical doctor who will monitor for adverse health effects.

2001 Upper Levels - Zinc		
Age	Infants and Children	Males and Females
0 to 6 months	4 mg	
7 to 12 months	5 mg	
1 to 3 years	7 mg	
4 to 8 years	12 mg	
9 to 13 years	23 mg	
14 to 18 years	34 mg	34 mg
Ages 19+		40 mg

Notes[37]

The immune system is adversely affected by even moderate degrees of zinc deficiency. Severe zinc deficiency depresses immune function. Zinc is required for the development and activation of T-lymphocytes, a kind of white blood cell that helps fight infection. When zinc supplements are given to individuals with low zinc levels, the numbers of T-cell lymphocytes circulating in the blood increase and the ability of lymphocytes to fight infection improves. Studies show that poor, malnourished children in India, Africa, South America, and Southeast Asia experience shorter courses of infectious diarrhea after taking zinc supplements. Amounts of zinc provided in these studies ranged from 4 mg a day up to 40 mg per day and were provided in a variety of forms (zinc acetate, zinc gluconate, or zinc sulfate). Zinc supplements are often given to help heal skin ulcers or bed sores (30), but they do not increase rates of wound healing when zinc levels are normal.

The effect of zinc treatments on the severity or duration of cold symptoms is controversial. A study of over 100 employees of the Cleveland Clinic indicated that zinc lozenges decreased the duration of colds by one-half, although no differences were seen in how long fevers lasted or the level of muscle aches. Other researchers examined the effect of zinc supplements on cold duration and severity in over 400 randomized subjects. In their first study, a virus was used to induce cold symptoms. The duration of illness was significantly lower in the group receiving zinc gluconate lozenges (providing 13.3 mg zinc) but not in the group receiving zinc acetate lozenges (providing 5 or 11.5 mg zinc). None of the zinc preparations affected the severity of cold symptoms in the first 3 days of treatment. In the second study, which examined the effects of zinc supplements on duration and severity of natural colds, no differences were seen between individuals receiving zinc and those receiving a placebo (sugar pill). Recent research suggests that the effect of zinc may be influenced by the ability of the specific supplement formula to deliver zinc ions to the oral mucosa. Additional research is needed to determine whether zinc compounds have any effect on the common cold.

Iron deficiency anemia is considered a serious public health problem in the world today. Iron fortification programs were developed to prevent this deficiency, and they have been credited with improving the iron status of millions of women, infants, and children. Some researchers have questioned the effect of iron fortification on absorption of other nutrients, including zinc. Fortification of foods with iron does not significantly affect zinc absorption. However, large amounts of iron in supplements (greater than 25 mg) may decrease zinc absorption, as can iron in solutions. Taking iron supplements between meals will help decrease its effect on zinc absorption.

Iodine

The only function of iodine involves the synthesis of thyroid hormone. Approximately 60% of the total body pool of iodine is stored in the thyroid gland. The remainder is found in the blood, ovary, and muscle. Thyroid hormone is necessary for regulation of human growth and development.[38]

Iodine is absorbed intestinally from dietary sources or dermally from topical iodine applications or from iodine vapors produced as by-products of industrial activity. Iodine vapor is also emitted from cleansing agents used commercially in sterilization processes and from fossil fuel combustion such as occurs in automobile engines. Currently, the most common source of exposure to iodine is from automobile exhaust. In the 1970's, the amount of iodine measured in the environment reached levels that were a cause for concern prompting the dairy industry to discontinue use of iodine-containing agents in sterilization of milking equipment to reduce the iodine content of milk.[38]

Food Sources[38]

Although most foods do not contain iodine, one teaspoon of iodized salt consumed daily is more than sufficient to satisfy physiological requirements for this nutrient. Other dietary sources of iodine include drinking water, seafood (clams, lobster, oysters, sardines and ocean fish) and dairy products from feed additives as well as from disinfectants used on dairy farms. The iodine content of fruits and vegetables is dependent upon soil content. More detailed information on food sources of iodine is provided below.

Deficiency[38]

Iodine deficiency was frequently observed in landlocked regions of the US at the beginning of the 20th century necessitating iodine fortification of salt, an inexpensive and widely used seasoning. The development of iodine deficiency is no longer a problem, since landlocked regions receive produce grown in coastal areas where soil is rich in iodine. Signs of iodine deficiency include hypothyroidism, lethargy, and weight gain. The clinical presentation of iodine deficiency is goiter. Goiter can also develop from high intakes of goitrogens, naturally occurring substances in foods which decrease iodine availability or interfere with its tissue utilization. Dietary sources of goitrogens include cabbage, turnips, rapeseed oil (canola oil), peanuts, cassava, and soybeans. Goitrogens are inactivated by heating, roasting or cooking.

Cretinism is a condition which develops in the fetus from iodine deficiency during pregnancy. This condition is characterized by mental retardation and dwarfism. Neonates are routinely screened for adequate thyroid hormone levels in developed countries and is being adopted in developing countries.

Toxicity

Chronic excessive intakes of iodine may compromise thyroid function and also contribute to development of goiter and hypothyroidism due to feedback inhibition of thyroid hormone synthesis. Grave's disease develops in response to an overactive thyroid and is not a condition associated with iodine toxicity.

The upper limit of safety established for iodine by the Food and Nutrition Board of the Institute of Medicine is approximately 1,100 mcg daily for adults.

Dietary Reference Intakes[38]

Age	Iodine mcg		
Infants			
0-6 months	110		
7-12 months	130	Females	
Children		9-13 years	120
1-3 years	90	14-18 years	150
4-8 years	90	19-30 years	150
Males		31-50 years	150
9-13 years	120	51-70 years	150
14-18 years	150	> 70 years	150
19-30 years	150	Pregnancy	
31-50 years	150	≤ 18 years	220
51-70 years	150	19-30 years	220
> 70 years	150	31-50 years	220

Selenium

Selenium is a component of glutathione peroxidases which are primarily responsible for reducing peroxide free radicals that include lipid peroxide formation in cell membranes. Reduction of peroxides formed by oxidation of membrane phospholipids breaks the auto-oxidative chain reaction that damages cell membranes. Selenium-dependent antioxidant protection of cell membrane phospholipids is synergistic with vitamin E. Selenium also has a role in prostaglandin synthesis by protecting the oxidative state of lipid intermediates formed during cyclooxygenase reactions which determines the balance of the end products and whether proaggregatory, pro-inflammatory or anti-aggregatory, anti-inflammatory responses will dominate.[39]

Food Sources[39]

Selenium is commonly found in Brazil nuts, seafood, kidney, liver, meat, poultry, whole grain pasta, sunflower seeds, oatmeal, soy nuts, other nuts, eggs and low-fat dairy products.

Food sources provide selenium in either the inorganic forms selenite or selenate or in an organic form where it displaces sulfur in methionine or cysteine. Soil selenium content determines the amount of selenium concentrated in plant sources which can vary as much as 200-fold between crops grown in different regions. Since produce and grain products consumed in the US are obtained from various regions, the average selenium intake from plant sources is similar between different geographical areas. Processing of grains decreases the selenium content of the grain products. Meat and poultry are more reliable selenium sources because livestock feed is supplemented with selenium.

Deficiency[39]

Clinical selenium deficiency is rarely observed in humans. Marginal intakes may reduce activities of selenium-dependent peroxidases. Changes in these enzyme activities have been associated with development of Keshan Disease (cardiomyopathy) and Kashin-Beck Disease (chondrodystrophy) in children in selenium-deficient regions of China. Selenium deficiency can also develop in malnourished patients dependent on enteral or parenteral nutrition for long periods of time. Muscle pain, weakness, and tenderness have been reported by these patients. Selenium supplementation can correct this type of deficiency.

Dietary Reference Intakes[39]

Selenium(mcg/day)				
Infants				
0 - 6 months 15		Females		
7 - 12 months	20	9 - 13 years	40	
Children		14 - 18 years	55	
1 - 3 years	20	19 - 30 years	55	
4 - 8 years	30	31 - 50 years	55	
Males		51 - 70 years	55	
9 - 13 years 40		> 70 years	55	
14 - 18 years	55	Pregnancy		
19 - 30 years	55	< 18 years	60	
31 - 50 years	55	19 - 30 years	60	
51 - 70 years	55			
> 70 years	55			

Toxicity

The upper limit of safety for selenium established by the Food and Nutrition Board of the Institute of Medicine is 400 micrograms daily for adults. Excessive amounts of selenium (> 750 mcg/day) can cause nausea, vomiting, diarrhea, loss of hair and nails, tenderness and swelling of the fingers, fatigue, irritability, skin lesions, tooth damage and nervous system disturbances.

Supplementation that provides > 3 times the DRI is more likely to cause toxicity than what is consumed from dietary sources. Organic selenium supplements (selenomethionine and selnocycsteine) are better absorbed than inorganic forms. Symptoms of selenium toxicity include dermatitis, loose hair, brittle nails, and peripheral neuropathy.

Copper

Copper is a component of prolyl and lysyl hydoxylases, enzymes involved in collagen synthesis. Because of this, connective tissue-rich tissues such as capillaries, scar tissue, and bone matrix are most sensitive to copper status. Copper also functions at the catalytic site of the antioxidant enzyme superoxide dismutase. Additionally, the copper-containing plasma protein ceruloplasmin is integral to iron metabolism since it catalyzes oxidation of the mineral, which is required for its binding to proteins involved in absorption, transport, and storage. The redox potential of copper ions gives it a key role in energy metabolism as a component of the cytochromes that participate in electron transport.[40]

Approximately one third of the total body pool of copper is localized in skeletal muscle. Another third is found in brain and liver. The remaining amount of total body copper is found in bone and other tissues. Since copper is excreted primarily in the bile, diseases of the liver and gall bladder may affect copper balance.[40]

Copper absorption is regulated by changes in the total body pool. The increase in absorptive efficiency observed when total body copper decreases is mediated by an intestinal copper-binding protein that is also involved with mucosal storage of zinc. Consequently, high dose zinc supplements (150 mg/day) can dramatically contribute to copper deficiency by decreasing the amount of protein available to bind copper. High dose vitamin C supplements (1500 mg/day) may also decrease copper absorption because the reduced form of the mineral, which is increased in the presence of vitamin C, is less well-absorbed than the oxidized form.

Food Sources[40]

Copper is found in foods such as organ meats, seafood, nuts, seeds, whole grains, legumes, chocolate, cherries, dried fruits, milk, tea, chicken, and potatoes.

Deficiency[40]

Although severe copper deficiency is rarely observed, marginal copper status is not uncommon. High dose supplements of zinc, vitamin C, and iron are contributing causes of marginal copper deficiency. Microcytic hypochromic anemia in the presence of normal serum ferritin is the primary clinical feature of marginal copper deficiency. This anemia, which is hematologically identical to iron-deficiency anemia, develops as a result of abnormalities in iron utilization. Skeletal abnormalities, reproductive difficulties, impaired nervous tissue function, and changes in hair and skin pigmentation have been observed in severe copper deficiency. A role for copper in the maintenance of bone mass has been determined from observations of osteoporosis in preterm infants born with inadequate copper reserves.

Dietary Reference Intakes[40]

Copper(mcg)				
Infants				
0 - 6 months	200			
7 - 12 months	220	**Females**		
Children		9 - 13 years	700	
1 - 3 years	340	14 - 18 years	890	
4 - 8 years	440	19 - 30 years	900	
Males		31 - 50 years	900	
9 - 13 years	700	51 - 70 years	900	
14 - 18 years	890	> 70 years	900	
19 - 30 years	900	**Pregnancy**		
31 - 50 years	900	< 18 years	1,000	
51 - 70 years	900	19 - 30 years	1,000	
> 70 years	900	31 - 50 years	1,000	

Toxicity

Copper toxicity is unlikely unless exposure to large amounts occurs as a result of industrial contamination or inappropriate use of supplements. Large dose copper supplements (10-20 mg/day) may contribute to liver damage, abnormalities in red blood cell formation, weakness, and nausea.[40]

Copper toxicity is the primary abnormality associated with Wilson's Disease. This inborn error of metabolism initially impacts the central nervous symptom causing tremors, dystonia, dysarthria, dysphagia, chorea, drooling, mental retardation and lack of coordination. Treatment involves a copper-restricted diet and long-term oral penicillamine therapy. Penicillin binds copper and reduces its absorption.[40]

The upper limit of safety established for copper by the Food and Nutrition Board of the Institute of Medicine is approximately 900 mcg daily for adults.[40]

Manganese

Manganese is a cofactor for enzymes involved in hydrolysis, phosphorylation, decarboxylation, and transamination. It also promotes activities of transferases such as glycosyltransferase, and of glutamine synthetase and superoxide dismutase.[41]

Food Sources[41]

Wheat germ, nuts, seeds, whole grains, oysters, sweet potatoes, tofu, chocolate, brewed tea and dark molasses are good sources of manganese. Fruits and vegetables such as pineapple, grape juice and tomato juice provide moderate levels of manganese. Dairy products and meat provide little manganese.

Deficiency[41]

Manganese Deficiency in humans has not been documented, but has been induced experimentally in animals. Poor growth and abnormal reproduction have been observed in rats and mice. No reported cases of manganese toxicity resulting from dietary intake have been reported. Manganese Toxicity has been observed from inhalation manganese-containing dust by workers in mines and steel mills manifested by adverse effects on the central nervous system.[41]

The Daily Reference Intakes[41]

	Manganese (mg)		
Infants			
0-6 months	0.003	Females	
7-12 months	0.6	9-13 years	1.6
Children		14-18 years	1.6
1-3 years	1.2	19-30 years	1.8
4-8 years	1.5	31-50 years	1.8
Males		51-70 years	1.8
9-13 years	1.9	70	1.8
14-18 years	2.2	Pregnancy	
19-30 years	2.3	18 years	2.0
31-50 years	2.3	19-30 years	2.0
51-70 years	2.3		
>70 years	2.3		

Toxicity

The upper limit of safety for manganese established by the Food and Nutrition Board of the Institute of Medicine is approximately 11 mg daily for adults. See table below for more age- and gender specific guidelines.[41]

Chromium

Chromium was first identified as a component of the "glucose-tolerance factor" which is required for maintenance of normal blood glucose. As part of this factor, chromium acts synergistically with insulin to facilitate cellular uptake of blood glucose. Chromium may also have a role in other insulin-dependent activities such as protein and lipid metabolism. [42] Research does not support claims that chromium piccolinate supplements facilitate weight loss, build muscles or decrease body fat. However, chromium supplementation has been found to improve glucose tolerance in elderly adults who have low blood chromium levels. Tissue chromium depletion has been observed with age and may be responsible for abnormalities in glucose metabolism that often develop with age.[42] When complexed with organic compounds, chromium is more efficiently absorbed as an inorganic salt. Milled grains or other processed foods have considerably less chromium content than their unprocessed counter-parts. Foods cooked with acid-based sauces in stainless steel pans may obtain additional chromium from some types of cookware.[42]

Food Sources[42]

Dietary sources of chromium include whole grains, potatoes, oysters, liver, seafood, , cheese, chicken, and meat. Brewer's yeast is a rich source of organic chromium complexes.

Deficiency[42]

Diets composed primarily of processed foods may not provide sufficient amounts of chromium. Since chromium is lost in urine, sweat, bile, and hair, excessive physical exercise or tissue injury may also deplete tissue chromium levels.

Chromium deficiency is characterized by insulin resistance, hyperglycemia and lipid abnormalities. Clinically, this deficiency has only been reported with long-term administration of parenteral nutrition when chromium is not added to these solutions.

The Daily Reference Intakes[42]

Chromium (mcg)			
Infants			
0-6 months	.2		
7-12 months	5.5	Females	
Children		9-13 years	21
1-3 years	11	14-18 years	24
4-8 years	15	19-30 years	25
Males		31-50 years	25
9-13 years	25	51-70 years	20
14-18 years	35	>70 years	20
19-30 years	35	Pregnancy	
31-50 years	35	18 years	29
51-70 years	30	19-30 years	30
>70 years	30	31-50 years	30

Toxicity

No cases of chromium toxicity from excessive dietary intake have been reported. Chromium administered parenterally in high doses may cause skin irritation. The upper limit of safety for chromium has not been determined due to lack of data of adverse effects. The Food and Nutrition Board of the Institute of Medicine recommends intake of chromium should be from food only to prevent high levels of intake.

Molybdenum

Molybdenum is a cofactor of aldehyde oxidases which are involved in purine and pyrimidine detoxification. Xanthine oxidase is responsible for metabolism of uric acid. Molybdenum may also have a role in stabilizing the unoccupied glucocorticoid receptor.[42]

Food Sources[42]

Milk, dried beans, peas, nuts and seeds, eggs, liver tomatoes, carrots and meats are good sources of molybdenum.

Deficiency[42]

No cases of human molybdenum Deficiency have been reported. See table below for more age and gender specific guidelines.

Daily Reference Intakes[42]

Molybdenum(mcg)			
Infants			
0-6 months	2	Females	
7-12 months	3	9-13 years	34
Children		14-18 years	49
1-3 years	17	19-30 years	45
4-8 years	22	31-50 years	45
Males		51-70 years	45
9-13 years	34	> 70	45
14-18 years	43	Pregnancy	
19-30 years	45	< 18 years	50
31-50 years	45	19-30 years	50
51-70 years	45	31-50 years	50
70 years	45	> 70	50

Toxicity

No cases of human molybdenum toxicity have been reported. The upper limit of safety for molybdenum established by the Food and Nutrition Board of the Institute of Medicine is approximately 2,000 mcg daily for adults.

SUMMARY

Minerals are inorganic elements essential to life that act as control agents in body reactions and cooperative factors in energy production, body building and maintenance of tissues. They retain their identity (they cannot be changed into anything else), and they cannot be destroyed by heat, air, acid, or mixing (can be lost in cooking water).

Minerals require no digestion and are absorbed intact from the small intestines. They can become charged particles and can form compounds. Sodium and chloride are a familiar example of a compound i.e., sodium chloride (table salt).[1]

Like the water soluble vitamins, some minerals are readily absorbed into the blood, transported freely, and readily excreted by the kidneys. Some minerals must have carriers to be absorbed and transported just like the fat soluble vitamins.[1]

Minerals are divided into two categories - the major minerals and the trace minerals. The trace minerals are found in smaller amounts in the body, while the major minerals are found in larger amounts. The major minerals are calcium, sodium, chloride, potassium, sulfur, phosphorous and magnesium. The trace minerals are iron, zinc, iodine, copper, manganese, fluoride, chromium, selenium and others.[1]

As with all the other essential nutrients, minerals are vital to life. Determining adequate intake of each micronutrient individually can be an "arduous task". Computerized software can make the task manageable. However, individuals can be assured of obtaining all the micro nutrients in adequate amounts if their diets include 7 to 9 servings of fruits and veggies, whole grain, all natural products, and calcium through dairy products or supplements.

CHAPTER 8 - SAMPLE TEST

1. List two trace minerals and discuss the roles of each.

2. List two major minerals and discuss the roles of each.

3. Why would it be unwise to take three times the RDA of iron?

4. What are the number of servings of calcium in your diet? What are the recommended number of servings of calcium? Keep a food log again and determine the number of servings of calcium, fruits and vegetables in your diet.

5. What advice would you give to a client who tells you that he or she is taking three grams (3000 mg) of calcium per day?

REFERENCES

1. Shils ME. Modern Nutrition in Health and Disease. 9th ed. Baltimore: Williams & Wilkins, 1999.

2. Standing Committee on the Scientific Evaluation of Dietary Reference Intakes, Food and Nutrition Board, Institute of Medicine. Dietary Reference Intakes for Calcium, Phosphorus, Magnesium, Vitamin D and Fluoride. Washington DC: The National Academies Press, 1997.

3. Subar AF, Krebs-Smith SM, Cook A, Kahle LL. Dietary sources of nutrients among US adults. J Am Diet Assoc 1998;98:537-47.

4. National Osteoporosis Foundation. NOF osteoporosis prevention - risk factors for osteoporosis. 2003. http://www.nof.org/prevention/risk.htm.

5. Dawson-Hughes B, Dallal GE, Krall EA, Sadowski L, Sahyoun N, Tannenbaum S. A controlled trial of the effect of calcium supplementation on bone density in postmenopausal women. N Engl J Med 1990;323:878-83.

6. Elders PJ, Lips P, Netelenbos JC, et al. Long-term effect of calcium supplementation on bone loss in perimenopausal women. J Bone Min Res 1994;9:963-70.

7. Menopausal hormone therapy: Summary of a scientific workshop. Ann Intern Med 2003;138:361-364.

8. American College of Obstetricians and Gynecologists. Questions and answers on hormone therapy. American College of Obstetricians and Gynecologists Web site response to the WHI study results on estrogen and progestin hormone therapy. 2002. http://www.acog.org/from_home/publications/ press_releases/nr08-30-02.cfm.

9. Johnson AO, Semenya JG, Buchowski MS, Enwonwu CO, Scrimshaw NS. Correlation of lactose maldigestion, lactose intolerance, and milk intolerance. Am J Clin Nutr 1993;57:399-401.

10. Rao DR, Bello H, Warren AP, Brown GE. Prevalence of lactose maldigestion: Influence and interaction of age, race, and sex. Dig Dis Sci 1994;39:1519-24.

11. Coffin B, Azpiroz F, Guarner F, Mlagelada JR. Selective gastric hypersensitivity and reflex hyporeactivity in functional dyspepsia. Gastroenterology 1994;107:1345-51.

12. Hertzler SR, Huynh B, Savaiano DA. How much lactose is "low lactose". J Am Diet Assoc 1996;96:243-46.

13. Marsh AG, Sanchez TV, Midkelsen O, Keiser J, Mayor G. Cortical bone density of adult lacto-ovo-vegetarian and omnivorous women. J Am Diet Assoc 1980;76:148-51.

14. Reed JA, Anderson JJ, Tylavsky FA, Gallagher JCJ. Comparative changes in radial-bone density of elderly female lacto-ovo-vegetarians and omnivores. Am J Clin Nutr 1994;59:1197S-1202S.

15. Janelle KC, Barr SI. Nutrient intakes and eating behavior scores of vegetarian and non-vegetarian women. J Am Diet Assoc 1995;95:180-86.

16. Burckhardt P, Dawson-Hughes B, Heaney RP. Nutritional aspects of osteoporosis. Academic Press 2001. 17. 17. Spencer H, Menczel J, Lewin I, Samachson J. Effect of high phosphorus intake on calcium and phosphorus metabolism in man. J Nutr 1965;86:125-32.

18. Department of Health and Human Services. Nutrition and Your Health: Dietary Guidelines for Americans. Home and Garden Bulletin No. 232 2000;Fifth Edition.

19. Nutrition Business Journal. NBJ's supplement business report 2003. US consumer sales in $mil. San Diego, 2002:6.22.

20. Andon MB, Peacock M, Kanerva RL, De Castro JAS. Calcium absorption from apple and orange

juice fortified with calcium citrate malate (CCM). J Am Coll Nutr 1996;15:313-16.

21. Heaney RP, Saville PD, Recker RR. Calcium absorption as a function of calcium intake. J Lab Clin Med 1975;85:881-90.

22. Heaney RP, Recker RR, Hinders SM. Variability of calcium absorption. Am J Clin Nutr 1988;47:262-64.23.

23. http://dietary-supplements.info.nih.gov/factsheets/calcium.asp.

24. http://www.iom.edu/CMS/3788/3969.aspx.

25. http://www.feinberg.northwestern.edu/nutrition/factsheets/phosphorus.html.

26. http://dietary-supplements.info.nih.gov/factsheets/magnesium.asp.

27. Rude RK. Magnesium deficiency: A cause of heterogeneous disease in humans. J Bone Miner Res 1998;13:749-58. [PubMed abstract].

28. Wester PO. Magnesium. Am J Clin Nutr 1987;45:1305-12. [PubMed abstract].

29. Saris NE, Mervaala E, Karppanen H, Khawaja JA, Lewenstam A. Magnesium: an update on physiological, clinical, and analytical aspects. Clinica Chimica Acta 2000;294:1-26.

30. Institute of Medicine. Food and Nutrition Board. Dietary Reference Intakes: Calcium, Phosphorus, Magnesium, Vitamin D and Fluoride. National Academy Press. Washington, DC, 1999.

31. U.S. Department of Agriculture, Agricultural Research Service. 2003. USDA National Nutrient Database for Standard Reference, Release 16. Nutrient Data Laboratory Home Page, http://www.nal.usda.gov/fnic/foodcomp.

32. Vormann J. Magnesium: nutrition and metabolism. Molecular Aspects of Medicine 2003:24:27-37.

33. Feillet-Coudray C, Coudray C, Tressol JC, Pepin D, Mazur A, Abrams SA. Exchangeable magnesium pool masses in healthy women: effects of magnesium supplementation. Am J Clin Nutr 2002;75:72-8.

35. Xing JH and Soffer EE. Adverse effects of laxatives. Dis Colon Rectum 2001;44:1201-9.

36. http://www.ext.colostate.edu/pubs/foodnut/09356.html.

37. http://dietary-supplements.info.nih.gov/factsheets/cc/zinc.html.

38. http://www.feinberg.northwestern.edu/nutrition/factsheets/iodine.html.

39. http://www.feinberg.northwestern.edu/nutrition/factsheets/selenium.html.

40. http://www.feinberg.northwestern.edu/nutrition/factsheets/copper.html.

41. http://www.feinberg.northwestern.edu/nutrition/factsheets/manganese.html.

42. http://www.feinberg.northwestern.edu/nutrition/factsheets/chromium.html.

Chapter 9
Alternative Medicine

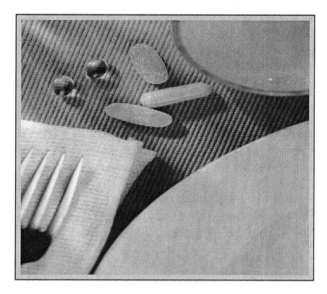

The information presented in this chapter will focus on alternative medicine therapies (which includes biologically based therapies (supplements) and energy based therapies.

Objectives

After reading and studying this chapter you should:

1. Discuss the origins of the National Center for Complimentary and Alternative Medicine (NCCAM).

2. Discuss biologically based therapies - supplements and botanicals in light of the Dietary Supplement Health and Education Act of 1994.

3. Discuss the role of the Office of Dietary Supplements (ODS).

4. Discuss practices by some supplement manufacturers that "taints" the entire industry.

5. Discuss the results of clinical trials completed by NCCAM.

6. Discuss energy based therapies and the results of NCCAM clinical trials.

7. Discuss how to make sense of the data and the decision making process for consuming supplements.

INTRODUCTION

Millions of Americans spend billions of dollars on alternative medicine. According to a nationwide government survey released in May 2004, 36 percent of U.S. adults aged 18 years and over use some form of complimentary alternative medicine which includes supplements. When prayer, specifically for health reasons, is included in the definition, the number of U.S. adults using some form of complimentary alternative medicine rises to 62 percent[1.]

Complimentary alternative medicine is defined as a group of diverse medical and health care systems, practices, and products, including supplements, that are not presently considered to be part of conventional medicine.

What is the science behind these alternative therapies? Advocates claim strong science exists and complain about the slow moving and overly cautious FDA, while scientists argue that Congress is advocating for unproven therapies rather than subjecting new treatments to evaluation.

This chapter will focus on discussion of complimentary alternative medicine, the origins and results of clinical trials funded by the National Center for Complimentary and Alternative Medicine. Biologically based therapies (supplements, herbs, etc.) and energy based therapies will also be discussed.

NCCAM

NCCAM

The National Center for Complimentary and Alternative Medicine (NCCAM) is the Federal Government's lead agency for scientific research on complimentary alternative medicine (CAM). NCCAM is dedicated to exploring complimentary and alternative healing practices in the context of rigorous science, training CAM researchers, and disseminating authoritative information to the public and professionals.[1] The office has a staff of approximately 75 employees with an annual budget of $121.5 million.

The origin of NCCAM began in 1992, when Senator Tom Harkin (D-Iowa), convinced bee pollen had cured his allergies, assigned $2 million of his discretionary funds to establish the Office of Unconventional Medicine, renamed the Office of Alternative Medicine (OAM).[2] Funds for OAM increased annually and in 1998 increased to $19.5 million. Also in 1998, Senator Harkin won a decisive battle when the NIH opened a new office - the National Center for Complimentary and Alternative Medicine (NCCAM) - with a $50 million budget.[2] As a sign that NCCAM was indeed a scientific entity to be dealt with, the renowned Dr. Stephen E. Straus was appointed the first director October 6, 1999.[2] When interviewed, Dr. Straus made it clear that the office would perform rigorous scientific studies and that the public and companies with vested interests in new alternative therapies "will have to accept that research may show that some new therapies will not be good; some therapies will not be safe; and some therapies will not be any more effective than present alternatives.[2]

Complimentary and Alternative Medicine

Complimentary alternative medicine is defined as a group of diverse medical and health care systems, practices, and products that are not presently considered to be part of conventional medicine. Conventional medicine is medicine as practiced by holders of M.D. (medical doctor) or D.O. (doctor of osteopathy) degrees and by their allied health professionals, such as physical therapists, psychologists, and registered nurses. Some health care providers practice both CAM and conventional medicine. Complimentary medicine is used *together with* conventional medicine. Alternative medicine is used *in place of* conventional medicine. Integrative medicine combines treatments from conventional medicine and CAM for which there is some high-quality evidence of safety and effectiveness.[3]

For a few dietary supplements, data have been deemed sufficient to warrant large-scale trials. For example, multicenter trials have concluded or are in progress on ginkgo (*Ginkgo biloba*) for prevention of dementia, glucosamine hydrochloride and chondroitin, a substance found in the cartilage around joints. Chondroitin in dietary supplements is made in the laboratory or from the cartilage of sharks and cattle.[3]

Over the past few decades, thousands of studies of various dietary supplements have been performed. To date, however, no single supplement has been proven effective in a compelling way. Nevertheless, there are several supplements for which early studies yielded positive, or at least encouraging, data. Good sources of information on some of them can be found at the Natural Medicines Comprehensive Database and a number of National Institutes of Health (NIH) Web sites. The NIH Office of Dietary Supplements (ODS) annually publishes a bibliography of resources on significant advances in dietary supplement research. Finally, the ClinicalTrials.gov database lists all NIH-supported clinical studies of dietary supplements that are actively accruing patients.[3]

Reviews of the data regarding some dietary supplements have been conducted, including some by the members of the Cochrane Collaboration. The Agency for Healthcare Research and Quality has produced a number of evidence-based reviews of dietary supplements, including garlic, antioxidants, milk thistle, omega-3 fatty acids. The Cochrane Database is accessible at www.cochrane.org/reviews.[3]

NCCAM Classifications

NCCAM classifies complimentary alternative therapies into five categories, or domains:[4]

1. Alternative Medical Systems

Alternative medical systems are built upon complete systems of theory and practice. Examples of alternative medical systems that have developed in Western cultures include homeopathic medicine and naturopathic medicine. Examples of systems that have developed in non-Western cultures include traditional Chinese medicine and Ayurveda.

2. Mind-Body Interventions

Mind-body medicine uses a variety of techniques designed to enhance the mind's capacity to affect bodily function. Some techniques that were considered complimentary alternative medicine in the past have become mainstream (for example, patient support groups and cognitive-behavioral therapy). Other mind-body techniques are still considered complimentary alternative medicine, including meditation, prayer, mental healing, and therapies that use creative outlets such as art, music, or dance.

3. Biologically Based Therapies

Biologically based therapies use substances found in nature, such as herbs, foods, and vitamins. Some examples include dietary supplements, herbal products, and the use of other so-called natural but as yet scientifically unproven therapies (for example, using shark cartilage to treat cancer).

4. Manipulative and Body-Based Methods

Manipulative and body-based methods are based on manipulation and/or movement of one or more parts of the body. Some examples include chiropractic or osteopathic manipulation, and massage.

5. Energy Therapies

Energy therapies involve the use of energy fields. They are of two types:

Biofield therapies are intended to affect energy fields that purportedly surround and penetrate the human body. The existence of such fields has not yet been scientifically proven. Some forms of energy therapy manipulate biofields by applying pressure and/or manipulating the body by placing the hands in, or through, these fields. Examples include qi gong, Reiki, and Therapeutic Touch. Bioelectromagnetic-based therapies involve the unconventional use of electromagnetic fields, such as pulsed fields, magnetic fields, or alternating-current or direct-current fields.

Biologically based therapies include, but are not limited to, botanicals, animal-derived extracts, vitamins, minerals, fatty acids, amino acids, proteins, prebiotics and probiotics found in foods such as yogurt or in dietary supplements, whole diets, and functional foods.[4]

In contrast to dietary supplements, functional foods are components of the usual diet that may have biologically active components (e.g., polyphenols, phytoestrogens, fish oils, carotenoids) that may provide health benefits beyond basic nutrition. Examples of functional foods include soy, nuts, chocolate, and cranberries. These foods' bioactive constituents are appearing with increasing frequency as ingredients in dietary supplements. Functional foods are marketed directly to consumers. Sales increased from $11.3 billion in 1995 to about $16.2 billion in 1999. Unlike dietary supplements, functional foods may claim specific health benefits.[11] The Nutrition Labeling and Education Act (NLEA) of 1990 delineates the permissible labeling of these foods for health claims.[4] See section on labeling for more details.

Since the NIH began the office of Internal Medicine in 1992, nine large clinical trials have been completed. These trials deal with biogically based therapies and energy based methods. Five trials dealt with supplements, including one trial that dealt with herbal remedies for hot flashes. One trial dealt with diets, one study dealt with acupuncture and one study dealt with Tai Chi.[5] The results of these trials will be discussed in the corresponding sections.

BIOLOGICALLY BASED THERAPIES-SUPPLEMENTS

A dietary supplement is any product that contains vitamins, minerals, herbs or other botanicals, amino acids, enzymes, and/or other ingredients intended to supplement the diet. The U.S. Food and Drug Administration has special labeling requirements for dietary supplements and treats them as foods, not drugs. Supplements must meet all of the following conditions. It is a product (other than tobacco) that is intended to supplement the diet and that contains one or more of the following: vitamins, minerals, herbs or other botanicals, amino acids, or any combination of the above ingredients. It is intended to be taken in tablet, capsule, powder, softgel, gelcap, or liquid form. It is not represented for use as a conventional food or as a sole item of a meal or the diet. It is labeled as being a dietary supplement.[6]

More than one half of the U.S. adult population use dietary supplements. In 1996 alone, consumers spent more than $6.5 billion on dietary supplements; by the year 2000 that figure rose to over $15 billion. The reason for this explosion is the passage of the Dietary Supplement and Health Education Act of 1994 (DSHEA) by Congress.[1]

According to a survey of physicians—primarily orthopedic surgeons, rheumatologists and sports medicine practitioners—60 percent of those polled felt there was not enough FDA oversight of the dietary supplement industry to warrant recommending supplements.[7] It's for that reason the implementation of good manufacturing practices is a crucial first step to the future of the industry—it will restore some of the luster of dietary supplements among health care professionals who are making disease-state treatment recommendations, stated Michael Johnsen, in Drug Store News, on April 11, 2005.[7]

The FDA is developing GMPs for dietary supplements. However, until they are issued, companies must follow existing manufacturing requirements for foods. Drug products must be approved by the FDA as safe and efficacious prior to marketing. In contrast, manufacturers of dietary supplements are responsible for ensuring that their products are safe. While the FDA monitors adverse effects after dietary supplement products are on the market, newly marketed dietary supplements are not subject to premarket approval or a specific postmarket surveillance period. Supplement makers also hope that GMPs will help sway opinion among public, policy makers concerning dietary supplements. "Once we have that in place, then the aura of the whole horrible, unregulated dietary supplement industry, may begin to disappear, indicates Pharmavite spokesman Doug Jones.[8]

It's this stigma of an unregulated industry promoting "snake oil treatments" that are no more effective than a placebo that keeps dogging the industry. Despite numerous sound clinical trials that support substantial health benefits for one ingredient or another, the sheer number of inconclusive studies combined with the industry's share of less-than-reputable suppliers has painted the industry with a negative brush.[8]

Background - DSHEA

Before 1994, The Food and Drug Administration regulated dietary supplements as foods to ensure that they were safe and wholesome, and that their labeling was truthful and not misleading. Ensuring safety involved evaluation of all new ingredients, including those used in dietary supplements. The FDA notes that under the DSHEA law supplements are no longer regulated like other products such as drugs, additives, cosmetics, foods (animal and human), medical devices, and radiation emitting consumer products (microwaves).

President Clinton, on October 25, 1994, signed the DSHEA "acknowledging that millions of consumers believe dietary supplements offer health benefits and that consumers want a greater opportunity to determine whether supplements may help them". With the passage of the DSHEA, supplement manufacturers were given "carte blanche" to market supplements without regulation. The Council of Responsible Nutrition, an organization of manufacturers of dietary supplements hailed this act as a "landmark change". "Landmark change it is!"[9]

Before 1994, the original definition of a supplement was a product that contained one or more of the essential nutrients. After DSHEA, the definition of a supplement was changed to any product intended for ingestion as a supplement to the diet. This definition now includes liquid, pill, capsule, or tablet forms of vitamins, minerals, herbs, botanicals and other plant derived substances, amino acids and concentrates, metabolites, constituents and extracts of these substances. Again, according to the FDA, dietary supplements are not drugs. The FDA definition of a drug is an article, which may or may not be derived from plants that are intended to diagnose, cure, mitigate, treat or prevent disease. Before marketing, drugs must undergo *clinical* studies to determine their effectiveness, safety, possible interactions with other substances, and appropriate dosages. The FDA reviews these data and authorizes usage before marketing. The FDA does not authorize or test dietary supplements. Under DSHEA Congress amended the Federal Food, Drug, and Cosmetic Act (FD&C Act) to include provisions that apply only to dietary supplements and dietary ingredients of dietary supplements. As a result of these provisions, dietary ingredients used in dietary supplements are no longer subject to the premarket safety evaluations required of other new food ingredients or for new uses of old food ingredients.[9]

In its 1998 statement, the FDA warns that dietary supplements are not replacements for conventional diets. The FDA also warns that It must not be assumed that "all natural means safe", (poisonous mushrooms are all natural); it must not be assumed that what is stated on the label is actually in the bottle; and just because the accompanying literature makes claims about the safety and health advantages of the supplement, it must not be assumed that these claims are true.[10]

According to the FDA, it is critical that consumers also understand health claims made by supplement manufacturers. Supplement manufacturers are not allowed to make claims about the use of a dietary supplement to diagnose, prevent, mitigate, treat, or cure a disease. They can, however, make statements about classical nutrient deficiency diseases as long as these statements disclose the prevalence of the disease in the United States. Unlike health claims, nutritional support statements need not be approved by the FDA. The FDA must simply be notified no later than 30 days after a product bears the claim. Beginning in March of 1999, a new statement on the label must read: "This statement has not been evaluated by the FDA. This product is not intended to diagnose, treat, cure, or prevent any disease".[10]

Since the DSHEA, supplement manufacturers do not have to provide information to the FDA to get a new product on the market, unlike all other food additives or drugs. The DSHEA does require manufacturers to include the words "dietary supplement" on product labels. Also required is one of the following two options:[9]

> 1. The manufacturer may submit to the FDA, at least 75 days before the product is expected to go on the market, information that supports their conclusion that a new ingredient can reasonably be expected to be safe. The information the manufacturer submits becomes publicly available 90 days after the FDA receives it;
>
> 2. The second option is the manufacturer can petition the FDA, asking to establish the conditions under which the new dietary ingredient would reasonably be expected to be safe.

Under the DSHEA, the FDA can only step in when the supplement has been shown to be unsafe. For example, in June 1997, the FDA proposed, among other things, to limit the amount of ephedrine alkaloids in supplements and provide warnings because dangers such as dizziness, changes in blood pressure, changes in heart rate, chest pain, heart attack, stroke, hepatitis, seizures, psychosis, and death occurred.

Office of Dietary Supplements (ODS)

The Dietary Supplement Health and Education Act of 1994 (Public Law 103-417, DSHEA), authorized the establishment of the Office of Dietary Supplements (ODS) at the NIH.[11] The ODS was created in 1995 within the Office of Disease Prevention (ODP), Office of the Director (OD), NIH. DSHEA defined the purpose and responsibilities of ODS as follows:

> · To explore more fully the potential role of dietary supplements as a significant part of the efforts of the United States to improve health care.
>
> · To promote scientific study of the benefits of dietary supplements in maintaining health and preventing chronic disease and other health-related conditions.
>
> · To conduct and coordinate scientific research within NIH relating to dietary supplements.
>
> · To collect and compile the results of scientific research relating to dietary supplements, including scientific data from foreign sources.
>
> · To serve as the principal advisor to the Secretary and to the Assistant Secretary for Health and provide advice to the Director of NIH, the Director of the Centers for Disease Control and Prevention, and the Commissioner of the Food and Drug Administration on issues relating to dietary supplements.

One of the purposes in creating the ODS was to promote scientific research in the area of dietary supplements. Dietary supplements can have an impact on the prevention of disease and on the maintenance of health.[11] In the US, these ingredients are usually defined as including plant extracts, enzymes, vitamins, minerals, amino acids, and hormonal products that are available without prescription and are consumed in addition to the regular diet. Although vitamin and mineral supplements have been available for decades, their health effects have been the subject of detailed scientific research only within the last 15-20 years. It is important to expand this research to include the health effects of other bioactive factors consumed as supplements to promote health and prevent disease. Considerable research on the effects of botanical and herbal dietary supplements has been conducted in Asia and Europe where plant products have a long tradition of use. The overwhelming majority of these supplements, however, have not been studied using modern scientific techniques. Nor have they been extensively studied in population groups that may be at risk for chronic diseases.

For many reasons, therefore, it is important to enhance research efforts to determine the benefits and risks of dietary supplements.[10]

FDA Issues Dietary Supplements Final Rule

In June of 2007, the FDA issued a final rule establishing regulations to require current good manufacturing practices (cGMP) for dietary supplements. "This rule helps to ensure the quality of dietary supplements so that consumers can be confident that the products they purchase contain what is on the label," said Commissioner of Food and Drugs Andrew C. von Eschenbach, M.D. "In addition, as a result of recent amendments to the Federal Food, Drug, and Cosmetic Act, by the end of the year 2007 the industry will be required to report all serious dietary supplement related adverse events to the FDA."[12] The regulations establish the cGMP needed to ensure quality throughout the manufacturing, packaging, labeling, and storing of dietary supplements. The final rule includes requirements for establishing quality control procedures, designing and constructing manufacturing plants, and testing ingredients and the finished product. It also includes requirements for record keeping and handling consumer product complaints.[12]

"The final rule will help ensure that dietary supplements are manufactured with controls that result in a consistent product free of contamination, with accurate labeling," said Robert E. Brackett, Ph.D., director of FDA's Center for Food Safety and Applied Nutrition.[12] Under the final rule, manufacturers are required to evaluate the identity, purity, strength, and composition of their dietary supplements. If dietary supplements contain contaminants or do not contain the dietary ingredient they are represented to contain, FDA would consider those products to be adulterated or misbranded.[12] The aim of the final rule is to prevent inclusion of the wrong ingredients, too much or too little of a dietary ingredient, contamination by substances such as natural toxins, bacteria, pesticides, glass, lead and other heavy metals, as well as improper packaging and labeling. The final rule includes flexible requirements that can evolve with improvements in scientific methods used for verifying identity, purity strength, and composition of dietary supplements.[12]

Exceptions

As a companion document, FDA also is issuing an interim final rule that outlines a petition process for manufacturers to request an exemption to the cGMP requirement for 100 percent identity testing of specific dietary ingredients used in the processing of dietary supplements. Under the interim final rule the manufacturer may be exempted from the dietary ingredient identity testing requirement if it can provide sufficient documentation that the reduced frequency of testing requested would still ensure the identity of the dietary ingredient.[12]

The final CGMP and the interim final rule became effective August 24, 2007. According to the FDA, "to limit any disruption for dietary supplements produced by small businesses, the rule has a three-year phase-in for small businesses." Companies with more than 500 employees have until June 2008 to comply, companies with less than 500 employees have until June 2009 to comply, and companies with fewer than 20 employees have until June 2010 to comply with the regulations.[12]

Supplement Industry Practices

Robert Park, Author of Voodoo Science – the Road from Foolishness to Fraud, says DSHEA is his candidate for the worst piece of legislation ever passed.[7] Supplement manufacturers are not held to any rigorous standards indicates Robert Park.[2]   "Before 1994 manufacturers had to prove that the product was safe or at least that what you said on the label was in the bottle". "Manufacturers don't have to do that anymore". Under DSHEA testing is voluntary. "It's wonderful right now for companies that make supplements. "I would not be regulated. The only people I would have to answer to is my stock holders to see how much profit I am making. The FDA can only step in when the supplement has been shown to be unsafe.[2]

Marcia Angell, Harvard University, emphasizes that "large drug companies might not test for safety and efficacy if they didn't have to. But they have to. The government requires it.[2]

Tests performed by ABC's TV program 20/20 on over 100 bottles of supplements found that one in four did not have what the manufacturer stated on the label. Dr. Todd Cooperman of consumerlab.com provided the detailed analysis for the 20/20 investigation. According to Dr. Cooperman, the only way to know what's in a supplement pill is to test it. The investigation centered on three popular supplements: Chondroitin, SAM-e, and ginseng. Eight of the 15 bottles of chondroitin tested, failed – they did not have the amount that was stated on the label. Four bottles had less than 10% of what was stated on the label. To everyone's surprise, some of the most expensive brands of chondroitin had the least amount. Six of the thirteen bottles of SAM-e tested, failed. Most had less than half the amount listed on the bottle. One bottle had no SAM-e. Consumerlab.com tested SAM-e three times, in three different labs, using three different methods to be sure they weren't making a mistake. And five out of twenty-one bottles of ginseng tested, failed. EIGHT BOTTLES HAD QUINTOZENE in them, A PESTICIDE SPRAYED ON THE PLANT WHEN IT IS GROWING.[13]

It's not just consumerlab.com that found problems. The Good Housekeeping Institute tested SAM-e, Consumer Reports tested echinacia, and the Los Angeles Times tested St. John's Wort. All reported that what was stated on the label was not always in the bottle. According to Dr. Cooperman, until someone is checking the industry there is no incentive to fix the problem.[13]

"It's like a wild west show", states, Joe Graden, pharmacologist and radio talk show host of the People's Pharmacy. According to Dr. Graden, "Supplement manufacturers can get away with anything and many of them do. People are popping pills and they don't know what they're getting into. People think "it's natural, how bad can it be?" But supplements are chemicals just like drugs; in overdose they can cause side effects just like drugs; in wrong combinations they can cause complications, just like drugs. Your body can't tell the difference". Dr. Graden agrees with consumerlab.com: "Since there is no one policing the supplement industry, manufacturers are taking short cuts, which can lead to products that are not legitimate, and that's a dangerous scenario." Dietary supplements are the ultimate merger of self-improvement and free enterprise, with the promises and pitfalls of both, says By Jeff O'Connel, author of Beyond Balco: The Untold Dietary Supplement Scandal. When you purchase that bottle of pills or canister of powder, you may be walking out with a useful concoction or the equivalent of sawdust — or something truly harmful.[10]

ConsumerLab.com, a company that's tested more than 1,900 dietary supplements for quality and purity reported that "One of every four supplements tested had some problem." For example, Tod Cooperman's team analyzed Nature's Plus Ultra Chondroitin 600, a joint-health supplement that claims to be "the highest potency, most concentrated chondroitin supplement ever developed." But the lab results showed that the product didn't contain even trace amounts of chondroitin. In fact, eight of 11 chondroitin supplements failed to deliver on label claims. You can't even count on multi-vitamins: 52 percent of those didn't make the grade in ConsumerLab.com testing. Worse, many of these multivitamins contained excessive amounts of lead, prompting the nation's second-largest supplement retailer, Vitamin Shoppe, to pull one of its multivitamin formulations from store shelves last January.[14]

In many cases, the problem starts at the supplier. "Most of the small manufacturers don't test raw materials coming through the door," says Jeff Feliciano, formerly the director of research and quality assurance for Weider Global Nutrition. Instead, these firms rely on paperwork called a certificate of analysis. This is a supplier's written promise of an ingredient's quality and purity. Unfortunately, it's just that: a promise. "There's an old saying: Anyone with a printer can produce a certificate of analysis," says Warren Majerus, an auditor with a nonprofit organization that inspects supplement plants worldwide.[14]

To avoid the risk of putting damaged or worthless goods on retailers' shelves, many larger supplement companies have voluntarily adopted a policy of either testing raw materials in-house or sending them out to a reliable third party. "It's the only way to truly protect the reputation of your product and your customers' health," says Feliciano.[14] The FDA is now saying that "Manufacturers must confirm a "certificate of Analysis," says Vasilios Frankos, Ph.D., the director of the division of dietary-supplement programs at the FDA. Enforcing the guidelines could be difficult, however, considering that while the number of supplement makers increased between 2003 and 2006, the number of FDA investigators declined by 16 percent. To further complicate matters, the quality of raw materials isn't the only question mark — sometimes it's their identity.[14]

Batch Spiking[14]

"Random batch spiking" has a long history in the supplement business. It works like this: "The manufacturer sprinkles an illegal substance into an over-the-counter dietary supplement," says Feliciano. "The legal ingredients are claimed on the label, but they don't disclose the drug."

"Drugs like this don't typically show up on lab tests, unless someone's looking for them," says Lockwood. "The idea is to use them to quickly build a customer base and steal market share by making a product that works 'better' than its competitors."

That sales strategy is still in evidence. In May, the FDA advised consumers to discontinue the use of two "male-enhancement" supplements: True Man and Energy Max. In a chemical analysis, the FDA discovered that both products contained "undeclared analog ingredients." An analog is defined by the FDA as a chemical that has a similar structure to a prescription drug. True Man contained an analog of sildenafil, the active ingredient in Viagra; Energy Max contained an analog of vardenafil, the active ingredient in Levitra.[14]

Chris Lockwood, formerly the senior category director of diet, energy, food, and beverage at the supplement retailer GNC and now a doctoral candidate in exercise physiology at the University of Oklahoma says that even if all the ingredients are safe (and listed), you still may not be swallowing what you expected. "Fairy dusting" is the name of this industry trick, says Lockwood. Say the hot item of the moment is whey-protein isolate, which is a more pure form of protein than the less expensive whey-protein concentrate. The marketing department at Company X tells its R & D team, "This new product has to contain whey-protein isolate. That's what consumers are buying." But when the formulators crunch the numbers they realize they can afford to use only 1 gram (g) of isolate for every 40 g concentrate. To keep the whey-protein isolate from standing out as the bottom entry in the ingredients list, they bunch the huge amount of concentrate and the tiny amount of isolate together into a "proprietary protein blend" whose collective heft places it near the top of the list. "This creates the impression that the canister is loaded with something that's really only present in near-trace amounts," says Lockwood.[14]

Of course, many people simply fall prey to bogus marketing copy. Last January, marketers of four diet products — Xenadrine EFX, CortiSlim, One-A-Day WeightSmart, and TrimSpa — agreed to settle charges of false advertising made by the Federal Trade Commission, and paid $25 million in claims. Investigators found that before-and-after subjects had lost weight by dieting and exercising, not by popping pills. According to the FTC, this company's own research showed that members of a placebo group lost more weight than the supplement takers did.[14]

If a quarter of all dietary supplements failed to match label claims when tested by ConsumerLab.com, that means three-fourths did live up their promises. Indeed, many U.S. companies make high-quality dietary supplements. "Big companies refuse to participate in any of this renegade activity," says Feliciano. "They have all sorts of defense systems in place. You'll often find four or five Ph.D.'s working in quality control, and these are big-money positions. When they sign off on something, they're legally responsible."

The problem is the bottom third of what is a huge industry. "There are guys tarnishing the reputation of the whole industry because they're making potentially dangerous products in their home kitch-ens," says a former researcher at Yale University school of medicine, who requested anonymity since he now consults with supplement companies on product formulations. What's more, these lower-tier manufacturers often thrive on loopholes in the Dietary Supplement Health and Education Act (DSHEA). The DSHEA doesn't require supplement companies to prove their products are safe and effective before bringing them to the market. Instead, supplements are allowed to be stocked on shelves as long as the product label doesn't claim the supplement diagnoses, treats, cures, or prevents any disease, and its ingredients are naturally occurring. A second stipulation is a bit deceptive. It means that if a natural compound can be chemically synthesized in a lab and isn't classified as a controlled substance, it can legally be used as an ingredient and sold over the counter.

BALCO[14]

One of the first chemists to do just that was Patrick Arnold, the man best known for synthesizing "The Clear," the designer steroid given to Barry Bonds by the Bay Area Laboratory Co-Operative (BALCO). In the mid-1990s, Arnold discovered — or rather, rediscovered — the active ingredient in andros-tenedione, the infamous Mark McGwire supplement. This ingredient can be found in the bark of Scotch pine trees, so it's naturally occurring, and at the time it wasn't a controlled substance.

Arnold knew that "andro," which falls into a category called pro-hormones, was just one chemical step removed from the hormone testosterone. "The concept is that if ingested, you'll provide your body with more compounds that can be converted to testosterone," says Lockwood. "But these hormone precursors could just as easily be converted to estrogen."

In January 2005, the Drug Enforcement Agency added specific pro-hormones to its list of anabolic steroids classified as Schedule III controlled substances. These legal definitions, however, are cast narrowly, in the form of a list containing the names of specific molecular structures. The result: more loopholes.

Underground chemists take advantage of the gap between the chemical and legal definitions of a steroid. So they set out to tweak molecules that are still anabolic and still steroids, yet haven't been categorized as such by the DEA. These new substances are often referred to as pro-steroids. "It's more accurate to consider these types of products to be 'junk steroids,' " says Feliciano. "They're put on the market without toxicology tests, human studies, or concern for consumers' health. And although these products may imply or even state that they contain drug-like agents for which you don't need a prescription, you can be sure these claims have never been proven — and just as unsure about the supplement's true contents."

NCCAM Clinical Trial Results - Supplements[5]

Six of the nine trials completed by the NCAAM were looking at the effects of biologically based therapies.

1. St. John's Wort and Depression (April 2002)
2. Echinacea for the Prevention and Treatment of Colds in Adults (July 2005)
3. Glucosamine/Chondroitin Arthritis Intervention Trial (GAIT) (February 2006)
4. Garlic Does Not Appear to Lower "Bad" Cholesterol (February 2007)
5. Shark Cartilage Supplement Does Not Extend the Lives of Lung Cancer Patients (June 2007)4. 6. Herbal Supplement Fails to Relieve Hot Flashes (December 2006)

The clinical trail on the herbal supplement will be discussed in the section on "botanicals".

St. John's Wort and Depression (April 2002)[15]

Results of the St. John's Wort clinical trial found that an extract of the herb St. John's wort was no more effective for treating major depression of moderate severity than placebo, according to research published in the April 10, 2002 issue of the Journal of the American Medical Association.[4] The randomized, double-blind trial compared the use of a standardized extract of St. John's wort (Hypericum perforatum) to a placebo for treating major depression of moderate severity. The multi-site trial, involving 340 participants, also compared the FDA-approved antidepressant drug sertraline (Zoloft®) to placebo as a way to measure how sensitive the trial was to detecting antidepressant effects. "Many Americans use dietary supplements like St. John's wort for depression without consulting a physician," says principal investigator Jonathan R.T. Davidson, M.D., professor of psychiatry and director of the Anxiety and Traumatic Stress Program at Duke University Medical Center. "We felt there was a need to conduct a trial that could help us determine where St. John's wort fits in the overall management of depression." "Overall, we found that patients taking either St. John's wort or placebo had similar rates of response according to scales commonly used for measuring depression," says Dr. Davidson". Critics of the study point to the study design which looked at moderate and major forms of depression – not mild forms. However, Dr. Straus, M.D., NCCAM Director defends the study design: "Studies indicate that people with major forms of depression are more likely to use a supplement. These studies are difficult to complete, and at the end of the day someone is going to criticize you no matter what design you use".

Echinacea for the Prevention and Treatment of Colds in Adults[16]

On July 28, 2005, *The New England Journal of Medicine* published the results of a study of Echinacea for the prevention and treatment of the common cold that was funded by the National Center for Complementary and Alternative Medicine (NCCAM). The research was conducted by Dr. Ronald Turner, of the University of Virginia School of Medicine, and collaborators at Clemson University in South Carolina. The research team tested three preparations of the roots of a species of Echinacea which prior smaller studies had found to benefit adults with the common cold. The study was designed to test if Echinacea would help prevent or treat cold symptoms, since this is how Echinacea is often used by consumers. In this study, the researchers found that none of the three preparations at the 900 mg per day dose had significant effects on whether volunteers became infected with the cold virus or on the severity or duration of symptoms among those who developed colds. Critics of this study believe the dose of *E. angustifolia* used was too low.

Efficacy of Glucosamine and Chondroitin Sulfate May Depend on Level of Osteoarthritis Pain (Feb., 2006)[17]

In a study published in the *New England Journal of Medicine[7]*, the popular dietary supplement combination of glucosamine plus chondroitin sulfate did not provide significant relief from osteoarthritis pain among all participants. However, a smaller subgroup of study participants with moderate-to-severe pain showed significant relief with the combined supplements. "This rigorous, large-scale study showed that the combination of glucosamine and chondroitin sulfate appeared to help people with moderate-to-severe pain from knee osteoarthritis, but not those with mild pain," said Stephen E. Straus, M.D., NCCAM Director. "It is important to study dietary supplements with well-designed research in order to find out what works and what doesn't work." "Because of the small size of the moderate-to-severe pain subgroup, the findings in this group for glucosamine plus chondroitin sulfate should be considered preliminary and need to be confirmed in a study designed for this purpose," said Dr. Clegg, Professor of Medicine and Chief of Rheumatology at the University of Utah, School of Medicine. It is important to note that all of the products used in the study were subject to the FDA's pharmaceutical regulations and evaluated and manufactured by an FDA-licensed clinical research pharmacy center. The glucosamine and chondroitin sulfate used were tested for purity, potency, quality, and consistency among batches. Products were retested for stability throughout the study. The dosages selected were based on the prevailing doses in the scientific literature. The team of researchers continued their research with a smaller study to see whether glucosamine and chondroitin sulfate can alter the progression of osteoarthritis, such as delaying the narrowing of the joint spaces. About one-half of the participants in the larger study were eligible to enroll in this ancillary study.

Garlic Does Not Appear to Lower "Bad" Cholesterol (February 2007)[18]

A study from Stanford University casts doubt on the effectiveness of garlic to lower LDL (low density lipoprotein) cholesterol levels in adults with moderately high cholesterol. LDL cholesterol is widely known as "bad cholesterol," and is believed to be a leading contributor to heart disease. Christopher Gardner, Ph.D., and colleagues conducted a randomized, placebo-controlled trial studying whether three different formulations of garlic could lower LDL cholesterol. The study participants were randomly divided into four groups to receive raw garlic, a powdered garlic supplement, an aged extract supplement, or a placebo. The 169 participants who completed the study had their cholesterol levels checked monthly for the duration of the 6-month trial. None of the formulations of garlic had a statistically significant effect on the LDL cholesterol levels. The authors caution that these results should not be generalized for all populations or all health effects. An accompanying editorial in the journal Archives of Internal Medicine points out that LDL cholesterol levels are only one factor contributing to heart disease, and that this trial did not investigate garlic's effects on other risk factors, such as high blood pressure.

Powdered Shark Cartilage for Advanced Breast and Colorectal Cancer (July 2005)[19]

Results of a study funded by the National Center for Complementary and Alternative Medicine (NC-CAM) and the National Cancer Institute (NCI) indicate that adding powdered shark cartilage (Benefin®) to standard cancer therapy did not benefit patients with advanced breast or colorectal cancer. The study, a randomized, placebo-controlled, double-blind clinical trial, enrolled 88 patients and assessed overall survival, side effects and quality of life. The study results were published in the July 1, 2005 issue of the journal Cancer. The researchers designed and carried out this study because laboratory and animal studies of some forms of shark cartilage had suggested anti-cancer properties, specifically, an ability to slow growth of new blood vessels critical to the growth of new tumors. Other studies are continuing with different preparations of shark cartilage and different cancers. In this study, it was difficult for patients to follow the study protocol. All patients were to receive standard care for their cancer and were randomized to receive either the Benefin® shark cartilage product or an identical-smelling placebo. The study required participants to mix the powder with juice or water and drink it 3 to 4 times a day. Half of the patients in both groups stopped taking the study product after 1 month. Poor patient adherence, difficulty with enrolling the target of 600 patients, and the lack of apparent evidence of benefit of the product resulted in the decision to stop the study early.

BIOLOGICALLY BASED THERAPIES - BOTANICALS

A botanical is a plant or plant part valued for its medicinal or therapeutic properties, flavor, and/or scent. Herbs are a subset of botanicals. Products made from botanicals that are used to maintain or improve health may be called herbal products, botanical products, or phytomedicines. To be classi-fied as a dietary supplement, a botanical must meet the definition of a supplement previously de-scribed.[20]

Botanicals are sold in many forms: as fresh or dried products; liquid or solid extracts; and tablets, capsules, powders, and tea bags. For example, fresh ginger root is often found in the produce section of food stores; dried ginger root is sold packaged in tea bags, capsules, or tablets; and liquid preparations made from ginger root are also sold. A particular group of chemicals or a single chemical may be isolated from a botanical and sold as a dietary supplement, usually in tablet or capsule form. An example is phytoestrogens from soy products.[20]

Common preparations include teas, decoctions, tinctures, and extracts. A tea, also known as an infusion, is made by adding boiling water to fresh or dried botanicals and steeping them. The tea may be drunk either hot or cold. Some roots, bark, and berries require more forceful treatment to extract their desired ingredients. They are simmered in boiling water for longer periods than teas, making a decoction, which also may be drunk hot or cold. A tincture is made by soaking a botanical in a solution of alcohol and water. Tinctures are sold as liquids and are used for concentrating and preserving a botanical. They are made in different strengths that are expressed as botanical-to-extract ratios (i.e., ratios of the weight of the dried botanical to the volume or weight of the finished product). An extract is made by soaking the botanical in a liquid that removes specific types of chemicals. The liquid can be used as is or evaporated to make a dry extract for use in capsules or tablets.[20]

Standardization is a process that manufacturers may use to ensure batch-to-batch consistency of their products. In some cases, standardization involves identifying specific chemicals (also known as markers) that can be used to manufacture a consistent product. Dietary supplements are not required to be standardized in the United States. In fact, no legal or regulatory definition exists for standardization in the United States as it applies to botanical dietary supplements. Because of this, the term "standardization" may mean many different things. Some manufacturers use the term standardization incorrectly to refer to uniform manufacturing practices; following a recipe is not sufficient for a product to be called standardized. Therefore, the presence of the word "standard-ized" on a supplement label does not necessarily indicate product quality.[20]

Many people believe that products labeled "natural" are safe and good for them. This is not neces-sarily true because the safety of a botanical depends on many things, such as its chemical makeup, how it works in the body, how it is prepared, and the dose used.[20]

The action of botanicals range from mild to powerful (potent). A botanical with mild action may have subtle effects. Chamomile and peppermint, both mild botanicals, are usually taken as teas to aid digestion and are generally considered safe for self-administration. Some mild botanicals may have to be taken for weeks or months before their full effects are achieved. For example, valerian may be effective as a sleep aid after 14 days of use but it is rarely effective after just one dose. In contrast a powerful botanical produces a fast result.   Kava, as one example, is reported to have an immediate and powerful action affecting anxiety and muscle relaxation.

The dose and form of a botanical preparation also play important roles in its safety. Teas, tinctures, and extracts have different strengths. The same amount of a botanical may be contained in a cup of tea, a few teaspoons of tincture, or an even smaller quantity of an extract. Also, different preparations vary in the relative amounts and concentrations of chemical removed from the whole botanical. For example, peppermint tea is generally considered safe to drink but peppermint oil is much more concentrated and can be toxic if used incorrectly. It is important to follow the manufacturer's suggested directions for using a botanical and not exceed the recommended dose without the advice of a health care provider.[20]

It is difficult to determine the quality of a botanical dietary supplement product from its label. The degree of quality control depends on the manufacturer, the supplier, and others in the production process. Scientists use several approaches to evaluate botanical dietary supplements for their potential health benefits and safety risks,[20]

NCCAM Clinical Trial Results

The herbal supplement black cohosh, whether used alone or with other botanicals, did not relieve hot flashes in women in the Herbal Alternatives (HALT) for Menopause Study. HALT, co-funded by NCCAM and the National Institute on Aging, did find that women using menopausal hormone therapy received significant relief from their hot flashes and night sweats.[21]

The year-long, randomized, double-blind trial compared several herbal regimens and menopausal hormone therapy to placebo. The study included 351 women, ages 45 to 55, who were approaching menopause or were postmenopausal. HALT was conducted at the Seattle-based Group Health Center for Health Studies. Each participant was experiencing at least two hot flashes and/or night sweats daily at the study's start.[21]   Researchers found no significant difference between the number of daily hot flashes and/or night sweats in any of the herbal supplement groups compared to the placebo group. After one year, the average difference was fewer than 0.6 symptoms per day. However, the average difference at one year in symptoms between the menopausal hormone therapy and placebo group was significant—4.06 fewer symptoms per day among women receiving hormones.[21]

BIOLOGICALLY BASED THERAPIES - ERGOGENIC AIDS

Ergogenic aids are any external influences which can positively affect physical or mental performance. These include mechanical aids, pharmacological aids, physiological aids, nutritional aids, and
psychological aids.[31] Ergogenic aids may directly influence the physiological capacity of a particular
body system thereby improving performance, remove psychological constraints which impact performance, and increase the speed of recovery from training and competition. These can be as
simple as water used before and after exercising to aid in hydration, to something as advanced as
anabolic steroids.[31]

Numerous ergogenic aids that claim to enhance sports performance are used by amateur and professional athletes. Approximately 50 percent of the general population have reported taking some
form of dietary supplements, while 76 to 100 percent of athletes in some sports are reported to use
them.[32] New products with ergogenic claims appear on the market almost daily. Most are classified as
supplements, which means the contents of the product and the claims on the label have not been
evaluated by the U.S. Food and Drug Administration and may not have any scientific basis.[32]

Anabolic Steroids

Anabolic steroids are testosterone derivatives with three mechanisms of action. First, anticatabolic
effects reverse the actions of glucocorticoids and help metabolize ingested proteins, converting a
negative nitrogen balance into a positive one. Second, anabolic effects directly induce skeletal muscle
synthesis. Third, there is a "steroid rush"—a state of euphoria and decreased fatigue that allows the
athlete to train harder and longer.[5] Many early studies used physiologic doses, or doses only two to
three times these amounts, and provided mixed results. More recent reviews,[5] controlling for various measurement methods, have concluded that anabolic steroids do indeed cause increased strength
and muscle mass. A randomized, double-blind, 10-week study[6] of 40 men examined the effect of
supraphysiologic testosterone doses. The participants were divided into four groups: those given a
placebo with or without weight training, and those given 600-mg testosterone enanthate with or
without weight training. Diet and training times were controlled. Fat-free mass, muscle size and
strength increased more than placebo in both groups taking testosterone than in the groups taking
placebo. The subjects in the exercise plus testosterone group had a 9 percent increase in mass and
23 percent increase in bench-press strength, compared with 3 percent and 9 percent, respectively, in
the subjects in the exercise plus placebo group.[33] These doses were comparable with the doses that
many athletes who use steroids take.

Anabolic steroids have many adverse effects, most related to the unwanted androgenic effects.
Some of the adverse effects are potentially serious and irreversible. Anabolic steroids such as
testosterone and its derivatives are prescription medications with clearly defined indications. Procur-
ing and using them without a prescription is illegal. Most sports organizations have rules that ban the
use of anabolic steroids for any reason.[32]

Creatine

Creatine monohydrate is a commonly used supplement, accounting for about US $400 million in
annual sales in the United States alone. Athletes in the former Soviet Union may have been ingesting

creatine to enhance performance as early as the 1970s, but the popularity of creatine with athletes increased substantially in the early 1990s by the revelation that Olympic gold medal winners Linford Christie and Sally Gunnell used creatine. Moreover, scientific publications reporting that dietary creatine supplementation could increase muscle creatine stores and improve the performance of brief, high-power exercise lent credence to the anecdotal evidence of creatine benefits. Unlike many dietary supplements, much research has been conducted on creatine, but its efficacy as an ergogenic aid remains controversial.[34]

Creatine is a non-essential compound that can be obtained in the diet or synthesized by the liver, pancreas, and kidneys. Creatine exists in free and phosphorylated forms (i.e., phosphocreatine or PCr), and approximately 95% of the body's creatine is stored in skeletal muscle, where its primary function is as an energy buffer. During times of increased energy demand, phosphocreatine (PCr) donates its phosphate to adenosine diphosphate (ADP) to produce adenosine triphosphate (ATP). Exercise tasks like sprinting and weight lifting that involve brief, intense efforts rely heavily on the ATP-PCr energy system. It is the only fuel system in the muscles that can produce energy at sufficiently high rates to accomplish these tasks. But the ATP-PCr energy system can provide ATP at maximal rates for only seconds before PCr stores are depleted. Consequently, it has been hypothesized that people who increase their muscle creatine levels by ingesting creatine supplements have a greater energy reserve available to support this type of activity. In addition to increasing muscle creatine stores, creatine supplementation may increase phosphocreatine resynthesis, although this has not been shown in every case.[35,36,37]

Several hundred studies have examined the effects of creatine supplementation on exercise performance and have been summarized and reviewed.[37,38,39] Initially, studies focused on the effects of creatine supplementation on exercise performance using laboratory tests and not on the performance of sport-specific or field tests. In controlled laboratory tests (e.g., cycling), creatine supplementation appears to improve performance of short-term (<30 s) high-intensity exercise, particularly when there are repeated bouts. There is less convincing evidence that creatine supplementation can enhance exercise performance during exercise of longer durations (>90 s). It makes intuitive sense that creatine may not prove ergogenic in longer exercise tasks given the relatively small contribution of phosphocreatine to energy production during tasks 1.5 to 3 minutes in length. However, even when creatine supplementation did not improve the endurance component of prolonged cycle ergometry it did improve sprint performance within and after the endurance phase. Therefore, it is possible that creatine supplementation may prove useful during sprinting episodes within and at the end of certain prolonged events such as cycling races.

Several studies have evaluated the ergogenic effects of creatine supplementation on sport-specific performance and on field tests. However, the finding of improved sports performance resulting from creatine supplementation is not consistent.[40]

Many studies have not reported an ergogenic effect of creatine supplementation. In addition to the obvious implication that creatine supplementation is not a reliable ergogenic aid, these inconclusive findings have been attributed to various factors, including: 1) low sample size relative to the high variability of muscle creatine increases following supplementation, 2) consumption of meat (which contains creatine) by placebo-supplemented subjects, 3) type of exercise studied, and 4) duration of exercise test and rest period between bouts of exercise.[37,38]

To provide an unbiased review of the research on creatine supplementation and exercise performance, several investigators have performed meta-analyses, which compare and statistically analyze the results of selected published studies. In such meta-analyses, statistical "effect size" is calculated based on the magnitude of change (improvement), a weight is placed on the study results
based on factors such as sample size, and studies are selected with strict criteria such as including
only studies with randomized, placebo-controlled designs. For example, Misic and Kelley compared
29 studies that met their criteria and concluded that creatine supplementation did not enhance anaerobic
performance.[41]   A different conclusion was reached by Branch, who included 100 studies in his meta-
analysis of the effects of short-term creatine supplementation on body composition and performance.[42] Branch found a significant increase in body mass and lean body mass and an improvement
in repetitive bouts of laboratory-based isometric, isokinetic, and isotonic resistance exercise lasting
30 s or less, but not in running or swimming performance. The results of Branch are in agreement
with many narrative review articles as well as the ACSM creatine roundtable, which suggests a
benefit of creatine to exercise lasting 30 seconds or less.[43]

Despite the literature clearly showing that a brief (5 day) high-dose creatine-loading phase is sufficient to saturate muscles with creatine, survey data indicate that athletes often ingest creatine supplements for weeks or months, rather than for several days before an athletic event. Juhn et al. reported that baseball and football players most often ingest creatine in the off-season, which is the
time of year when athletes undergo training to increase strength and/or body mass for the forthcom-
ing competitive season.[44] Thus, rather than ingesting creatine acutely to improve performance at a
particular athletic event, many athletes use creatine chronically in an effort to increase muscle
strength, muscle size, and body mass during training.

Weight gain is the most consistent adverse effect reported.[34] In studies that investigated side effects,
no other adverse effects were found, including no changes in electrolyte concentrations, muscle
cramps or strains.[7] Researchers[45] examined the renal function of patients who had been using creatine for as long as five years and found no detrimental effects.[45] It must be noted, however, that most
research to date has examined creatine use of three months or less, leaving questions about long-
term use unanswered. (Note: See chapter 10 - Table 3 for further details on the study of patients
using oral creatine for as long as five years with no detrimental effects).

Caffeine

Caffeine has been previously discussed in Chapter 5 as a catabolic factor. The recent introduction of
caffeine (or guarana) to 'energy drinks', confectionery and sports foods/supplements has increased
the opportunities for athletes to consume caffeine, either as part of their everyday diet or for specific
use as an ergogenic aid.

In January 2004, caffeine was removed from the 2004 World Anti-Doping Agency Prohibited List,
allowing athletes who compete in sports that are compliant with the WADA code to consume caffeine,
within their usual diets or for specific purposes of performance, without fear of sanctions. Caffeine
has numerous actions on different body tissues. The actions may vary between individuals and
include both positive and negative responses. Effects include the mobilization of fats from adipose
tissue and the muscle cell, changes to muscle contractility, alterations to the central nervous system

to change perceptions of effort or fatigue, stimulation of the release and activity of adrenaline, and effects on cardiac muscle.[33]

Recent evidence has changed the perspective on two of the widely promoted effects of caffeine: That caffeine enhances endurance performance because it promotes an increase in the utilization of fat as an exercise fuel and 'spares' the use of the limited muscle stores of glycogen; and that caffeine-containing drinks have a diuretic effect and cause an athlete to become dehydrated. In fact, studies now show that the effect of caffeine on 'glycogen sparing' during submaximal exercise is short-lived and inconsistent - not all athletes respond in this way. Therefore, it is unlikely to explain the enhancement of exercise capacity and performance seen in prolonged continuous events and exercise protocols. In addition, caffeine-containing drinks such as tea, coffee and cola drinks provide a significant source of fluid in the everyday diets of many people and any effect of caffeine on urine losses is minor - particularly in people who are habitual caffeine users.[33]

There is evidence that caffeine enhances endurance and provides a small but worthwhile enhancement of performance over a range of exercise protocols. These include short duration high intensity events (1-5 min), prolonged high intensity events (20-60 min), endurance events (90 min + continuous exercise), ultra-endurance events (4 hours +), and prolonged intermittent high intensity protocols (team and racquet sports). These effects are seen in non-users. The effect on strength/power and brief sprints (10-20 sec) is unclear. The mechanism underpinning performance benefits is unclear, but it is likely to involve alterations to the perception of effort or fatigue, as well as direct effects on the muscle. Most studies of caffeine and performance have been undertaken in laboratories. Studies that investigate performance effects in elite athletes under field conditions or during real-life sports events are scarce and need to be undertaken before specific recommendations for caffeine supplementation protocols can be made.[33]

Antioxidants

Although regular exercise produces many positive health benefits, it also causes an increased production of free radicals. Indeed, intense or prolonged exercise can cause radical-mediated injury to skeletal muscles, particularly in untrained individuals. Further, radicals probably contribute to muscular fatigue during endurance events. Therefore, it is not surprising that there is strong interest in the effects of antioxidant supplements on exercise performance.[46]   Numerous animal studies indicate that antioxidant supplements can delay muscular fatigue. Nonetheless, most animal studies have used antioxidant treatments that cannot be used in humans, so these results should not be directly extrapolated to humans.

Only a few studies have examined the effects of antioxidant supplementation on muscular endurance in humans. Further, many of the studies were flawed, and most studies have investigated the effects of a single antioxidant rather than the combined effects of several antioxidants. Although several human studies indicate that supplementation with vitamin E, and/or vitamin C reduce exercise-induced radical injury, there is limited evidence that antioxidant supplementation can improve human athletic performance. However, because of the paucity of research on this topic, additional studies are required before a firm conclusion can be reached about the effects of antioxidant treatment on human exercise performance.

There is little scientific support for antioxidant supplementation in athletes who consume a well-balanced diet that is rich in fruits and vegetables. Further, over-consumption of antioxidants may have potentially harmful side effects, because high levels of some antioxidants can be toxic. For example, extreme doses of vitamin E have been reported to impair muscular performance in animals. Therefore, athletes considering the use of antioxidant supplements should seek the advice of a well-trained nutritionist prior to adding these supplements to their diet.[46]

Energy Drinks

Energy drinks are canned or bottled beverages sold in convenience stores, grocery stores, and bars and nightclubs (in mixed drinks). Most energy drinks are carbonated drinks that contain large amounts of caffeine and sugar with additional ingredients, such as B vitamins, amino acids (e.g. taurine), and herbal stimulants such as guarana.[47]

Energy drinks are marketed primarily to people between the ages of 18 and 30 as a stimulant, which is why energy drinks have names that convey strength, power, and speed, and sexuality. Although sales of energy drinks in the United States were $3.5 billion in 2005, according to Beverage Digest, the category was only recently created with the launch of the Red Bull Energy Drink.[47]

One of the biggest concerns is the unknown effects of the combination of ingredients in energy drinks. Many ingredients are believed to work synergistically with caffeine to boost its stimulant power. For instance, one can of Red Bull contains 1000 mg of taurine. A German double-blind study compared a taurine and caffeine drink, a caffeine-only drink, and a placebo drink. Stroke volume—the volume of blood ejected with each beat of the heart—was increased only in the group taking the taurine-and-caffeine drink. Taurine appears to play an important role in muscle contraction (especially in the heart) and the nervous system.   Red Bull also contains 600 mg of glucuronolactone, a substance that is naturally found in the body. There is a lack of published information on the health effects of glucuronolactone supplementation in humans or on the safety of this combination.   Energy drinks contain sugar (although sugar-free energy drinks are now available), because it is a quick source of energy. B vitamins are sometimes added to energy drinks in small amounts. It makes energy drinks appear healthy, although they probably contribute little. B vitamins are needed to convert food into energy. Some energy drinks contain guarana, a South American herb that is an additional source of caffeine.

Energy Drinks Should Not Be Mixed With Alcohol.[47] Red Bull and vodka has become a popular mixed drink at bars because it has a reputation for reducing the depressant effects of alcohol (e.g. fatigue) while enhancing the "feel good" buzz. But while people may not feel impaired, their blood alcohol concentration is still high. People may consume larger amounts of alcohol as a result. A study compared the effects of alcohol alone to an alcohol plus energy drink combination. Researchers found that the alcohol plus energy drink significantly reduced subjective alcohol-related symptoms such as headache, weakness, dry mouth, and impairment of motor coordination, even though breath alcohol concentration and objective tests of motor coordination and reaction time didn't reflect this. The caffeine in energy drinks is also dehydrating, which may slow the body's ability to metabolize alcohol.[47]

Energy drinks should not be confused with sports drinks such as Gatorade, which are consumed to help people stay hydrated during exercise. Sports drinks also provide carbohydrates in the form of sugar and electrolytes that may be lost through perspiration.[47]

Amino Acid Supplements

Protein and amino acid supplements are popular with body builders and strength training athletes. Although protein is needed to repair and build muscles after strenuous training, most studies have shown that athletes ingest a sufficient amount without supplements. See section on protein quality for further details on choosing a protein source.

Although selected amino acid supplements are purported to increase growth hormone, studies using manufacturer recommended amounts have not found an increase in growth hormone and muscle mass. Ingesting high amounts of single amino acids is contraindicated because they can affect the absorption of other essential amino acids and produce nausea or impair both training and performance.

Energy Bars

Today, anyone who feels the need for a nutritional boost might keep a few of the energy, or meal-replacement bars, stashed in a gym bag, purse or briefcase.   Not all bars are created equal. There are literally hundreds of choices. Some are very high in calories, mainly from sugar and fat. Some even resemble candy bars with a few extra nutrients, so it is important to read the nutrition label. Some bars are high in carbohydrates, some are high protein bars. Other bars are breakfast bars, meal replacement bars, diet bars, even brain bars that claim to help you think more clearly. So when choosing an energy bar keep the following in mind. Look for bars that are low in fat (less than 5 grams per bar), high in fiber (3 to 5 grams per bar), high in protein (7 to 10 grams per bar). If your watching your weight, look for a bar with fewer than 150 calories. Limit yourself to one bar a day and drink plenty of water with it to help achieve the feeling of being full. The bars can be pricey, ranging from $1.50 to $3.50 per bar. A less expensive alternative is a snack of peanut butter with graham crackers. It has the same calories, protein, carbs and fat that are found in some energy bars at a fraction of the cost.[47]

Most nutritionists emphasize that even when consuming energy bars, don't let them crowd whole foods out of your diet. For a quick snack, you may be better off eating an apple or a banana. Before an athletic competition, a bagel or graham crackers can produce a response in blood glucose levels similar to some energy bars, and they cost a lot less.[48]

ENERGY BASED THERAPIES

The **veritable** energies employ mechanical vibrations (such as sound) and electromagnetic forces, including visible light, magnetism, monochromatic radiation (such as laser beams), and rays from other parts of the electromagnetic spectrum. They involve the use of specific, measurable wavelengths and frequencies to treat patients.[22]

In contrast, **putative** energy fields (also called biofields) have defied measurement to date by reproducible methods. Therapies involving putative energy fields are based on the concept that human beings are infused with a subtle form of energy. This vital energy or life force is known under different names in different cultures, such as qiIn traditional Chinese medicine, the vital energy or life force proposed to regulate a person's spiritual, emotional, mental, and physical health and to be influenced by the opposing forces of yin and yang. In traditional Chinese medicine a whole medical system that originated in China. It is based on the concept that disease results from disruption in the flow of qi and imbalance in the forces of yin and yang. It aims to integrate the body, mind, and spirit to prevent and treat disease. Therapies used include herbs, massage, and yoga and elsewhere as prana, etheric energy, fohat, orgone, odic force, mana, and homeopathic resonance.[3] Vital energy is believed to flow throughout the material human body, but it has not been unequivocally measured by means of conventional instrumentation. Nonetheless, therapists claim that they can work with this subtle energy, see it with their own eyes, and use it to effect changes in the physical body and influence health.[22]

Practitioners of energy medicine believe that illness results from disturbances of these subtle energies (the biofield is an energy field that is proposed to surround and flow throughout the human body and play a role in health). Biofields have not been measured by conventional instruments. Reiki and qi gong are examples of therapies that involve biofields. For example, more than 2,000 years ago, Asian practitioners postulated that the flow and balance of life energies are necessary for maintaining health and described tools to restore them.[22]

Acupuncture is a family of procedures that originated in traditional Chinese medicine. Acupuncture is the stimulation of specific points on the body by a variety of techniques, including the insertion of thin metal needles though the skin. It is intended to remove blockages in the flow of qi and restore and maintain health. Acupressure is a type of acupuncture that stimulates specific points on the body using pressure applied by the hands.[22]

In the aggregate, these approaches are among the most controversial of CAM practices because neither the external energy fields nor their therapeutic effects have been demonstrated convincingly by any biophysical means. Yet, energy medicine is gaining popularity in the American marketplace and has become a subject of investigations at some academic medical centers. A recent National Center for Health Statistics survey indicated that approximately 1 percent of the participants had used Reiki, a therapy in which practitioners seek to transmit a universal energy to a person, either from a distance or by placing their hands on or near that person.[22]

NCCAM Clinical Trial Results

Acupuncture provides pain relief and improves function for people with osteoarthritis of the knee and serves as an effective complement to standard care. "For the first time, a clinical trial with sufficient rigor, size, and duration has shown that acupuncture reduces the pain and functional impairment of osteoarthritis of the knee," said Stephen E. Straus. "These results also indicate that acupuncture can serve as an effective addition to a standard regimen of care and improve quality of life for knee osteoarthritis sufferers. The findings of the study—the longest and largest randomized, controlled phase III clinical trial of acupuncture ever conducted—were published in the December 21, 2004, issue of the *Annals of Internal Medicine*.[5] Overall, those who received acupuncture had a 40 percent decrease in pain and a nearly 40 percent improvement in function compared to baseline assessments.[23]

The randomized, controlled trial of *Tai Chi* (April 2007), led by Michael Irwin, M.D., at the University of California, Los Angeles, included 112 healthy adults ages 59 to 86.[24] Each person took part in a 16-week program of either tai chi or health education with 120 minutes of instruction weekly. Tai chi combines aerobic activity, relaxation, and meditation, which the researchers note have been reported to boost immune responses. After the tai chi and health education programs, with periodic blood tests to determine levels of varicella virus immunity, people in both groups received a single injection of VARIVAX, the chickenpox vaccine approved for use in the United States. Nine weeks later, the investigators did blood tests to assess each participant's level of varicella immunity, comparing it to immunity at the start of the study. Tai chi alone was found to increase participants' immunity to varicella, and tai chi combined with the vaccine produced a significantly higher level of immunity, about a 40 percent increase, over the vaccine alone. The study also showed that the tai chi group's rate of increase in immunity over the course of the study was double that of the health education group. Finally, the tai chi group reported significant improvements in physical functioning, bodily pain, vitality and mental health.[24]

MAKING SENSE OF THE DATA

With the abundance of conflicting information available about dietary supplements, it is more important than ever to sort the reliable information from the questionable. Scientific evidence supporting the benefits of some dietary supplements (e.g., vitamins and minerals) is well established for certain health conditions, but others need further study. Whatever the choice, supplements should not replace prescribed medications or the variety of foods important to a healthful diet. Dietary supplements may help "support" a healthy eating plan, but cannot undo the ill effects of not eating healthy.[25]

Although certain products may be helpful to some people, there may be circumstances when these products can pose unexpected risks. Many supplements contain active ingredients that can have strong effects in the body. It is important to understand that if a chemical (supplements are chemicals) has an effect in the body, then it must have a side effect. Side effects can range from "minor" to very serious.[25]

Taking a combination of supplements, taking them in combination with medicine, or substituting them in place of prescribed medicines could lead to harmful, even life-threatening results. Also, some supplements can have unwanted effects before, during, and after surgery. It is important to let your doctor and other health professionals know about the vitamins, minerals, botanicals, and other products you are taking, especially before surgery.[25] Here a few examples of dietary supplements believed to interact with specific drugs:
- Calcium and heart medicine (e.g., Digoxin), thiazide diuretics (Thiazide), and aluminum and magnesium-containing antacids.
- Magnesium and thiazide and loop diuretics (e.g., Lasix®, etc.), some cancer drugs (e.g., Cisplatin, etc.), and magnesium-containing antacids.
- Vitamin K and a blood thinner (e.g., Coumadin).
- St. John's Wort and selective serotonin reuptake inhibitor (SSRI) drugs (i.e., antidepressant drugs and birth control pills).

Choosing a Supplement

When choosing a supplement remember "safety first.[26] Some supplement ingredients, including nutrients and plant components, can be toxic based on their activity in the body. Do not substitute a dietary supplement for a prescription medicine or therapy. Think twice about chasing the latest headline. Sound health advice is generally based on research over time, not a single study touted by the media.

Be wary of results claiming a "quick fix" that depart from scientific research and established dietary guidance. Learn to spot false claims. Remember: "If something sounds too good to be true, it probably is." Some examples of false claims on product labels: Quick and effective cure-all; can treat or cure disease; "totally safe; all natural; definitely no side effects; limited availability; no-risk, money-back guarantees; or requires advance payment.

More is not always better. Some products can be harmful when consumed in high amounts, for a long time, or in combination with certain other substances. The term "natural" doesn't always mean safe. Do not assume that this term ensures wholesomeness or safety. For some supplements, "natural" ingredients may interact with medicines, be dangerous for people with certain health conditions, or be harmful in high doses. For example, tea made from peppermint leaves is generally considered safe to drink, but peppermint oil (extracted from the leaves) is much more concentrated and can be toxic if used incorrectly.[26]

Is the product worth the money? Resist the pressure to buy a product or treatment "on the spot." Some supplement products may be expensive or may not provide the benefit you expect. For example, excessive amounts of water-soluble vitamins, like vitamin C and B vitamins, are not used by the body and are eliminated in the urine.[26]

In addition, there are a few independent organizations that offer "seals of approval" that may be displayed on certain dietary supplement products. These indicate that the product has passed the organization's quality tests for things such as potency and contaminants. These "seals of approval" do not mean that the product is safe or effective; they provide assurance that the product was properly manufactured, that it contains the ingredients listed on the label and that it does not contain harmful levels of contaminants. These organizations include: Consumerlab.com approved quality product seal (http://www.consumerlab.com/seal.asp); NSF International dietary supplement certification (http://www.nsf.org/business/dietary_supplements/index.asp?program=DietarySups); U.S. Pharmacopeia dietary supplement verification program (http://www.usp.org/USPVerified/ dietarySupplements/).

Consumerlab.com[27]

ConsumerLab.com, founded in 1999 by Dr. Tod Cooperman, has independently tested over 2,000 products. It publishes results of its tests at www.consumerlab.com — which receives over 2.5 million visits per year. Products tested are purchased independently by Consumerlab at the retail level (stores, mail order, online, etc.). CL does not accept product samples from manufacturers for *Product Reviews* and CL may select samples at any time during the year (to avoid sampling bias). Products are selected to reflect popular brands in the market as well as a selection of smaller brands. Blinded tests are conducted by academic and commercial laboratories selected for their expertise in the type of testing needed for each product. These facilities are generally FDA inspected, follow GLP (good laboratory practice) protocols, are accredited by outside groups and/or participate in method validation programs.

Consumerlab has been criticized because it tests only one sample and also "sells" its seal of approval to manufacturers that wish to have their product tested. Consumerlab scientists counter this criticism by obtaining samples from retails stores and not from the manufacturer directly.

NSF International Dietary Supplement Certification

Since 1944, NSF International, an independent, not-for-profit organization, has been testing products. The NSF Mark can be found on millions of consumer, commercial, and industrial products today. Products evaluated and certified by NSF International include bottled water, food equipment, home water treatment products, home appliances, plumbing and faucets, and even pool and spa components. The NSF Mark provides the consumer with assurance that the product has been thoroughly and independently tested.

NSF became involved in the testing of dietary supplements because of the growth of the diet industry over the past decade and the fact that these products do not receive the same regulation as prescription or over-the-counter drugs. Given the fast pace at which many dietary supplements enter the marketplace and the many reports that have been published suggesting that some of these products do not actually contain the ingredients or ingredient quantities indicated on the product's label, consumers today have cause to be concerned.

NSF does not simply evaluate test data submitted by manufacturers. They start by auditing each production facility separately. Samples of the products produced at each plant are then tested by accredited laboratories to determine if the actual contents of the tested products match those printed on the label.

There are three main components of the NSF dietary supplements certification program:

1. Determining if the ingredients in the tested products match what is shown on the product's label.
2. Determining if any ingredients are present in the tested products that are not disclosed on the label.
3. Determining if any contaminants are present in the tested products.

For a complete list of approved dietary supplements visit www. nsf.org online products database.

To help minimize the risk that a dietary supplement or sports nutrition product contains a substance banned by one of the major sports organizations, NSF developed the Certified for Sport™ program. Under this program, products are tested to ensure they contain the identity and quantity of dietary ingredients declared on the product label. In addition, the program helps ensure the product does not contain unacceptable quantities of contaminants for the recommended serving size listed on the product label. Exceeding recommended serving sizes may increase risk, so athletes should be sure to follow the serving size instructions indicated for the product.

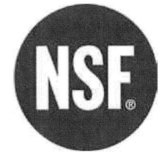

The list of prohibited substances includes all banned substances identified by leading sports organizations, such as the World Anti-Doping Agency (WADA), the National Football League (NFL) and Major League Baseball (MLB). The certification program certifies products and inspects facilities for a range of substances, including: Stimulants, narcotics, steroids, diuretics, beta-2-Agonists, beta blockers, masking agents, and other substances. The list of banned substances for which testing is performed is updated regularly based on the scientific ability to detect a banned substance and through input from the international sports community. For a list of products that are currently certified to meet the requirements of the program, please visit our www.nsf.org online products database.

To help address concerns about the contents and claims for functional foods, NSF expanded its Dietary Supplements Certification Program to include the evaluation of products classified as functional foods and beverages. The new Dietary Supplements and Functional Foods Certification Program provides test methods and evaluation criteria to certify that a functional food product does not contain unacceptable quantities of contaminants such as lead, pesticides, prescription drugs or other dangerous substances; that it complies with nutrition labeling requirements; and that it has been manufactured in accordance with current GMPs for quality, safety, and sanitation. For a current list of NSF-Certified functional foods and beverages, visit www.nsf.org   online products database.

NSF and Bottled Water

There are at least a dozen different types of bottled water available. Bottled water products are normally categorized according to the source of the water and the method(s) used by the bottler to treat it. Bottled water products are generally required to undergo disinfection. Bottlers who obtain water from a source which has not previously been disinfected, such as a spring or well, will usually use ozone or ultraviolet technologies to disinfect the water, as these processes do not normally leave a residual taste or odor in the water, like chlorine does. Bottled water companies can also purchase their source water from an approved potable water source, such as a municipal water supply.

Some bottling companies choose to further treat their bottled water products, using treatment processes such as filtration, reverse osmosis, or distillation. Although federal laws do not require the bottler to list any naturally occurring compounds on the product label, such as sulfates, sodium, or radon, if a bottler chooses to add any ingredients to the water, such as minerals, fluoride, or flavorings, this must be stated on the label. Any naturally occurring or added ingredients cannot exceed the maximum levels permitted by the applicable FDA or state regulations.

The FDA has established "Standards of Identity" for bottled water products sold in the U.S. Some of the more common types of bottled water are listed below:

Artesian Water: This is water that originates from a confined aquifer that has been tapped and in which the water level stands at some height above the top of the aquifer.

Fluoridated: This type of water contains fluoride added within the limitations established in the FDA Code of Federal Regulations. This category includes water classified as "For Infants" or "Nursery."

Ground Water: This type of water is from an underground source that is under a pressure equal to or greater than atmospheric pressure.

Mineral Water: Mineral water contains at least 250 parts per million total dissolved solids (TDS). It comes from a source tapped at one or more bore holes or spring, and originates from a geologically and physically protected underground water source. No minerals may be added to this water.

Purified Water: This type of water has been produced by distillation, deionization, reverse osmosis, or other suitable processes. Purified water may also be referred to as "demineralized water." It meets the definition of "purified water" in the United States Pharmacopoeia.

Sparkling Water: Sparkling water contains the same amount of carbon dioxide that it had at emergence from the source. The carbon dioxide may be removed and replenished after treatment.

Spring Water: This type of water comes from an underground formation from which water flows naturally to the Earth's surface.

Sterile Water: This type of water meets the requirements under "sterility tests" in the

United States Pharmacopoeia.

Well Water: Well water is taken from a hole tapping, etc. This hole may be bored, drilled, or otherwise constructed in the ground.

NSF International has been testing bottled water products for compliance with federal guidelines for many years. The NSF Bottled Water Certification Program is an annual, voluntary certification process that includes both extensive product evaluations as well as on-site audits of bottling facilities. Their testing program provides for annual unannounced plant inspections covering every aspect of a bottler's operation, from the source of the water, through the disinfection and treatment process, and including the container closure process. We also perform extensive product testing for over 160 chemical, inorganic, radiological, and microbiological contaminants.

For a complete list of NSF-certified bottled water products, please visit www.nsf.org bottled water online product database. If you would like further information about a particular brand or would like to receive a copy of the individual test report, feel free to contact the bottler at the address or telephone number shown.

U.S. Pharmacopeia Dietary Supplement Verification Program[29]

States Pharmacopeia (USP) is an independent, not-for-profit organization and is the official standard-setting body for medicine and its standards are enforceable by the FDA. USP is the standards-setting authority for all prescription and over-the-counter medicines and other healthcare products manufactured and sold in the United States.   USP sets standards for the quality of these products and works with healthcare providers to help them reach the standards.
USP's standards are also recognized and used in more than 130 countries. These standards have been helping to ensure good pharmaceutical care for people throughout the world for more than 185 years.

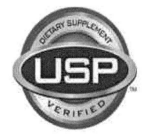

Unlike drugs (which are required by law to be tested by USP), supplement manufacturers can "voluntarily" request to have their products tested. The USP Verified Dietary Supplement Mark is awarded to finished dietary supplements that pass USP's comprehensive verification processes. Manufacturers can display the mark on the label of USP Verified products. The mark represents that USP has rigorously tested and verified the supplement to assure: what's on the label is in fact in the bottle—all the listed ingredients in the declared amount; the supplement does not contain harmful levels of contaminants; the supplement will break down and release ingredients in the body; the supplement has been made under good manufacturing practices.

Visit http://www.usp.org/USPVerified/dietarySupplements/supplements.html to obtain a list of verified products containing the USP Verified Dietary Supplement Mark.

When to take a Supplement

Before taking any supplement, consider homeostasis. Homeostasis is "the maintenance of constant internal conditions". The human body, a homeostatic system, is constantly reacting to external and internal forces so as to maintain limits set by the body. Taking large amounts of any nutrient can result in pertabations in the homeostatic condition (causing disruption or disorder) forcing the body to react by producing opposing chemicals to bring about homeostasis. There comes a point when the body cannot produce the needed opposing chemicals and the disease state begins.

Whether the chemical is Vitamin C, nitrogen or vitamin A, too much or too little can disrupt homeostasis. So before consuming any supplement, consumers must ask the following questions:

Is the product safe?

If safe, is it effective?

If effective, is it necessary for health?

If necessary, am I willing to risk the side effects (5% die, 2% suffer liver damage, etc.)?

Most consumers of supplements (or drugs) do not believe that they will suffer the side effects (its always someone else that suffers the side effects). But consumers must ask themselves if they are willing to suffer the side effects before consuming any chemicals.

Choosing a Multivitamin

Major health and nutrition organizations (Tufts University, University of CA Berkeley, CSPI) recommend taking a multivitamin the reason being most people do not obtain all the essential nutrients needed on a daily basis. These same organizations quickly point out that a multivitamin cannot

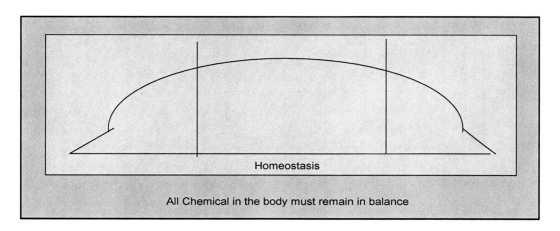

Homeostasis

All Chemical in the body must remain in balance

"undo" the harmful effects of an unhealthy diet and they caution Americans not to fall prey to marketing that indicates otherwise.

The following are suggestions when choosing (and ingesting) a multivitamin:

1. Since the passage of the 1994 DSHEA there are no regulatory agencies overseeing the supplement industry. There are, however, several certifying agencies that consumers can look to for quality assurance (NSF, USP and Consumerlab.com).

2. Multivitamin: Look for USP on the label or NSF (National Science Foundation). Take with food.

3. Look for 100% of the DV for Vitamin D, B vitamins, and 20 micrograms of vitamin K ,

copper, zinc, iodine, selenium, chromium.

4. Look for 5,000 IU's of Vitamin A with 40% in the form of beta carotene. More than 6,000 IUs of vitamin A increases the risk of fractures in people over 50

5. If calcium supplement is necessary take a separate supplement.

6. Iron: pre-menopausal women look for 100% of DV of iron. Men and post-menopausal women need only 45% of DV. Individuals with Hemochromatosis must avoid supplements with iron.

7. Words you do not need to see on the bottle: high potency; senior formula, stress formula, starch-free, natural, or slow-release, enzymes, hormones, amino acids, PAVA, ginseng or other herbs.

8. Strict vegetarians: B12, zinc, iron, and calcium.

9. Women of childbearing age: 400 IUs folate.

SUMMARY

This chapter focused on discussion of complimentary alternative medicine, the origins and results of clinical trials funded by the National Center for Complimentary and Alternative Medicine. Biologically based therapies (supplements, herbs, etc.) and energy based therapies will also be discussed.

Millions of Americans spend billions of dollars on alternative medicine.   According to a nationwide government survey released in May 2004, 36 percent of U.S. adults aged 18 years and over use some form of complimentary alternative medicine which includes supplements. When prayer specifically for health reasons is included in the definition, the number of U.S. adults using some form of complimentary alternative medicine in the rises to 62 percent[1].

Complimentary alternative medicine is defined as a group of diverse medical and health care systems, practices, and products, including supplement, that are not presently considered to be part of conventional medicine.

What is the science behind these alternative therapies? Advocates claim strong science exists and complain about the slow moving and overly cautious FDA, while scientists argue that Congress is advocating for unproven therapies rather than subjecting new treatments to evaluation.

The National Center for Complimentary and Alternative Medicine (NCCAM) is the Federal Government's lead agency for scientific research on complimentary alternative medicine (CAM). The origin of NCCAM began in 1992, when Senator Tom Harkin (D-Iowa), convinced bee pollen had cured his allergies, assigned $2 million of his discretionary funds to establish the Office of Unconventional Medicine, renamed the Office of Alternative Medicine (OAM).[2] Funds for OAM increased annually and in 1998 increased to $19.5 million. Also in 1998, Senator Harkin won a decisive battle when the NIH opened a new office - the National Center for Complimentary and Alternative Medicine (NCCAM) - with a $50 million budget.[2] As a sign that NCCAM was indeed a scientific entity to be dealt with, the renowned Dr. Stephen E. Straus was appointed the first director October 6, 1999.[2] When interviewed, Dr. Straus made it clear that the office would perform rigorous scientific studies and that the public and companies with vested interests in new alternative therapies "will have to accept that research may show that some new therapies will not be good; some therapies will not be safe; and some therapies will not be any more effective than present alternatives. [2]

Over the past few decades, thousands of studies of various dietary supplements have been performed. To date, however, no single supplement has been proven effective in a compelling way. Nevertheless, there are several supplements for which early studies yielded positive, or at least encouraging, data. Good sources of information on some of them can be found at the Natural Medicines Comprehensive Database and a number of National Institutes of Health (NIH) Web sites. The NIH Office of Dietary Supplements (ODS) annually publishes a bibliography of resources on significant advances in dietary supplement research. Finally, the ClinicalTrials.gov database lists all NIH-supported clinical studies of dietary supplements that are actively accruing patients.[3]

NCCAM classifies complimentary alternative therapies into five categories, or domains:[4]
1. Alternative Medical Systems
2. Mind-Body Interventions
3. Biologically Based Therapies
4. Manipulative and Body-Based Methods
5. Energy Therapies

Biologically based therapies include, but are not limited to, botanicals, animal-derived extracts, vitamins, minerals, fatty acids, amino acids, proteins, prebiotics and probiotics found in foods such as yogurt or in dietary supplements., whole diets, and functional foods.[4]

A dietary supplement is any product that contains vitamins, minerals, herbs or other botanicals, amino acids, enzymes, and/or other ingredients intended to supplement the diet. The U.S. Food and Drug Administration has special labeling requirements for dietary supplements and treats them as foods, not drugs must meet all of the following conditions. It is a product (other than tobacco) that is intended to supplement the diet and that contains one or more of the following: vitamins, minerals, *herbs or other botanicals, amino acids, or any combination of the above ingredients. It is intended to be taken in tablet, capsule, powder, softgel, gelcap, or liquid form. It is not represented for use as a conventional food or as a sole item of a meal or the diet. It is labeled as being a dietary supplement.[6]

According to a survey of physicians—primarily orthopedic surgeons, rheumatologists and sports medicine practitioners—60 percent of those polled felt there was not enough FDA oversight of the dietary supplement industry to warrant recommending supplements.[7] It's for that reason the implementation of good manufacturing practices is a crucial first step to the future of the industry—it will restore some of the luster of dietary supplements among health care professionals who are making disease-state treatment recommendations, stated Michael Johnsen, in Drug Store News, on April 11, 2005.[7]

It's this stigma of an unregulated industry promoting "snake oil treatments" that are no more effective than a placebo that keeps dogging the industry. Despite numerous sound clinical trials that support substantial health benefits for one ingredient or another, the sheer number of inconclusive studies combined with the industry's share of less-than-reputable suppliers has painted the industry with a negative brush.[8]

President Clinton, on October 25, 1994, signed the DSHEA "acknowledging that millions of consumers believe dietary supplements offer health benefits and that consumers want a greater opportunity to determine whether supplements may help them". With the passage of the DSHEA, supplement manufacturers were given "carte blanche" to market supplements without regulation. The Council of Responsible Nutrition, an organization of manufacturers of dietary supplements hailed this act as a "landmark change". "Landmark change it is!"[9]

Before 1994, the original definition of a supplement was a product that contained one or more of the essential nutrients. After DSHEA, the definition of a supplement was changed to any product intended for ingestion as a supplement to the diet. This definition now includes liquid, pill, capsule, or tablet forms of vitamins, minerals, herbs, botanicals and other plant derived substances, amino acids and concentrates, metabolites, constituents and extracts of these substances. Again, according to the FDA, dietary supplements are not drugs. The FDA definition of a drug is an article, which may or may not be derived from plants that are intended to diagnose, cure, mitigate, treat or prevent disease. Before marketing, drugs must undergo *clinical* studies to determine their effectiveness, safety, possible interactions with other substances, and appropriate dosages. The FDA reviews these data and authorizes usage before marketing. The FDA does not authorize or test dietary supplements. Under DSHEA congress amended the Federal Food, Drug, and Cosmetic Act (FD&C Act) to include provisions that apply only to dietary supplements and dietary ingredients of dietary supplements. As a result of these provisions, dietary ingredients used in dietary supplements are no longer subject to the premarket safety evaluations required of other new food ingredients or for new uses of old food ingredients.[9]

In its 1998 statement, the FDA warns that dietary supplements are not replacements for conventional diets. The FDA also warns that It must not be assumed that "all natural means safe", (poisonous mushrooms are all natural); it must not be assumed that what is stated on the label is actually in the bottle; and just because the accompanying literature makes claims about the safety and health advantages of the supplement, it must not be assumed that these claims are true.[10]

Under the DSHEA, the FDA can only step in when the supplement has been shown to be unsafe. For example, in June 1997, the FDA proposed, among other things, to limit the amount of ephedrine alkaloids in supplements and provide warnings because dangers such as dizziness, changes in blood pressure, changes in heart rate, chest pain, heart attack, stroke, hepatitis, seizures, psychosis, and death occurred.

The DSHEA authorized the establishment of the Office of Dietary Supplements (ODS) at the NIH.[11] The ODS was created in 1995 within the Office of Disease Prevention (ODP), Office of the Director (OD), NIH. One of the purposes in creating the ODS was to promote scientific research in the area of dietary supplements. Dietary supplements can have an impact on the prevention of disease and on the maintenance of health.[11] In the US, these ingredients are usually defined as including plant extracts, enzymes, vitamins, minerals, amino acids, and hormonal products that are available without prescription and are consumed in addition to the regular diet. Although vitamin and mineral supplements have been available for decades, their health effects have been the subject of detailed scientific research only within the last 15-20 years. It is important to expand this research to include the health effects of other bioactive factors consumed as supplements to promote health and prevent disease. Considerable research on the effects of botanical and herbal dietary supplements has been conducted in Asia and Europe where plant products have a long tradition of use. The overwhelming majority of these supplements, however, have not been studied using modern scientific techniques. Nor have they been extensively studied in population groups that may be at risk for chronic diseases. For many reasons, therefore, it is important to enhance research efforts to determine the benefits and risks of dietary supplements.[10]

Robert Park, Author of Voodoo Science – the Road from Foolishness to Fraud, says DSHEA is his candidate for the worst piece of legislation ever passed.[7] Supplement manufacturers are not held to any rigorous standards indicates Robert Park.[2]   "Before 1994 manufacturers had to prove that the product was safe or at least that what you said on the label was in the bottle". "Manufacturers don't have to do that anymore". Under DSHEA testing is voluntary. "It's wonderful right now for companies that make supplements. "I would not be regulated. The only people I would have to answer to is my stock holders to see how much profit I am making. The FDA can only step in when the supplement has been shown to be unsafe.[2]

Marcia Angell, Harvard University, emphasizes that "large drug companies might not test for safety and efficacy if they didn't have to. But they have to. The government requires it.[2]

Tests performed by ABC's TV program 20/20 on over 100 bottles of supplements found that one in four did not have what the manufacturer stated on the label. EIGHT BOTTLES HAD QUINTOZENE in them, A PESTICIDE SPRAYED ON THE PLANT WHEN IT IS GROWING.[13]

It's not just consumerlab.com that found problems. The Good Housekeeping Institute tested SAM-e, Consumer Reports tested echinacia, and the Los Angeles Times tested St. John's Wort. All reported that what was stated on the label was not always in the bottle. According to Dr. Cooperman, until someone is checking the industry there is no incentive to fix the problem.[13]

"Random batch spiking" has a long history in the supplement business. It works like this: "The manufacturer sprinkles an illegal substance into an over-the-counter dietary supplement," says Feliciano. "The legal ingredients are claimed on the label, but they don't disclose the drug."

Many people simply fall prey to bogus marketing copy. Last January, marketers of four diet products — Xenadrine EFX, CortiSlim, One-A-Day WeightSmart, and TrimSpa — agreed to settle charges of false advertising made by the Federal Trade Commission, and paid $25 million in claims. Investigators found that before-and-after subjects had lost weight by dieting and exercising, not by popping pills. According to the FTC, this company's own research showed that members of a placebo group lost more weight than the supplement takers did.[14]

If a quarter of all dietary supplements failed to match label claims when tested by ConsumerLab.com, that means three-fourths did live up their promises. Indeed, many U.S. companies make high-quality dietary supplements. "Big companies refuse to participate in any of this renegade activity," says Feliciano. "They have all sorts of defense systems in place. You'll often find four or five Ph.D.'s working in quality control, and these are big-money positions. When they sign off on something, they're legally responsible."

With the abundance of conflicting information available about dietary supplements, it is more important than ever to sort the reliable information from the questionable. Scientific evidence supporting the benefits of some dietary supplements (e.g., vitamins and minerals) is well established for certain health conditions, but others need further study. Whatever the choice, supplements should not replace prescribed medications or the variety of foods important to a healthful diet. Dietary supplements may help "support" a healthy eating plan, but cannot undo the ill effects of not eating healthy.

When choosing a supplement remember "safety first.[26] Be wary of results claiming a "quick fix" that depart from scientific research and established dietary guidance. Look for a certification logo on the supplement. Before taking any chemical, consumers must ask themselves: Is the product safe; if safe is it effective; if effective is it necessary for health; and am I willing to suffer the side effects.

CHAPTER 9 - SAMPLE TEST

1. Define "Complimentary Alternative Medicine" and discuss the role NCCAM plays.

2. Discuss the classifications of "Complimentary Alternative Medicine".

3. Discuss the Dietary Supplement Healthy and Education Act of 1994 and how it changed an entire industry.

4. Describe the role of the "Office of Dietary Supplements".

5. Summarize the results of the NCCAM published data.

6. Define botanicals and discuss problems associated with these types of supplements.

7. List the three organizations that offer seals of approval displayed on dietary supplements.

8. Discuss details on how to choose a supplement and what to look for when buying a supplement.

REFERENCES

1. http://nccam.nih.gov/about/ataglance/.
2. Aronson, A. et al. The alternative fix. Frontline (production of WGBH Boston). 2003.
3. http://nccam.nih.gov/health/backgrounds/biobasedprac.htm.
4. http://nccam.nih.gov/health/whatiscam/.
5. http://nccam.nih.gov/research/results/.
6. http://ods.od.nih.gov/factsheets/DietarySupplements.asp.
7. Johnsen, M. Drug Store News. April, 2005.
8. http://findarticles.com/p/articles/mi_m3374/is_5_27/ai_n13629730.
9.http://www.cfsan.fda.gov/~dms/dietsupp.html.
10. http://www.fda.gov/FDAC/features/1998/598_guid.html.
11. http://dietary-supplements.info.nih.gov/.
12. http://www.fda.gov/bbs/topics/NEWS/2007/NEW01657.html.
13. Walters, B. What's Really in the Bottle. ABC/20-20, Dec. 2005.
14. O'Connell, J. Beyond Balco: The Untold Dietary Supplement Scandal. Men's Health, Jan. 2008.
15 http://nccam.nih.gov/research/results/stjohnswort/
16. http://nccam.nih.gov/research/results/echinacea_rr.htm
17. http://nccam.nih.gov/research/results/gait/
18. Gardner CD, Lawson LD, Block E, et al. Effect of raw garlic vs. commercial garlic supplements on plasma lipid concentrations in adults with moderate hypercholesterolemia: a randomized clinical trial. *Archives of Internal Medicine.* 2007;167(4):346-353.
19. http://nccam.nih.gov/research/results/sharkcartilage_rr.htm.
20. http://nccam.nih.gov/health/backgrounds/biobasedprac.htm.
21. http://nccam.nih.gov/health/blackcohosh/.
22. http://nccam.nih.gov/health/backgrounds/energymed.htm.
23. http://nccam.nih.gov/research/results/acu-osteo.htm.
24. http://nccam.nih.gov/research/results/spotlight/081407.htm.
25. http://nccam.nih.gov/health/bottle/.
26. chttp://ods.od.nih.gov/Health_Information/ODS_Frequently_Asked_Questions.aspx.
27. http://www.consumerlab.com/.
28. http://www.nsf.org.
29. http://www.usp.org/aboutUSP/.
30. http://fcs.tamu.edu/food_and_nutrition/nutrifacts/issue17.pdf.
31. Wikipedia, the free encyclopedia.
32. http://www.aafp.org/afp/20010301/913.html
33. http://www.ais.org.au/nutrition/SuppFactSheets.asp
34. http://www.gssiweb.com/Article_Detail.aspx?articleid=626Poortmans JR, Francaux M. Long-term creatine supplementation does not impair renal function in healthy athletes. Med Sci Sports Exerc 1999;31: 1108-10.
35. Greenhaff, P. L., Bodin, K., Söderlund, K. & Hultman, E. (1994). Effect of oral creatine supple-mentation on skeletal muscle phosphocreatine resynthesis. *Am. J. Physiol.* 266, E725-730.
36. Vandebuerie, F., Vanden Eynde, B., Vandenberghe, K. & Hespel, P. (1998). Effect of creatine

loading on endurance capacity and sprint power in cyclists. *Int. J. Sports Med.* 19, 490-495.

37. Kreider, R. B. (2003). Effects of creatine supplementation on performance and training adaptations. *Mol. Cell. Biochem.* 244, 89-94.

38. Lemon, P. W. (2002). Dietary creatine supplementation and exercise performance: why inconsistent results- *Can. J. Appl. Physiol.* 27, 663-681.

39. Rawson, E. S. & Volek, J. S. (2003). The effects of creatine supplementation and resistance training on muscle strength and weight-lifting performance. *J. Strength Cond. Res.* 17, 822-831.

40. Skare, O. C., Skadberg & Wisnes, A. R. (2001). Creatine supplementation improves sprint performance in male sprinters. *Scand. J. Med. Sci. Sports* 11, 96-102.

41. Misic, M. & Kelley, G. A. (2002). The impact of creatine supplementation on anaerobic performance: A meta-analysis. *Am. J. Med. Sports* 4, 116-124.

42. Branch, J. D. (2003). Effect of creatine supplementation on body composition and performance: a meta-analysis. *Int. J. Sport Nutr. Exerc. Metab.* 13, 198-226.

43. College of Sports Medicine roundtable. The physiological and health effects of oral creatine supplementation. *Med. Sci. Sports Exerc.* 32, 706-717.

44. Juhn, M. S., O'Kane, J. W. & Vinci, D. M. (1999). Oral creatine supplementation in male collegiate athletes: a survey of dosing habits and side effects. *J. Am. Diet. Assoc.* 99, 593-595.

45. Poortmans JR, Francaux M. Long-term creatine supplementation does not impair renal function in healthy athletes. Med Sci Sports Exerc 1999;31: 1108-10.

46. http://www.gssiweb.com/Article_Detail.aspx?articleid=299.
http://altmedicine.about.com/od/completeazindex/a/energy_drinks.htm.

47. http://www.wpxi.com/health/1576714/detail.html.

48. http://www.medicinenet.com/script/main/art.asp?articlekey=51787.

Chapter 10
Nutrition Research

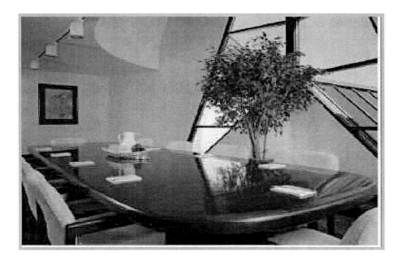

Over the last thirty years, the commercialization of science in the United States and around the world has increased dramatically. The revolution in genetics, patent protections for bioengineered molecules, laws strengthening intellectual property rights, and the 1980 Bayh-Dole Act authorizing licensing and patenting of results from federally-sponsored research created new incentives for scientists, clinicians, and academic institutions to join forces with for-profit industry in an unprecedented array of entrepreneurial activities.

In this chapter we will take an in-depth look at the current trends in nutrition research.

Objectives

After reading and studying this chapter you should:

1.   Discuss the latest trends in nutrition research and the possible conflicts of interest involved between for-profit corporations and non-profit corporations.

2.   Discuss the findings by Center for Science in the Public Interest (CSPI) concerning the 170 non-profit organizations and their ties to for-profit corporations.

3.   Discuss the issues involved with "Scientists Behaving Badly" and provide details about marketing versus research.

4.   Discuss the steps involved in critical analysis of research in nutrition.

INTRODUCTION

When conducting research, scientists follow what is known as the "scientific method". This method relies on identifying a problem to be solved or asks a specific question to be answered. The next step is to formulate a hypothesis (a possible solution) to the problem or answer to the question and make a prediction that can be tested through research. A study design is decided upon, the research is completed and the data is collected. The data must then be analyzed and the results interpreted. The original hypothesis is either supported by the data or is not supported. Scientists typically raise more questions so future research projects always exist.[1]

The findings from a research study are submitted to a board of reviewers composed of other scientists who rigorously evaluate the study to assure that the scientific method was followed. This process is known as "peer-review". Findings are considered preliminary until other scientists confirm or disprove them through other studies (replication). The findings are not accepted until they are replicated many times by other researchers.[1]

Many experts today question whether the adherence to the "scientific method" still exists. Over the last thirty years, the commercialization of science in the United States and around the world has increased dramatically. The revolution in genetics, patent protections for bioengineered molecules, laws strengthening intellectual property rights, and the 1980 Bayh-Dole Act authorizing licensing and patenting of results from federally-sponsored research created new incentives for scientists, clinicians, and academic institutions to join forces with for-profit industry in an unprecedented array of entrepreneurial activities.[2]

Not only are experts questioning adherence to the scientific method, but the American public is concerned about the fact that many physicians and scientists have financial ties to the drug and device industries and most people want the news media to do a better job disclosing these ties whenever experts are quoted.[2]

CONFLICT OF INTEREST

In response to the commercialization of science and the growing problem of conflicts of interest, the Integrity in Science Project was developed by Center for Science in the Public Interest (CSPI). CSPI is a non-profit organization that accepts no funds from government, corporations, or special interest groups.[3] To guard against corporate-funded and/or questionable science dominating the regulatory process, the Integrity in Science project selectively investigates and reports on the make-up of the federal government's more than 1,000 scientific advisory committees. The project also selectively monitors and issues reports about key non-government advisory bodies like the National Academies of Science, which Congress and regulatory agencies often turn to for advice.[3] Because these advisory committees provide critical guidance and scientific information for government agencies charged with protecting the public health and safety, it is imperative that these committees meet all the fairness and balance requirements of the Federal Advisory Committee Act. Every member of these committees must disclose conflicts of interest to the general public.[3]

The Integrity in Science project challenges committee members who have represented corporations with a stake in the outcome of a scientific study or regulatory proceeding. When such members are appointed to committees for their scientific expertise, the project also intervenes to ensure that equal representation is given to independent scientists and representatives of the public interest.[3]

Nonprofit Ties to Corporations

Nonprofit organizations traditionally have championed independent thinking and action in American society, a pillar of our democracy. Be they health charities, health-professional associations, or universities, they are usually, considered to be objective and serving the public interest. And, indeed, over the years, organizations as disparate as the American Heart Association and World Wildlife Fund have made enormous contributions in their sphere of interest.[4] In recent decades, though, a new factor has crept, often secretly, onto the scene. Corporations, with their own motivations, have learned that they can influence public opinion and public policy more effectively by working through seemingly independent organizations rather than under their own names. Their power to persuade is significantly enhanced when they can get an apparently independent nonprofit organization to advocate on their behalf. That's one reason we have seen tobacco, soft drink, and other besieged companies cozying up to nonprofit groups. People would be far more skeptical of a Corporate Polluters Lobbying Association than an industry-funded Harvard University Center on Important Issues. As one advertising company stated, "Gatorade uses the expert opinion of a university PhD—much better than just having someone from the company say it. Similarly, companies hope that a nonprofit's or university's good name will help improve their reputations. Call it "innocence by association.[4] Most nonprofit groups welcome corporate support. The funds allow them to have a higher public profile (which may translate into increased donations), hire new staff, and expand their programs. However, notwithstanding insistence by both the donors and the recipients that such grants come with no strings attached, a price usually is paid for accepting corporate largesse. That payment may be in the currency of credibility and independence. Medical-professional organizations and health charities are among the biggest recipients of industry funding. Drug and other companies open up their wallets to such groups to publicize and give credibility to the companies' high-profit products.[4]

CSPI, in *Lifting the Veil of Secrecy,* states that although many have cheered partnerships between industry and the research community, it is also acknowledged that they entail conflicts of interest that may compromise the judgment of trusted professionals, the credibility of research institutions and scientific journals, the safety and transparency of human subjects research, the norms of free inquiry, and the legitimacy of science-based policy.[4]

There is strong evidence that researchers' financial ties to chemical, pharmaceutical, or tobacco manufacturers directly influence their published positions in supporting the benefit or down playing the harm of the manufacturers' product. A growing body of evidence indicates that pharmaceutical industry gifts and inducements bias clinicians' judgments and influence doctors' prescribing practices. There are well-known cases of industry seeking to discredit or prevent the publication of research results that are critical of its products. Studies of life-science faculty indicate that researchers with industry funding are more likely to withhold research results in order to secure commercial advantage. Increasingly, the same academic institutions that are responsible for oversight of scientific integrity and human subjects protection are entering financial relationships with the industries whose product-evaluations they oversee.[4]

According to the Center for Science in the Public Interest (CSPI) more than 170 disease-related charities, health-professional societies, and university-based institutions enjoy the largesse of food, agribusiness, chemical, pharmaceutical, and other corporate interests[1]. But that generosity may exact too high a price on integrity in science.[4] One such example is the relationship between Coca-Cola and the American Academy of Pediatric Dentistry (AAPD). Before a large 2003 donation, the AAPD recognized the connection between sugary drinks and dental disease. When AAPD president David Curtis defended the Coke deal, he told reporters that the "scientific evidence is certainly not clear" on the role soft drinks play. "What a difference a million dollars makes", states Michael Jacobson, executive director of CSPI.[4]

Other nonprofit groups with questionable corporate ties include the American Dietetic Association (ADA), International Society for Regulatory Toxicology and Pharmacology, and the Society for Women's Health Research (SWHR). The ADA accepts outright donations from food companies. It also lets companies fund fact sheets: The National soft Drink Association "sponsors" the association's fact sheet on soft drinks; McDonalds sponsors "Nutrition on the Go", and so on. The International Society for Regulatory Toxicology and Pharmacology is sponsored by Dow Agrosciences, Eastmak Kodak, Gillette, Merck, Procter & Gamble, RJ Reynolds Tobacco, and other corporations that have an interest in weakening government regulation of chemicals. The Society for Women's Health Research (SWHR) criticized the way the National Institutes of Health publicized a major new study that found hormone replacement therapy (HRT) increased the risk of breast cancer and heart attacks in women. Wyeth, which markets Prempro, the most widely used HRT drug is a major contributor to SWHR. Wyeth underwrote the expenses for SWHR's April 2002 black-tie fund-raising dinner and a week later gave SWHR $250,000 at a special event.[4]

The report, *Lifting the Veil of Secrecy*, by CSPI also identified over 30 university-based research centers that draw substantial financial support from companies or corporate trade associations. Examples include several university centers on forestry funded by timber or paper industries and several centers on nutrition funded by food and agribusiness companies. These centers let corporations put an academic sheen on industry-funded research.[4]

TAKING SIDES

Taking Sides presents current issues in a debate-style format designed to stimulate student interest and develop critical thinking skills. Each issue is framed with an issue summary, an issue introduction, and a postscript. The pro and con essays represent the arguments of leading scholars and commentators in their fields.[5] Dr. Marion Nestle, author of Taking Sides - Food and Nutrition, provides further examples of situations in which food company alliances with nutrition academic and practioners raise questions of conflicts of interest.[5]

According to Dr. Nestle, financial relationships among food companies and nutrition professionals are not a new phenomenon.[5] A survey in the United States in the mid 1970s identified frequent payments by food companies to nutrition and agriculture faculties for consulting services, lectures, membership on advisory boards, and representation at congressional hearings.[7] More recently, a British study reported that 158 out of 246 members of national committees on nutrition and food policy consult for or receive funding from food companies.[8] Such relationships are so pervasive that it is virtually impossible for nutrition academics not to be recipients of food industry largesse in one way or another. As with sponsorship by tobacco or drug companies, such connections cannot help but raise questions about the ability of nutrition experts to provide independent opinions on matters of diet and public health. "I often hear nutrition colleagues state that the only way to improve the dietary intake of populations is to engage in partnerships and alliances with companies to produce more nutritious food, says Dr. Nestle.[9] "Although alliances do not necessarily imply an endorsement of the partner's products, they may well give the appearance of doing so."

The following examples taken from Dr. Nestle's commentary describe food company alliances with nutrition academics and practiners and raises further questions of conflicts of interest. In 2000, the Journal of Nutrition Education listed eight 'corporate patron friends' and four 'corporate sustaining friends who make an annual financial contribution to support the goals of the society and its journal'. In 2001, the more research-oriented Journal of Nutrition listed 11 food and drug companies as sustaining associates of its parent society, and the American Journal of Clinical Nutrition listed 28 such companies. The sponsors include companies such as Coca-Cola, Gerber, Nestle, Carnation, Monsanto, Procter & Gamble, Roche Vitamins, Slim-Fast Foods, and The Sugar Association, as well as others that make infant formula, nutritional supplements, functional foods, diet products, sugar-sweetened breakfast cereals, and genetically modified crops, all with nutritional attributes currently under active debate.

The New England Journal of Medicine and The Journal of the American Medical Association, which publish the 'hottest' of nutrition research, each receive around $20 million annually from drug company advertising, leading critics to charge that they 'are beholden to drug makers for their economic viability'.[12] The Journal of the American Dietetic Association reported $3 million in advertising in 1999, mainly from food and supplement companies.[13] To avoid suggestions that advertisers might influence the content of what gets published, journals sensitive to the issue deliberately attempt, but not always successfully, to isolate their editorial functions from interference from the business side of the publication.[14,15]

Food companies also support the publication of papers from sponsored conferences. In 2000, for example, companies such as Wyeth Nutritionals, Bristol-Myers Squibb, Mead Johnson, and the International Nut Council helped support publication of supplements to the American Journal of Clinical Nutrition. Such supplements tend to highlight the benefits of particular foods or diets in which the sponsors have some interest. This journal places the letter 's' on supplement page numbers, suggesting to knowledgeable readers that the sponsored articles may not have been subjected to the usual rigors of peer-review.[6]

Sponsorship of professional meetings can generate substantial revenue. The American Dietetic Association, for example, reported income of nearly $900 000 from its 1998 annual meeting. Thus, nutrition societies may actively seek corporate sponsorship, and companies willingly comply. Food, beverage, and supplement companies buy space at exhibits, place advertisements in program books, underwrite coffee breaks, meals, and receptions, sponsor research awards and student prizes, and provide bags, pens, and other meeting souvenirs. In return, they receive thanks in program books and get meeting participants to accept items with corporate logos both of which are forms of advertising. In the USA, the annual meeting of the American Society for Nutritional Science features a Kellogg-sponsored breakfast meeting for heads of university nutrition departments, and research sessions sponsored by such entities as the Dairy Council and the National Cattlemen's Beef Association.[6]

The American Dietetic Association acknowledged session sponsorship in its 2000 annual meeting from more than 40 food companies and trade associations, nearly all with commercial interests in the topic under discussion. The Mars company, for example, sponsored a session on phytochemicals in chocolate, Slim-Fast on obesity prevention and treatment, and Gatorade (Quaker Oats) on ergogenic aids in athletes.[6]

Does sponsorship influence the content of conference sessions? When one looks to other industries the answer is a resounding "yes". Studies of pharmaceutical industry practices show that physicians who accept travel funds, meals, or gifts, or who attend sponsored conferences are more likely to write prescriptions for the sponsor's medications. Dr. Nestle describes one investigative report revealing the deliberate nature of this strategy by vitamin companies. It describes how a vitamin manufacturer used a medical conference to generate interest in vitamins as agents of health, and notes that the company's influence on conference content was largely invisible, mainly because critics of the products had been excluded from the debate.[16] Although sponsorship of journals and conferences may not directly influence editorial content or the opinions of conference speakers, it may well do so in more subtle ways or give the appearance of doing so.[17]

Does industry sponsorship of research influence research results? A 1996 survey found nearly 30% of university faculty accepted industry funding. Another survey found 34% of the primary authors of nearly 800 papers in molecular biology and medicine to be involved in patents, to serve on advisory committees, or to hold shares in companies that might benefit from the research.[18] Indeed investigators who supported the use of drug or tobacco products were more likely to have financial relationships with such companies than neutral or critical authors. Such studies do not suggest that industry-sponsored research is always biased, just that there is a higher probability that it will draw more favorable results.[19]

Another example of this conflict of interest occurred In 1988, when the American Heart Association

(AHA), a longtime distinguished champion of research and education promoting low-fat and other dietary approaches to prevention of coronary heart disease, embarked on a program to label foods as 'heart-healthy'. The program would identify foods that met certain standards for fat, saturated fat, cholesterol, and sodium with a logo consisting of a red heart with a white checkmark and the words 'American Heart Association Tested & Approved'. Initially, the AHA planned to collect fees from companies and charging $40,000 for testing as well as an annual educational fee that ranged from $50,000 to $1 million depending on the size of the company. The proposal immediately ran into opposition from the United States Department of Agriculture. Officials became concerned that identifying single foods as heart-healthy distorted the nutritional principle that dietary patterns, not single foods, are associated with disease prevention. Officials of the Food and Drug Administration (FDA) charged that the program might interfere with the agency's efforts to develop new labeling rules.[20] Nevertheless, AHA invited 2300 makers of margarines, crackers, and frozen foods to apply for endorsement. The first 'Heart Check' foods appeared on shelves in early 1990, but representatives of seven states and two leading nutrition societies wrote to the FDA opposing the program on the grounds that promoting the health benefits of single foods was misleading.[21] When nearly two-thirds of the companies that had joined the program withdrew from participation, the AHA ended the program and agreed to return the fees it had collected.[22]

In 1994, however, the AHA tried another approach. This time, companies were to pay an initial fee of $2500 and an annual renewal fee of $650 for a seal of approval. By October 1997, 55 companies were participating, with 643 products certified. Examples include more than 50 Kellogg's products. The company advertised that it was pleased to provide consumers with 'guidance on selecting heart healthy foods', among which were such unlikely items as high-sugar Frosted Flakes, Fruity Marshmallow Krispies, and Low-Fat Pop-Tarts.[23] The current program requires a $7500 fee per product and $4500 for annual renewals, with a discount if more than 25 products are submitted in one year. Because the rules preclude endorsement of medical foods, dietary supplements, alcoholic beverages, and products owned by tobacco companies, Kellogg's Cocoa Frosted Flakes is 'heart smart', but the equivalent cereal from Post (owned by Philip Morris) is not. The program also permits advertisements extolling 'cholesterol free, fat free' Florida Grapefruit Juice as a means to fight heart disease.[24]

Another example of conflict of interest stems from the American Dietetic Association. The American Dietetic Association (ADA) represents the interests of about 70,000 nutritionists holding credentials as Registered Dietitians. Food companies employ many of its members, and its relations with the industry are especially close. ADA acknowledged donations of $735,000 from groups and individuals contributing $10,000 or more during the 1998, 1999 fiscal year, among which were 22 food product and trade associations. Overall, nearly 8% of the Association's $25 million annual income came from such grants that year. Reliance on such funding encourages perceptions that sponsorship prevents the ADA from ever criticizing the food industry. Indeed, ADA's stance on dietary advice is firmly pro industry. In 1993, the ADA collaborated with McDonald's on a campaign built around Happy Meals and toy food characters representing the major food groups.[25] The ADA journal also routinely carries a page of government nutrition news compiled by The Sugar Association.

The blurring of the distinction between food company marketing and dietary advice is most evident in the ADA's 70 or so information Fact Sheets each with its own corporate sponsor.[26] Although the ADA retains final editorial control, corporate sponsors or public relations agencies draft the content.[27]

In 2000, the ADA journal included a Kellogg's-sponsored Fact Sheet on vitamins during pregnancy, 'B smart for your heart and pregnancy with folic acid and vitamins B6 and B12'. Placed directly opposite was an advertisement for Kellogg's cereals, 'Have you heard the good news? Now many of your patients' favorite Kellogg's cereals are fortified with 100% of the Daily Value of folic acid, B6 and B12'. Such examples do not mean that the ADA ignores issues of conflicting interests. Indeed, its 1999 Code of Ethics includes a statement that 'the dietetic practitioner is alert to situations that might cause a conflict of interest or have the appearance of a conflict. The dietetics practitioner provides full disclosure when a real or potential conflict of interest arises'.[28] One journal editorial on the code correctly pointed out that 'in the world of nutrition research, a conflict of interest does not necessarily exist just because scientists receive support from a food/drug company or a government agency as long as the interests of the various groups do not conflict'. Another argued that adequate safeguards exist in the form of codes of ethics and peer review. Readers may well wonder, however, whether the Fact Sheets, or the ADA itself might express more critical views on some of the issues if they were independent of food company sponsorship.[6]

Dr. Nestle explains that the above examples were singled out for discussion not because they are necessarily more egregious than others, but because they more explicitly illustrate the potential conflicts of interests that can arise from sponsorship alliances. Given that food company sponsorship is not going to disappear, the question becomes one of establishing principles and policies that preserve genuine and perceived independence.[6]

Today, most scientists maintain that the first step in protecting against conflicting interests is disclosure of financial relationships. In the past, even when nutrition researchers were willing to disclose industry connections, they rarely were required to do so. This situation is now changing. Since 1998, the FDA has asked members of its review committees to state whether they have received stock, consulting fees, or other financial support from companies with interests in the agency's regulatory decisions, a requirement that many consider long overdue.[30] Leading science and medicine journals have begun to require financial disclosure statements from authors. The Lancet, for example, tells authors that 'the conflict of interest test' is a simple one. Is there anything that would embarrass you if it were to emerge after publication and you had not declared it? The Editor needs to be informed.[31] Nutrition publications such as the Journal of the American Dietetic Association, Journal of Nutrition, and Nutrition in Clinical Care have also instituted disclosure statements. The British Medical Journal set a gold standard. It requires its authors to submit an elaborate checklist in the hope that it will 'increase the number of authors who disclose competing interests'.[32]

Scientists Behaving Badly

Debates concerning questionable research practices and scientific integrity were linked in 1992 report by the National Academy of Sciences. The first group to provide empirical evidence based on self reports from large and representative samples of US scientists that document the occurrence of a broad range of misbehaviors was documented by C. Martinson, M. Anderson, and R de Vries. According to these researchers, we can no longer afford to ignore a wide range of questionable behavior that threatens the integrity of science. "Serious misbehavior in research damages the reputation of, and undermines public support for, science.[33] To protect the integrity of science, we must look beyond falsification, fabrication and plagiarism, to a wider range of questionable research practices," argue Brian C. Martinson, Melissa S. Anderson and Raymond de Vries.[33]

Scientists Behaving Badly was published in Nature (June, 2005). Martinson, et. al. surveyed several thousand scientists, based in the United States and funded by the National Institutes of Health (NIH), and asked them to report their own behavior. Their findings revealed a range of very questionable practices. The result of this research suggests that 'regular misbehaviors present greater threats to the scientific enterprise than those caused by high-profile misconduct cases such as fraud', reported the authors.[33] To assure anonymity, the survey responses were never linked to respondents' identities. Of the 3,600 surveys mailed to mid-career scientists, 3,409 were deliverable and 1,768 yielded usable data, giving a 52% response rate. Survey respondents were asked to report in each case whether or not ('yes' or 'no') they themselves had engaged in the specified behavior during the past three years. Overall, 33% of the respondents said they had engaged in at least one of the top ten behaviors during the previous three years. Among mid-career respondents, this proportion was 38%; in the early-career group, it was 28%. The research investigators believe that reliance on self reports actually underestimated the questionable behaviors despite assurances of anonymity. "It is now time for the scientific community to consider which aspects are most amenable to change, and what changes are likely to be the most fruitful in ensuring integrity in science," state the research authors. For more details outlining the research results published in this research visit http://www.biotech.bioetica.org/docta65.htm.[7]

Table 1 | Percentage of scientists who say that they engaged in the behaviour listed within the previous three years (n = 3,247)

Top ten behaviours	All	Mid-career	Early-career
1. Falsifying or 'cooking' research data	0.3	0.2	0.5
2. Ignoring major aspects of human-subject requirements	0.3	0.3	0.4
3. Not properly disclosing involvement in firms whose products are based on one's own research	0.3	0.4	0.3
4. Relationships with students, research subjects or clients that may be interpreted as questionable	1.4	1.3	1.4
5. Using another's ideas without obtaining permission or giving due credit	1.4	1.7	1.0
6. Unauthorized use of confidential information in connection with one's own research	1.7	2.4	0.8 ***
7. Failing to present data that contradict one's own previous research	6.0	6.5	5.3
8. Circumventing certain minor aspects of human-subject requirements	7.6	9.0	6.0 **
9. Overlooking others' use of flawed data or questionable interpretation of data	12.5	12.2	12.8
10. Changing the design, methodology or results of a study in response to pressure from a funding source	15.5	20.6	9.5 ***
Other behaviours			
11. Publishing the same data or results in two or more publications	4.7	5.9	3.4 **
12. Inappropriately assigning authorship credit	10.0	12.3	7.4 ***
13. Withholding details of methodology or results in papers or proposals	10.8	12.4	8.9 **
14. Using inadequate or inappropriate research designs	13.5	14.6	12.2
15. Dropping observations or data points from analyses based on a gut feeling that they were inaccurate	15.3	14.3	16.5
16. Inadequate record keeping related to research projects	27.5	27.7	27.3

Reprinted with permission from Brian C. Martinson, PhD and Nature Publishing Group.

RESEARCH VERSUS MARKETING

Cholesterol-lowering medications are the best-selling medicines in history and a "perfect" example of research versus marketing.[33] Used by more than 13 million Americans and an additional 12 million patients around the world, cholesterol-lowering medications produced $27.8 billion in sales in 2006. The drugs are thought to be so essential that, according to the official government guidelines from the National Cholesterol Education Program (NCEP), 40 million Americans should be taking them. Statins are sold by Merck (MRK) (Mevacor and Zocor), AstraZeneca (AZN) (Crestor), and Bristol-Myers Squibb (BMY) (Pravachol) in addition to Pfizer. And it's almost impossible to avoid reminders from the industry that the drugs are vital. A current TV and newspaper campaign by Pfizer, for instance, stars artificial heart inventor and Lipitor user Dr. Robert Jarvik. The printed ad proclaims that "Lipitor reduces the risk of heart attack by 36%...in patients with multiple risk factors for heart disease."[733]

The whole statin story is a classic case of good drugs pushed too far, argues Dr. Howard Brody, professor of family medicine at the University of Texas Medical Branch at Galveston. The drug business is, after all, a business. Companies are supposed to boost sales and returns to shareholders. The problem they face, though, is that many drugs are most effective in relatively small subgroups of sufferers. With statins, these are the patients who already have heart disease. But that's not a blockbuster market. So companies have every incentive to market their drugs as being essential for wider groups of people, for whom the benefits are, by definition, smaller. "What the shrewd marketing people at Pfizer and the other companies did was spin it to make everyone with high cholesterol think they really need to reduce it," says Dr. Bryan A. Liang, director of the Institute of Health Law Studies at the California Western School of Law and co-director of the San Diego Center for Patient Safety. "It was pseudo-science, never telling you the bottom-line truth, that the drugs don't help unless you have pre-existing cardiovascular disease." The marketing worked, Liang says, "even in the face of studies and people screaming and yelling, myself included, that it is not based on evidence."[33]

Dr. James M. Wright, a professor at the University of British Columbia and director of the government-funded Therapeutics Initiative looked at the data for the majority of patients who don't have heart disease. He found no benefit in people over the age of 65, no matter how much their cholesterol declines, and no benefit in women of any age. He did see a small reduction in the number of heart attacks for middle-aged men taking statins in clinical trials. But even for these men, there was no overall reduction in total deaths or illnesses requiring hospitalization—despite big reductions in "bad" cholesterol. "Most people are taking something with no chance of benefit and a risk of harm," says Wright.[33]

For one thing, many researchers harbor doubts about the need to drive down cholesterol levels in the first place. Those doubts were strengthened on Jan. 14, when Merck and Schering-Plough (SGP) revealed results of a trial in which one popular cholesterol-lowering drug, a statin, was fortified by another, Zetia, which operates by a different mechanism. The combination did succeed in forcing down patients' cholesterol further than with just the statin alone. But even with two years of treatment, the further reductions brought no health benefit.[33]

The second crucial point is hiding in plain sight in Pfizer's own Lipitor newspaper ad. The dramatic 36% figure has an asterisk. Read the smaller type. It says: "That means in a large clinical study, 3% of patients taking a sugar pill or placebo had a heart attack compared to 2% of patients taking Lipitor." The numbers in that sentence mean that for every 100 people in the trial, which lasted 3 1/3 years, three people on placebos and two people on Lipitor had heart attacks. The difference credited to the drug? One fewer heart attack per 100 people. So to spare one person a heart attack, 100 people had to take Lipitor for more than three years. The other 99 got no measurable benefit. Or to put it in terms of a little-known but useful statistic, the number needed to treat (or NNT) for one person to benefit is 100.[33]

Compare that with today's standard antibiotic therapy to eradicate ulcer-causing H. pylori stomach bacteria. The NNT is 1. Give the drugs to 11 people, and 10 will be cured. When Wright and others explain to patients without prior heart disease that only 1 in 100 is likely to benefit from taking statins for years, most are astonished.[73] There are reasons to believe the overall benefit for many patients is even less than what the NNT score of 100 suggests. That NNT was determined in an industry-sponsored trial using carefully selected patients with multiple risk factors, which include high blood pressure or smoking. In contrast, the only large clinical trial funded by the government, rather than companies, found no statistically significant benefit at all. Results claiming small benefits are always uncertain, says Dr. Nortin M. Hadler, professor of medicine at the University of North Carolina at Chapel Hill and a longtime drug industry critic. "Anything over an NNT of 50 is worse than a lottery ticket; there may be no winners," he argues. Several recent scientific papers peg the NNT for statins at 250 and up for lower-risk patients, even if they take it for five years or more. "What if you put 250 people in a room and told them they would each pay $1,000 a year for a drug they would have to take every day, that many would get diarrhea and muscle pain, and that 249 would have no benefit? And that they could do just as well by exercising? How many would take that?" asks drug industry critic Dr. Jerome R. Hoffman, professor of clinical medicine at the University of California at Los Angeles.[33] Drug companies and other statin proponents readily concede that the number needed to treat is high. "As you calculated, the NNT does come out to about 100 for this study," said Pfizer representatives in a written response to questions. But statin promoters have several counterarguments. First, they insist that a high NNT doesn't always mean a drug shouldn't be widely used. After all, if millions of people are taking statins, even the small benefit represented by an NNT over 100 would mean thousands of heart attacks are prevented.[33]

That's a legitimate point, and it raises a tough question about health policy. How much should we spend on preventative steps, such as the use of statins or screening for prostate cancer, that end up benefiting only a small percentage of people? "It's all about whether we think the population is what matters, in which case we should all be on statins, or the individual, in which case we should not be," says Dr. Peter Trewby, consultant physician at Darlington Memorial Hospital in Britain. "What is of great value to the population can be of little benefit to the individual. It's like buying a raffle ticket for a community charity," says Dr. Trewby. It's for a good cause, but you are unlikely to win the prize.[7]

In its written response, Pfizer did not challenge this key assertion: that the drugs do not reduce deaths or serious illness in those without heart disease. Instead, the company repeated that statins reduce the "risk of death from coronary events" and added that Wright's analysis was not published in a peer-reviewed scientific journal. "The industry is highly regulated and that every message in ads and marketing accurately reflects Lipitor's labeling and the data from the clinical trials."[33]

In an eagerly awaited trial completed in 2006, the companies compared Zetia plus a statin with a statin alone in patients with genetically high cholesterol. But the drugmakers delayed announcing the results, prompting scientific outrage and the threat of a congressional investigation. The results, finally revealed on Jan. 14, 2007 showed the combination of Zetia and a statin reduced LDL levels more than the statin alone. But that didn't bring added benefits. In fact, the patients' arteries thickened more when taking the combination than with the statin alone. Skip Irvine, a spokesman for the joint venture, says the study was small and insists there's a "strong relationship between lowering LDL cholesterol and reducing cardiovascular death." [33]

Why the mismatch? Some of the blame goes to the way results are presented. A 36% decline in heart attacks sounds more dramatic and important than an NNT of 100. "It comes as a shock to see the NNT," says Dr. Barnett S. Kramer, director of the office of medical applications of research at the National Institutes of Health. Drug companies take full advantage of this; they advertise the big percentage drops in, say, heart attacks, while obscuring the NNT. But when it comes to side effects, they flip-flop the message, dismissing concerns by saying only 1 in 100 people suffers a side effect, even if that represents a 50% increase. "Many physicians don't know the NNT," says Dr. Darshak Sanghavi, a pediatric cardiologist and assistant professor of pediatrics at the University of Massachu-setts Medical School and a fan of using NNTs.[33] If we knew for sure that a medicine was completely safe and inexpensive, then its widespread use would be a no-brainer, even with a high NNT of 100. But an estimated 10% to 15% of statin users suffer side effects, including muscle pain, cognitive impairments, and sexual dysfunction. And the widespread use of statins comes at the cost of billions of dollars a year, not just for the drugs but also for doctors' visits, cholesterol screening, and other tests. Since health-care dollars are finite, "resources are not going to interventions that might be of benefit," says Dr. Beatrice A. Golomb, associate professor of medicine at the University of California at San Diego School of Medicine.[33]

To statin critics, Americans have come to rely too much on easy-to-grasp health markers. People like to have a metric, such as cholesterol levels, that can be monitored and altered. "Once you tell people a number, they will be fixated on the number and try to get it better," says University of Texas' Brody. Moreover, "the American cultural norm is that doing something makes us feel better than just watching and waiting," says Barry. That applies to doctors as well. They are being pushed by the national guidelines, by patients' own requests, and by pay-for- performance rules that reward phy-sicians for checking and reducing cholesterol. "I bought into it," Brody says. Not to do so is almost impossible, he adds. "If a physician suggested not checking a cholesterol level, many patients would stomp out of the office claiming the guy was a quack." Yet Brody changed his mind. "I now see it as myth that everyone should have their cholesterol checked," he says. "In hindsight it was obvious. Duh! Why didn't I see it before?"[33]

What would work better? Perhaps urging people to switch to a Mediterranean diet or simply to eat more fish. In several studies, both lifestyle changes brought greater declines in heart attacks than statins, though the trials were too small to be completely persuasive. Being physically fit is also important. "The things that really work are lifestyle, exercise, diet, and weight reduction," says UCLA's Hoffman. "They still have a big NNT, but the cost is much less than drugs and they have benefits for quality of life."[33]   To complicate the picture, cholesterol is just one of the risk factors for coronary disease. Dr. Ronald M. Krauss, director of atherosclerosis research at the Oakland Re-search Institute, explains that higher LDL levels do help set the stage for heart disease by contributing to the buildup of plaque in arteries. But something else has to happen before people get heart disease. "When you look at patients with heart disease, their cholesterol levels are not that much higher than those without heart disease," he says. Compare countries, for example. Spaniards have LDL levels similar to Americans', but less than half the rate of heart disease. The Swiss have even higher cholesterol levels, but their rates of heart disease are also lower. Australian aborigines have low cholesterol but high rates of heart disease.[33] If cholesterol lowering itself isn't a panacea, why is it that statins do work for people with existing heart disease? In his laboratory at the Vascular Medicine unit of Brigham & Women's Hospital in Cambridge, Mass., Dr. James K. Liao began pondering this question more than a decade ago. The answer, he suspected, was that statins have other biological effects.[33] Since then, Liao and his team have proved this theory. First, a bit of biochemistry. Statin drugs work by bollixing up the production of a substance that gets turned into cholesterol in the liver, thus reducing levels in the blood. But the same substance turns out to be a building block for other key chemicals as well. In the body, these additional products are signaling molecules that tell genes to turn on or off, causing both side effects and benefits.[33]

Add it all together, and "current evidence supports ignoring LDL cholesterol altogether," says the University of Michigan's Hayward. In a country where cholesterol lowering is usually seen as a matter of life and death, these are fighting words. A prominent heart disease physician and statin booster fumed at a recent meeting that "Hayward should be held accountable in a court of law for doing things to kill people," Hayward recounts. NECP's Cleeman adds that, in his view, the evidence against Hayward is overwhelming.[33] But while the new analyses may rile those who have built careers around the need to reduce LDL, they also point the way to using statins more effectively. Surprisingly, both sides in the debate agree on the general approach. *For anyone worried about heart disease, the first step should always be a better diet and increased physical activity.* Do that, and "we would cut the number of people at risk so dramatically" that far fewer drugs would be needed, says Krauss. For those people who still might benefit from treatment, a recent analysis by Hayward shows that statins might better be prescribed based on patients' risk of heart disease, not on their LDL cholesterol levels. The higher the risk, the better the drugs seem to work. "If two patients have the same risk, the evidence says they get the same benefit from statins, whatever their LDL levels," Hayward says.[733]

Ways to fine-tune this approach may be coming soon. The company that first sequenced the human genome, Celera Group (CRA), has found a genetic variation that predicts who benefits from the drugs. Perhaps 60% of the population has it, says Dr. John Sninsky, vice-president of discovery research, and for everyone else, the NNT is sky-high. "It does not relate at all to your cholesterol level," Sninsky adds.[33] If the drugs were used more rationally, drugmakers would take a hit. But the nation's health and pocketbook might be better off. Could it happen? Will data on NNTs, the weak link to cholesterol, and knowledge of genetic variations change what doctors do and what patients believe? Not until the country changes the incentives in health care, says UCLA's Hoffman. "The way our health-care system runs, it is not based on data, it is based on what makes money."[7]

CRITICAL ANALYSIS OF CURRENT RESEARCH

While many professionals in the nutrition field perform research and use statistics to analyze results, many more read the results of research and apply it to the real world. Therefore it is vitally important to be able to critically analyze a research report to determine if the methods and results are valid and if they apply to you as a professional. This section will look at each of the major sections of the research report and will provide ideas for what to look for, how to apply the information, and how to determine if a specific study is worth incorporating into your work.[34]

Study Design

Table 2 summarizes the different types of studies and outlines the limitations associated with each. Simply put, the two major types of studies are descriptive and analytical.[35]

Descriptive studies are concerned with describing general characteristics of associations with a disease (smoking and lung cancer). *Descriptive* studies focus on whole populations or individuals[1].

Correlational studies (also known as population studies) refer to associations of whole populations. Correlation should not infer cause and effect. For example, humans have toe nails, finger nails, and die. Inferring cause and effect would suggest that finger nails and toe nails kill. Absurd, yes. But many individuals in the media and in science are making such "absurd" leaps. Another example of such a leap was a correlational study suggested a link between meat consumption and colon cancer.[36] When looking at large populations of women in different countries and meat consumption, this study found a direct relationship between meat consumption and increased risk for colon cancer in women. Correlational studies are useful in formulating a hypothesis, but are limited because they only look at population averages. There is no way of knowing if women who develop colon cancer even eat meat. People with high meat consumptions may also have diets high in saturated fat or low in fiber, which can be a contributing factor for the increased rate of disease.

Case reports and case series *describe* characteristics of one or a number of individuals with a given disease. For example, in 1980 five young, previously healthy homosexual men were diagnosed with a type of pneumonia seen only in older men and women whose immune systems were suppressed.[37] This unusual circumstance suggested that these individuals suffered from an unknown disease (now known as AIDS).

A third type of *descriptive* study is the cross sectional survey. Individuals are asked to complete surveys with respect to personal and demographic characteristics. The frequency of diseases are then compared to age, gender, socioeconomic and lifestyle variables. For example, individuals with cancer often have lower serum beta-carotene levels than healthy individuals of the same age and gender. However, there is no way of knowing if the low beta-carotene levels are due to the cancer or to the dietary changes associated with the debilitating effects of the disease.

Analytical studies differ from descriptive studies in that the comparison is explicit; i.e. the investigator assembles groups of individuals for the specific purpose of systematically determining whether or not the risk of disease is different for individuals exposed or not exposed to the factor of interest.

Analytical studies are classified as observational or intervention studies (clinical trials). Observational studies include case-control studies or cohort studies (retrospective or prospective studies). In a case-control study, a group who has a certain disease is compared to a group without the disease. For example, participants in a study examining the effects of artificial sweeteners and bladder cancer were interviewed to obtain information on their history of consumption of foods with artificial sweeteners[4]. One group consisted of 536 people without cancer, and the other consisted of 592 hospitalized patients with bladder cancer. The investigators found a similar proportion of individuals who had used artificial sweeteners among both groups.

In a cohort study groups of individuals are classified on the basis of the presence or absence of exposure and then followed for a specified period of time to determine the development of the disease. A retrospective study looks back in time. It involves contacting people who were recently diagnosed with a disease (pancreatic cancer) and similar people who were not diagnosed with the same disease. Both groups are asked questions concerning the exposure (caffeine). Some studies may collect blood samples or other information about possible causes of the disease. Scientists then analyze the data to see if individuals with the disease ate differently than the group without the disease with respect to the exposure (caffeine).

Retrospective studies are the only way to study rare diseases since they do not require a lot of people or a long period of time. These studies are able to focus on a specific disease, and food or lifestyle that may affect the disease; *they are a first step in establishing a relationship between a certain disease and a food or chemical.* Examples of headlines from such studies are: "Study links caffeine to increased pancreatic cancer";[28] or "Study links use of aspartame to brain tumors".[29]

Retrospective studies can be inaccurate and may contain confounding variables (other variables that may be responsible for the observed effect). Known confounding variables can be adjusted for. In the above example of caffeine and pancreatic cancer, smoking is a known confounding variable; i.e., a larger percentage of coffee drinkers smoke, hence smoking must be controlled for in the study design. There may be unknown variables that produced the increased incidence of cancer, not the caffeine (coffee drinkers may not eat as many fruits and vegetables). Another serious flaw with this type of design is that it is difficult to establish what people ate in previous years and there is a potential for what is known as recall bias-people with a diagnosed disease are more apt to investigate their disease and may report differently than people without the disease.

A prospective study is one in which data is collected on a large group of people for an extended time period and disease frequency is determined. Examples of prospective studies include: The Nurses Health Study[7] which began in 1977 and includes over 120,000 female nurses; the Framingham Heart Study which is now in its third generation and began with 6,000 men and women.[8] In this type of study there is no recall bias because data is collected before the disease develops. Individuals are asked questions concerning their present habits; hence the data is apt to be more accurate. Data can be collected periodically and more than one disease can be studied.

An example of a serious problem with this type of study is a recent headline concerning tofu and an increased rate of dementia observed in middle-aged Japanese-American men. The cited study was part of the Honolulu Asian Aging Study.[9] The data was based on two interviews, 5 years apart, and the data was self-reported. The problem is that it is impossible to know whether tofu is responsible for the slight premature aging of the brain that was observed, of there is something else about men

Table 2
Types of Study Design

	Definition	Example	Limitations
Descriptive:			
1. Correlational (descriptive)	General characteristics of associations (exspoures) with a disease in whole populations.	Per capita consumption of meat and increased rate of colon cancer in women.	Used to form a hypothesis but no way of knowing if results relate to individuals.
2. Individuals a. Case series	Characteristics of individuals with a given disease.	Five young homosexual men with pneumonia seen only in older people.	Indicates an association but no way of knowing the cause.
b. cross sectional	Frequency of disease in individuals compared to age, gender, socioeconomic and lifestyle variables.	The Health Interview Survey periodically collects info from 100,000 US individuals and disease frequency is calculated. Low serum beta-carotene levels have been associated with cancer.	No way knowing if the exposure (low serum beta-carotene) was related to the cause of the disease.
Analytical:			
1. Observational a. Case control	Group with disease (case) under study are compared to group without the disease (control).	"Bladder cancer and artificial sweeteners". One group with bladder cancer compared to a group without cancer with respect to intake of artificial sweeteners.	No way of knowing if the variable under study (artificial sweeteners) was actually responsible for the cancer.
b. Cohort	Study groups are classified on presence or absence of exposure and followed to determine development of disease.	See below	See below
• retrospective	Looks back in time. People diagnosed with a disease and people who were not diagnosed are compared as to what they ate before diagnosis.	"Study links caffeine to pancreatic cancer". Individuals with pancreatic cancer and individuals without the cancer are asked about previous caffein intake and the groups are compared.	Indicates assoication but have recall bias, and may contain confounding variables (not the caffeine but coffee drinkers may not eat fruits and vegatbles, etc.).
• prospective	Data is collected on a large group of people for an extended period and disease frequency is determined.	Honolulu-Asia Aging Study. Asian men followed for five years. Tofu associated with premature aging of the brain.	Associations may be due to other factors. Men who ate the most tofu came from poorer families which may have affected brain function.
2. Clinical Trials	Researchers randomly assign large groups of people without a specific disease to either a treatment group or a control group.	HERS Trial indicated that 4 years of HRT did not reduce risk of heart disease.	No way of knowing why. Was it the design of the study, or are there no "heart" benefits from HRT?

who eat tofu that is responsible. Researchers adjusted for age, weight, education, alcohol, smoking, etc., but did not control for childhood environment. Men who ate the most tofu tended to come from poorer immigrant families, so they may have had a poor diet which may have affected brain development, not the tofu. Hence, results from this type of study must be viewed with skepticism.

The second type of analytical study is a clinical trial. Researchers randomly assign hundreds or thousands of people without a specific disease to either a treatment group or a control group. The treatment group is given a specific diet, or supplement, and the control group is given a "look alike" or inactive placebo. The groups are followed for several years and the disease rate in each group is compared. In this type of study the researchers decide how much of the nutrient will be given to the treatment group versus the control group. This ensures that there is a sizeable difference between the groups. There is no confounding because a trial randomly assigns people to one group. These studies are relatively easy to interpret.

Clinical trials take into account the "placebo effect". Placebo effect is the measurable, observable, or felt improvement in health not attributable to treatment. Some believe the placebo effect is psychological, due to a belief in the treatment or to a subjective feeling of improvement. In other words, if people believe a product will work, there is a distinct possibility that it will. In a study of 17 asthmatics, some subjects experienced a temporary decline in lung function after breathing in a solution that they were told would make breathing more difficult but was, in fact, ordinary saline solution. According to the researchers it is common to find a placebo effect of 30% or more in people with asthma[1]. Dr. Irving Kirsch, a psychologist at the University of Connecticut, analyzed 39 studies, done between 1974 and 1995, of depressed patients treated with drugs, psychotherapy, or a combination of both. He found that 50% of the drug effect is due to the placebo response.[40] Fifty-two percent of colitis patients treated with a placebo in 11 different trials reported feeling better - and 50% of the inflamed intestines actually looked better when assessed with a sigmoidoscope.[41] When placebos are given for pain management, the course of pain relief follows what you would get with an active drug. The peak relief comes about an hour after it's administered, as it does with the real drug.[41] Hence, in scientific research the placebo effect must be controlled for if the results are to be attributed to the product.

The limitations associated with clinical trials are that they are expensive to conduct and if the trial fails it's hard to know what happened. Was it the dose, the population studied, the trial period, or the sample size? In a 1996 trial, researchers reported unexpected findings when increased lung cancer risk was found in the beta-carotene group versus the control group.[42] Beta-carotene was chosen because results from observational studies indicated that people who ate more carotene-rich fruits and vegetables had a lower risk of lung cancer. It is not known why this specific trial produced such unexpected results. Perhaps it is something else in beta-carotene rich foods that prevent cancer!

Initial research from analytical studies indicated beneficial effects of hormone replacement therapy in reducing the risk of heart disease in women. In 1995, the Postmenopausal Estrogen/Progestin Interventions Trial (PEPI)[43] reported cholesterol-lowering abilities of estrogen replacement in older women. Based on this clinical trial physicians began recommending HRT. The PEPI study was limited however, in that it provided only a short-term look at the effects of hormones on blood pressure and cholesterol metabolism. The trial was not long enough to determine whether HRT actually prevented heart disease. In 1997 The New England Journal of Medicine published an observational study conducted by researchers at Brigham and Women's Hospital that tracked the history of about 60,000 menopausal nurses over a period of 18 years.[44]   The results indicated that, on average, women who took hormone supplements for up to 10 years lowered their death rate from all causes by 37%.   The FDA never approved HRT in reduction of heart disease in women because there was not enough evidence through clinical trials to indicate benefit.   There are now 5 clinical trials that have shown no benefit of HRT in reduction of heart disease in women.   The latest clinical trial was stopped because of an increase in heart attacks or deaths due to heart disease.[45] Physicians jumped on the band wagon prematurely and now many women are paying the price.

From all types of studies, including clinical trials, legal arguments are mounting in favor of several nutrients; folic acid in the prevention of neural tube defects, vitamin D in prevention of hip fractures, and calcium in the prevention of precancerous colon polyps.   Until all the legal arguments are in, and until there is consensus among the scientific community, it may be wise to "wait and see" before jumping on any band wagon.

Questions to be Answered

Here are some questions that aid in assessing the relevancy and accuracy of research studies.
   1. What is the study design?
   2. What are the limitations associated with this type of study?
   3. Was the research published in a peer-reviewed journal? Peer review refers to the process by which the editors of a journal ask experts in a study's subject to review the study (usually 7 to 10 other experts) to ensure it was conducted appropriately. If the study was poorly designed or comes up short, it is usually not published. However, peer-review is not a guarantee that the research is unbiased.
   4. How was the study conducted? What was the sample size and duration of the study? If a study reports that the tested product builds muscle in animals, it should not be assumed that the same results will be seen in humans. Studies reporting results seen on very small populations for short time periods may not be reliable. Also, the study must begin with unbias assumptions, populations, etc.
   5. Who paid for the study? Was the study funded by the same company that sells the product being touted as a new life saving discovery?
   6. Was there a control group? To obtain reliable data, the study should be a controlled double blind study in which the subjects (and persons actually involved in distributing the product) are not informed as to whether they are given the actual product being tested or a placebo. Without a control group, there is no way of knowing if the product is actually producing the wanted results or if other variables within the group caused the wanted results.
   7. How applicable is the research. You might be interested in a weight loss drug that definitely works, but if people are dying from the drug, you need to ask yourself if looking slimmer in your coffin is really what you want.
   8. Has the research been replicated many times? If the claims are based on a single study, the advice from experts is to wait for more reliable, unbiased research to reproduce the same results. The results of multiple studies should be compared to results conducted by other researchers from reputable institutions.

Even when the research is well designed, duplicated, and safety issues have been answered, the results may not be applicable to you. Were the subjects men or women; were they athletes, or sedentary individuals; were they healthy individuals, or individuals with diseases such as diabetes, cancer, or HIV? If you are different from the experimental group, then you should not assume that the results will apply to you.

The FDA warns that fraudulent products can often be identified by the types of claims:
   1. Claims that the product is a secret cure and use terms such as breakthrough, magical, miracle cure, and new discovery.
   2. Pseudomedical jargon such as detoxify, purify, and energize to describe a product's effects. These claims are vague and hard to measure. They make it easier for success to be claimed even though nothing has been accomplished.
   3. Claims that the product can cure a wide range of unrelated diseases. No product can do that.
   4. Claims that the product is backed by scientific studies, but with no list of references or references that

are inadequate. For instance, if a list of references is provided, the citations cannot be traced, or if they are traceable, they are out of date, irrelevant, or poorly designed.

5. Claims that the supplement has only benefits-no side effects. A product potent enough to help people will be potent enough to cause side effects.

6. Accusations that the medical profession, drug companies, and the government are suppressing information about a particular treatment. It would be illogical for large numbers of people to withhold information about potential medical therapies when they and their families might one benefit from them.

7. Products that claim to be patented to provide health benefits.

Table 3 summarizes several studies using the above techniques. In the first example Mead Johnson & Company[46] used researchers at the International Diabetes Center to complete research on their energy bar. Only ten subjects were involved in the study all with differing degrees of diabetes and ranged in age from 43 to 74 years of age. Mead Johnson & Company launched a marketing and sales campaign after this research was published and dietitians received free samples along with marketing materials claiming that their bar was a healthy choice for diabetics. But from the results of the actual research a "Snickers" bar had the same results.

In the next example researchers looked at the effects of oral creatine supplementation in young healthy athletes.[47] Again the sample size was small. Eight men and 1 woman were recruited and asked how often, how much, and for how long have they been taking creatine. The amount of reported intake ranged from one to eighty grams per day. One person reported taking creatine for 5 years but the article does not indicate how much creatine that person consumed. The results indicate that there were no detrimental effects of creatine supplementation. This study, published in the ACSM journal is of such poor quality and design one has to wonder how it was approved by ten peer-reviewers. It is clear that peer-review can no longer be a criteria for judging the merits of research.

Adherence to a low carb diet in the next example shows how research can be, not only funded by a for-profit organization, but also controlled by the organization.[48] The research for this project was funded by an unlimited grant from the Atkins Group and staff members at Duke University were actually trained by the Atkins Group. Participants in this research project were given supplements which biased the results. They were given an appetite suppressant and added nutrients known to reduce cholesterol levels.

The next two examples look at research completed at the university level by companies that have developed expensive equipment.[49,50] Are these devices really as accurate as the results claim? Are you confidence that the people making the equipment can also evaluate it? Most scientists are not confident about the results.

The final example provides details of a research project in which the product being tested is not the product being used in the research. German researchers "blew the whistle" on the research authors by publishing a letter to the editor of Human Nutrition and Metabolism indicating that the manufacturer of the study concentration reported producing an "enriched" product for the study.[51]

As these examples indicate, even peer-reviewed research is suspect in today's environment of marketing versus science. As professionals we have an obligation to take a critical look at all research before accepting the results.

Table 3 - Questions to Be Answered

Research	Study Design	Conducted	Peer-Review	Limitations	Who Paid	Control Group	Results/Applicable	Replication
Reader, M. et.al - Glycemic and insulinemic response of subjects with Type II diabetes after consumption of three energy bars	Randomized 3 way crossover	7 men, 3 women given 3 different energy bars	Yes, Journal of the American Dietetic Association	small sample, large variability in subject age and length of diabetes	Reseach was paid for byMead Johnson & Co that made one of the bars	No. Used each participant as their own control	The Snickers bar and the Mead Johnson bar produced similar results in insulin values after 90 min	NO. This is a research study that Mead Johnson Quodes im marketing their bar
Long-term oral creatine supplementatin does not impair renal function in healthy athletes	Descriptive (correlational)	8 men, 1 woman self reporting of oral creatine from one to five years. What is the definition of long term? One person reported taking creatine for five years	Yes, Medicine in Science & Sports (ACSM Journal)	small sample, self reporting.	Unknown	Yes. Used 85 male sedentary subjects self reporting that they were not taking creatine supplements	No renal damage	Other similar design studies
Effect of 60month adherence to a very low carbohydrate diet program	Descriptive (correlational)	51 people put on a 6 month low carbohydrate diet with no caloric restriction.	Yes, American Journal of Medicine	Adherence self reported.Physical activity uncontrolled so no way of knowing why people lost modest results.	Unlimited grant by Atkins group given to Duke Univeristy (Dr. Westman lab) and Atkins group trained the research staff	No	Participants were told they could eat unlimited amount of protein and fat. The total daily caloric intake averaged 1500 cal. Participants were given a diet formula with an appetite suppresant and an oil formula known to reduce choleterol levels	Other similar desing studies
A new handled device for measuring resting metabolic rate and oxygen consumption	Descriptive (correlational)	RMR was measured in 63 subjects (21 to 69) using the Body Gem	Yes, Journal of the American Dietetic Association	Body Gem was compared to the Douglas Bag (no other measurements)	Paid for by the makers of the Body Gem	No	No differences in measurement between the Douglas Bag and the Body Gem.	No independent, non bias research has been done
Evaluation of air displacement for assessing body composition of collegiate wrestlers.	Descriptive (correlational)	Body composition was measured using the Bod Pod and compared to hydrostatic weighing	Yes, Medicine in Science & Sports (ACSM Journal)	Bod Pod was measured agains hydrostatic measurement which has a margin or erro	Research conducted and paid for by the makers of the Body Gem	No	Bod Pod method provides similar results for body fat as hydrostatic weighing	No independent, non bias research has been done
A mixed fruit and vegetable concentrate increases plasma antioxidant vitamins and folate and lowers plasma homocystein in men	Descriptive (correlational)	Concentratin of homocysteine were measured in 32 men.	Yes, Human Nutrition and Metabolism	The concentrate given to the study participants were "enriched" with purePlus" beta caroline, ascorbic acid, vitamin E and folic acid, which was not stated in the article	Research paid for by the makers of "Juice Plus"	No	Plasma homocystein was reduced	No independent, non bias research has been done. The manufacturers of the study capsules "blew the whistle" the whistle"

REPUTABLE RESOURCES

So, as professionals, what sources can we trust to provide us with well designed research that is published without conflicts of interest? The answer is we have to do our "homework". Several universities have excellent health letters that summarize the latest nutrition data. In most instances these universities, along with Center for Science in the Public Interest, agree on the latest nutrition research findings. It is this "consensus", along with multiple research studies indicated similar results which provides credence to the reported results. As evidence accumulates scientists begin to integrate the findings which then become accepted among the nutrition community. Over the years, the picture of what is "true" gradually changes and dietary recommendations are then reviewed and changed.

CSPI (http://www.cspinet.org/integrity/press_releases.html) publishes weekly press releases identifying possible conflict of interest and is also an excellent resource.[4]

SUMMARY

When conducting research, scientists follow what is known as the "scientific method". This method relies on identifying a problem to be solved or asks a specific question to be answered. The next step is to formulate a hypothesis (a possible solution) to the problem or answer to the question and make a prediction that can be tested through research. A study design is decided upon, the research is completed and the data is collected. The data must then be analyzed and the results interpreted. The original hypothesis is either supported by the data or is not supported. Scientists typically raise more questions so future research projects always exist.[1] In response to the commercialization of science and the growing problem of conflicts of interest, the Integrity in Science Project was developed by Center for Science in the Public Interest (CSPI). CSPI is a non-profit organization that accepts no funds from government, corporations, or special interest groups.[3]

Taking Sides presents current issues in a debate-style format designed to stimulate student interest and develop critical thinking skills. Each issue is framed with an issue summary, an issue introduction, and a postscript. The pro and con essays represent the arguments of leading scholars and commentators in their fields.[5] Dr. Marion Nestle, author of Taking Sides - Food and Nutrition, provides further examples of situations in which food company alliances with nutrition academic and practioners raise questions of conflicts of interest.[5] Scientists Behaving Badly was published in Nature (June, 2005). Martinson, et. al. surveyed several thousand scientists, based in the United States and funded by the National Institutes of Health (NIH), and asked them to report their own behavior. Their findings revealed a range of very questionable practices. The result of this research suggests that 'regular misbehaviors present greater threats to the scientific enterprise than those caused by high-profile misconduct cases such as fraud', reported the authors.[33]

While many professionals in the nutrition field perform research and use statistics to analyze results, many more read the results of research and apply it to the real world. Therefore it is vitally important to be able to critically analyze a research report to determine if the methods and results are valid and if they apply to you as a professional.

CHAPTER 10 - SAMPLE TEST

1. What is the scientific method and discuss its applicability in today's current research environment.

2. What is meant by non-profit ties to corporations and what impact does this have on modern research in nutrition?

3. What does "Taking Sides" refer to and list several examples discussed by Dr. Nestle.

4. Discuss the ten top behaviors of scientists behaving badly.

5. What is the difference between research and marketing?   Provide details.

6. What are the steps involved in critical analysis of research?

7. Analyze a recent research paper using the steps involved in critical analysis.

REFERENCES

1. Whitney,E. Rolfes,S. Understanding Nutrition, 11th Ed. Thompson Wadsworth, 2008.

2. http://www.cspinet.org/integrity/about.html.

3. http://www.cspinet.org/integrity/challenging.html.

4. http://www.cspinet.org/integrity/liftingtheveil.html.

5. Nestle, M. Dixon, B. Taking sides - Food and Nutrition. McGraw-Hill/Duskin, 2003.

6. Nelson, Public Nutrition Commentary. Public Health Nutrition: 4(5), 1015,1022 DOI: 10.1079/PHN2001253.

7. Rosenthal B, Jacobson M, Bohm M. Feeding at the company trough. Congressional Record, August 26, 1976; H897,7.

8. Cannon G. The Politics of Food. London: Century Hutchinson, 1987.

9. Dietary Guidelines Alliance. Reaching Consumers with Meaningful Health Messages: A Handbook for Nutrition and Food Communicators. Chicago, IL: Dietary Guidelines Alliance, 1996.

10. Owen BM, Braeutigam R. The Regulation Game: Strategic Use of the Administrative Process. Cambridge, MA: Ballinger, 1978;7.

11. Nestle M. Food Politics: How the Food Industry Influences Nutrition and Health. Berkeley, CA: University of California Press, 2002 (in press).

12. Shell ER. The Hippocratic wars. New York Times Magazine, June 28, 1998; 3,8.

13. American Dietetic Association and American Dietetic Association Foundation. 1999 ADA/F Annual Report [Online]. Available: http://www.eatright.org/ (2000, 13 Apr).

14. Angell M. Is academic medicine for sale? N. Engl. J. Med. 2000; 342: 1516,8.

15. Altman LK. New England Journal of Medicine names third editor in a year. New York Times, May 12, 2000; A20.

16. Wazana A. Physicians and the pharmaceutical industry: is a gift ever just a gift? JAMA 2000; 283: 373,80.

17. Wilde P. Media coverage spurs fad for vitamin pills, after year-long industry effort. Nutrition Week, May 22, 1992;1,6.

18. Krimsky S, Rothenberg LS, Kyle G, Stott P. Financial interests of authors in scientific journals: a pilot study of 14 14 publications. Sci. Eng. Ehics 1996;2:395-410.

19. Bero LA, Barnes D. Industry affiliations and scientific conclusions [letter]. JAMA 1998; 280: 1142.

20. Parachini A. Food fight: Heart Association plan to label 'healthy' foods drawing fire from agencies, nutritionists. Washington Post, August 2, 1988; E1, E6.

21. State attorneys general support FDA position on AHA HeartGuide label. Nutrition Week, February 8, 1990; 1.

22. Angier N. Heart Association cancels its program to rate foods. New York Times, April 3, 1990; A1, C6.

23. Kellogg Company. Letter in press release addressed to Dear Health Professional. Battle Creek, MI, February, 1997.

24. Burros M. Additives in advice on food. New York Times, November 15, 1995; C1, C5. 1020 M Nestle

25. McDonald's Corporation. American Dietetic Association and McDonald's partner to teach kids the fundamentals of nutrition [news release]. Oak Brook, IL, February 24,1993.

26. American Dietetic Association. Nutrition Fact Sheets Online]. Available: http://www.eatright.org/

(1997, November 15; 2000, April 10).

27. Gallagher A. Taking a stand on emerging issues. J. Am. Diet. Assoc. 2000; 100: 410.

28. American Dietetic Association. Code of ethics for the profession of dietetics. J. Am. Diet. Assoc. 1999; 99: 109,13.

29. McNutt K. Conflict of interest. J. Am. Diet. Assoc. 1999; 99: 29,30.

30. Stolberg SG. New rules will force doctors to disclose ties to drug industry. New York Times, February 3, 1998; A12.

31. The Lancet. Writing for The Lancet [Online]. Available: http://www.thelancet.com/ (2000, 10 Apr).

32. British Medical Journal. Declaration of competing interest: guidance for authors [Online]. Available: http:// www.bmj.com/guides (1999, 17 Jul).

33. Nature. Vol 435(9). June 2005; http://www.biotech.bioetica.org/docta65.htm

34. http://allpsych.com/researchmethods/criticalanalysis.html

35. Hennekins CH, Buring JE. 1987. *Epidemiology in Medicine*. Boston,MA: Little, Brown and Company.

36. Armstrong BK, et al. 1975. Environment factors and cancer incidence and mortality in different countries. *Int J Cancer*,15:617.

37. Center for Disease Control. 1981. *Pneumocystic* pneumonia—Los Angeles. *M.M.W.R.*,30:250.

38. LaVecchiaC ,et al. 1987. Coffee consumption and risk of pancreatic cancer. *Int J Cancer*,40(3);309-13.

39. Gurney JG, et al. 1997. Aspartame consumption in relation to childhood brain tumor risk. *J Natl Cancer Inst*,89(14):1072-4.

40. Kirsh, I, Sapirstein, G. Listening to Prosac but hearing placebo: A meta-analysis of antidepressant medication. Prevention & Treatment. Vol 1, June 1998.

41. Talbot, M. The Placebo Prescription. New York Times Magazine, January 9, 2000.

42. Prior A, et al. 2000. Beta carotene: from biochemistry to clinical trials. Nutrition Review, 58(2pt1):39-53 Review.

43. The Writing Group for the PEPI Trial. 1995. Effects of estrogen or estrogen/progestin regimens on heart disease risk factors in postmenopausal women. The Postmenopausal Estrogen/Progestin Interventions (PEPI) Trial. *JAMA*,273(3):199-208.

44. Grostein, F, et al. 1997. Postmenopausal hormone therapy and mortality. New Eng J of Med, 336(25)1769-75.

45. Grady, D, Etal. 2000. Postmenopausal hormone therapy increases risk for venous thromboembolic disease. Ann Intern Med, 132(9):690-696.

46. Reader,M. B. O'Connell et.al. 2002. Glycemic and insulinemic response of subjects with type 2 diabetes after consumption of three energy bars. Journal of the ADA.Vol 102,8:1139.

47. Poortmans,J. M. 1999. Francaux. Long-term oral creatine supplementatin does not impair renal functin in halthy athletes. Med & Sci in Sports & Exercise. 0195-993108-1108.

48. Westman, E. W. Yancy, et.al. 2002. Effect of 6-month adherence to a very low carbohydrate diet program. Am. J Med. 113:30-36.

49. "A handheld device for measuring resting metabolic rate - Assessment and Treatment of Obesity". Nutrition Research Newsletter. May 2003. FindArticles.com. 25 Jan. 2008. http://findarticles.com/p/articles/mi_m0887/is_5_22/ai_102519790.

50. Utter,A. Gross,F. et al. *Evaluation of Air Displacement for Assessing Body Composition of Collegiate Wrestlers*. Medicine & Science in Sports & Exercise. 35(3):500-505, March 2003.

51. Letter to the editor: http://jn.nutrition.org/cgi/content/full/133/11/3725.

Nutrition for Professionals

Part 2

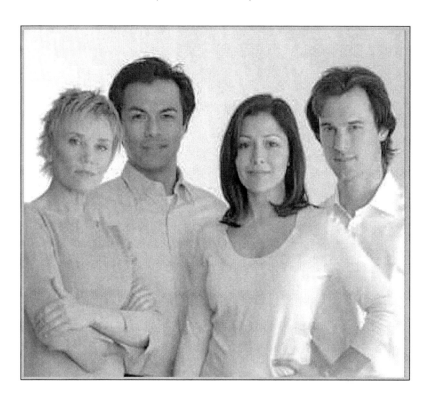

Incorporating Nutrition

Chapter 11
Prerequisites

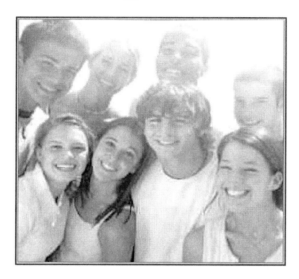

This chapter will focus on critically important considerations before embarking on a nutrition program. These considerations include legal issues, choosing an appropriate client base, discussion of a scope of practice, and discerning the skills necessary for successful implementation of a nutrition program.

Objectives

After reading and studying this chapter, you should:

1. Be able to describe the legal issues involved with implementing a nutrition program.

2. Discuss a scope of practice for implementing a safe and effective nutrition program.

3. Discuss the skills necessary for successful implementation of a nutrition program, including required coaching skills and the Stages of Readiness to Change.

INTRODUCTION

Forty-one states have laws that regulate the profession of dietetics and nutrition. Implementation of any nutrition program by professions other than dietetics requires a thorough understanding of these laws.

The question becomes why fitness professionals and not dietitians? After all, dietitians are the "nutrition experts." The reason lies in the fact that the dietetics profession is clinical in nature and not wellness driven. Dietitians have a degree in clinical nutrition and must obtain wellness/fitness education after receiving their dietetics degree. The basic educational requirement in a dietetics program is a bachelor's degree with a major in dietetics, foods and nutrition, food service systems management, or a related area. Students take courses in foods, nutrition, institution management, chemistry, biology, microbiology, and physiology. Other courses are business, mathematics, statistics, computer science, psychology, sociology, and economics. There are 227 ADA-approved bachelor's degree programs[1] and all are clinically based.

Fitness professionals are the "ideal" professionals to incorporate nutrition in conjunction with their fitness/wellness programming because of their fitness background.   They simply need to obtain a basic knowledge of nutrition. Upon having obtained the appropriate nutrition education, they can either work directly with a qualified professional or use materials developed by a qualified professional.

The need is too great for any one profession to solve the problem of obesity. The problem is not being resolved by the medical community or the dietetics community. "Allied health professionals must become involved if we are to resolve the obesity problem," states former Secretary of Health and Human Services, Tommy Thompson. Health care organizations are trying, but their main focus is, and always has been, illness; they are not equipped to take on the role of prevention. Tommy Thompson has asked all allied health professionals to take an active role in reducing obesity at the community level; hence fitness professionals can provide a solution to the growing obesity epidemic.[2]

The next step is for the fitness profession to encourage, rather than discourage, the implementation of nutrition programs by qualified fitness professionals. This chapter will discuss the types of regulations involved, outline a nutrition scope of practice for fitness professionals and provide details on the prerequisites required before implementing a nutrition program.

LEGAL CONSIDERATIONS

State regulations fall into the following categories: licensure; statutory certification; or registration. These terms are defined as:[1]

· Licensure - statutes include an explicitly defined scope of practice, and performance of the profession (nutrition / weight management) is illegal without first obtaining a license from the state. Hence it is illegal to provide nutrition or weight management in these states without a license. There is a provision, however, that allows a person to provide weight control services provided the program is developed and monitored by a licensed professional; and provided the individual does not change the program.

· Statutory Certification - limits use of particular titles to persons meeting predetermined requirements, while persons not certified can still practice the occupation or profession. Individuals in these states may provide weight management and nutrition services without being licensed; however, individuals may not use the term dietitian or licensed dietitian without adequate credentials.

· Registration - is the least restrictive form of regulation. Unregistered persons are permitted to practice the profession. Individuals in these states may provide weight management and nutrition services without being licensed.

However, the laws governing nutrition education are skewed and politically motivated. While most states have licensure laws providing details about qualifications required for individuals providing nutrition education, these same legal requirements provide clauses that allow individuals in health food stores to provide nutrition education with absolutely no qualifications. Also, there are no limitations on writing nutrition and diet books. So anyone can write a book dealing with nutrition with absolutely no nutrition background whatsoever.

Illinois is one example of a state with a "licensure" law. In 1991 Illinois passed The Dietetic and Nutrition Services Practice Act - which regulates and defines the scope of practice in nutrition.[4]

"Any person who practices, offers to practice, attempts to practice, or holds oneself out to practice dietetics or nutrition counseling without being licensed under this Act shall, in addition to any other penalty provided by law, pay a civil penalty to the Department in an amount not to exceed $5000 for each offense as determined by the Department. Exemptions: Any person licensed in the state of Illinois under any other ACT engaging in the practice for which he or she is licensed; the practice of nutrition services by a person who is employed by the U.S. government; any person providing oral nutrition information as an operator or employee of a health food store or business that sells health products, including dietary supplements, food, or food materials, or disseminating written nutrition information in connection with the marketing and distribution of those products; THE PRACTICE OF NUTRITION SERVICES BY ANY PERSON WHO PROVIDES WEIGHT CONTROL SERVICES, provided the nutrition program has been reviewed by, consultation is available from, and no program change can be initiated without prior approval by, an individual licensed under this ACT, a dietitian or nutrition counselor licensed in another state that has licensure requirements to be at least as stringent as the requirements by this Act, or a registered dietitian. The Illinois law goes on to itemize other details not relevant to this discussion."

Connecticut is an example of a state with a "certification" regulation. Under this law persons not certified can still practice the occupation or profession of nutrition, but may not use particular titles, such as dietitian, certified dietitian, or licensed dietitian.[6]

While states such as CT allow non-licensed professionals to provide weight management and nutrition services, it is not recommended for professional and legal reasons. As health professionals we take an oath to do nor harm. Providing nutrition services without adequate professional supervision could result in harm; and while it may be legal in some states, an individual could be held liable if an incident occurred because of inaccurate of damaging advice provided. Supervision from a sufficiently trained, licensed professional is required to maintain professional status among the fitness and nutrition community.

SCOPE OF PRACTICE

For the previously mentioned reasons all fitness professionals should provide a program under the direct supervision of a licensed dietitian; or provide a program that has been reviewed by, in consultation with, or directly approved by a sufficiently qualified, licensed dietitian/nutritionist.

The American Academy of Sports Dietitians and Nutritionists (AASDN) is a non-profit organization dedicated to providing fitness professionals with a scope of practice for implementing nutrition programs. The goal of this *National Nutrition Scope of Practice for Health and Fitness Professionals* is to eliminate confusion as to the scope and depth of nutrition information that can be administered legally, safely, ethically, and professionally by all health and fitness professionals nationwide.[6]

Why a specific scope of practice for health and fitness professionals? Frustration and confusion exists in the health and fitness profession when it comes to nutrition education, advice, and services that can be provided, not only legally, but professionally as well. Some fitness professionals provide nutrition education based solely on "anecdotal data", while other more qualified professionals are afraid to provide information because they have been told it is beyond their scope of practice.

The goal of this scope of practice is to provide health and fitness professionals with clear, concise, and professional standards for inclusion of nutrition in conjunction with fitness/wellness programs. These guidelines adhere to all state licensure laws and ADA guidelines.

In order to adhere to professional and legal issues, the *National Nutrition Scope of Practice for Health and Fitness Professionals* provides "standards" on several critical issues. One standard deals with supplements; another standard deals with minimal education requirements; and a third standard deals with working in conjunction with qualified professionals.

According to the scope of practice by AASDN, all fitness professionals must avoid conflicts of interest by not recommending, endorsing, or selling supplements of any kind. Fitness professionals are well aware of the legal issues associated with recommending and selling drugs and the serious consequences associated with drugs. Supplements, while legal, should be viewed with the same cautionary guidelines.

As discussed in detail in chapter 9, supplements are not regulated and have caused serious harm and even death. Law suits have been initiated and damages have been awarded against fitness professionals. A court awarded millions of dollars to the family of Anne Capati.[7] Ann arrived at her gym on October 1, 1998. Her new job as a director of a design group at The Limited was demanding, and 37 year old Anne, was proud of herself for being able to stick with her exercise regimen in spite of her long hours. She had already lost 15 pounds—weight she had trouble losing since the birth of her second child. Once in the gym, Anne complained to her trainer (40 year old August Casseus) that her head hurt; it had been throbbing for days. She began doing light squats as he instructed and after a few minutes she felt nauseated and dizzy. She put the weight bar down, vomited, and passed out. Anne was taken to the hospital. Anne's trainer told the emergency room doctor that Anne had been taken an ephedra based product. Anne died at 9:30 that evening leaving a husband and two children. Ten days later, Ann's husband, Doug, found a handwritten sheet of instructions in his wife's gym bag that listed a diet plan from Anne's trainer. The plan listed several supplements, including Thermadrene. That night Doug researched ephedra on the internet and found that ephedra had been implicated in other deaths. Ann had hypertension and should have never taken an ephedra based product. There was a warning on the label not to take the product if you had health problems. In June of 1999 Doug filed a $40 million wrongful-death suit against Crunch Fitness, August Casseus, The Vitamin Shoppe and four manufacturers of ephedra products.

So who was found responsible? The courts found the Crunch club liable and awarded millions of dollars to the Capati family. The court also found the personal trainer liable and again awarded the family millions of dollars. Why? The court determined that when an individual enters a health club there is an assumption of safety; and when a person hires a personal trainer the same assumption exists. Even though there was a warning on the label, both the club and personal trainer were held liable. Other lawsuits have been filed and large sums of money awarded. For this reason, AASDN scope of practice recommends that fitness professionals remove themselves from any association with supplements and drugs.

According to AASDN, the practice of nutrition in conjunction with fitness programming must also include minimal education requirements. Fitness professionals can obtain the proper education through collegiate courses, continuing education courses and a certification in nutrition.

Also for legal reasons, AASDN recommends that implementation of nutrition in conjunction with fitness programming must include programs that have been developed by, or reviewed by, and in consultation with, a licensed dietitian/nutritionist. No program change can be initiated without prior approval by a licensed dietitian/nutritionist. No program can be modified or altered in any way without approval by a licensed dietitian/nutritionist. This standard recommends that all health/fitness professionals use only materials developed by a qualified, licensed professional. Those materials can not be changed without proper approval from the qualified professional. The health/fitness professional, in conjunction with the licensed nutrition professional, may provide clients with more specialized services including educational information through lectures, articles, and classes. Also in conjunction with a licensed professional, they may provide energy calculations, analyze food intake, and provide pre-approved menu plans for the apparently healthy, exercising population.

Nothing in the standards authorizes the health/fitness professional to diagnose disease, or make nutritional recommendations for individuals requiring special dietary needs. Nothing in the standards authorizes the health/fitness professional to provide such services without direct approval and in consultation with a licensed dietitian/nutritionist.

Choosing a Qualified Dietitian

Choosing a qualified professional to oversee fitness programs is of utmost importance. It must not be assumed that all dietitians have the appropriate background to institute a wellness program, or have the appropriate background to oversee health and fitness programs. Dietitians are allowed to advertise a wellness "specialty" on the ADA website but are not required to indicate any experience or education. Hence, it should not be assumed that a dietitian has knowledge or experience in wellness or fitness. Dietitians wishing to work in a wellness venue must obtain further education upon graduation.   It is also recommended that dietitians obtain a fitness certification. Visit www.aasdn.org for more details.

REQUIRED SKILL - COACHING

Working with clients requires a working knowledge of coaching skills. This section will not make you a coaching expert; but it will provide you with some "Essentials of Coaching for Fitness Professionals".[4]

You've obviously heard about coaching by this point in your career. There are business coaches, career coaches, relationship coaches—you name the field, there seems to be a coach for it. But what is coaching? The definition is a concisely worded description of this powerful concept: Coaching is a co-creative partnership between a qualified coach and a willing client that supports the client through desired life changes.[4]

The key to this definition is the term "co-creative". In coaching, you are not the expert in your client's life. You work with your client to discover solutions to their wellness challenges as they emerge through discussion and exploration. Therefore, coaching is very different from athletic or personal training, nutrition consulting, or traditional therapy or counseling.[4]

In personal training, athletic training, or nutrition consulting sessions, you are the expert, you have the information or answers, and you educate your client by passing on that information or those answers. The client is more like a sponge waiting to soak up your expertise, not a creative partner who is equally involved in the informing process.[4]

For example: A nutrition consultant might use an intake food diary of a client to work up a list of possible areas for improvement, such as reducing saturated fat intake. The nutrition consultant would then decide that the client's next session would be geared toward educating the client about saturated fat and its health effects, in hopes that the client would see the benefit in reducing the amount of saturated fat she eats. Whereas in coaching, the coach would see an elevated intake of saturated fats, and then ask the client what, if anything, he/she is willing to change about it. If the client did not see that an elevated saturated fat intake was harmful, or did not feel a need to change that part of his/her lifestyle, the coach might ask if the client were open to being educated about the effects of saturated fat, but if the client said "no," nothing would be done at that time. The coach could broach the topic again at an appropriate time when the client expressed an interest in making a healthy change regarding fat intake.[4]

Just a special note here about coaching in a wellness profession. Because you are already an established expert in your profession—whether it be nutrition, fitness, or athletic training—you are endowed with the knowledge that a lot of your coaching clients will seek as they make and set wellness goals. In life or business coaching, the coach does not have a high level of expertise in the wellness arena. If their clients want help with health related issues, their clients must set goals to seek out and retain help from wellness experts such as yourself. But since you're the coach, when and how do you decide to provide the wellness expertise that your client needs? The answer is easy: You only provide information that your client requests in relation to goals. If your client expresses a desire to work with a trainer, and you are a trainer, you can offer your services. If he/she needs specific information about cholesterol, you can provide that to. But these requests for your expertise MUST come from the client, and they must be spelled out in the weekly coaching goals. You must almost play "split personality" as you coach a client that you are also providing with wellness direction. But being a wellness coach gives you a special opportunity that other coaches do not have—the chance to be that much more involved in your client's progress. You don't have to refer to a different professional and hope for the best—you ARE the referred professional! This alone sets wellness coaching apart from other types of coaching. [4]

Counseling vs. Coaching

Coaching is different from psychological counseling or "therapy" in three very important ways. One, in counseling or therapy it is assumed that something is "wrong" with the client. Two, a counselor or therapist is assumed to "know what's wrong and how to fix it" based on a body of knowledge that the client can be compared against. And three, counseling and therapy look to the PAST to try to help explain WHY a client acts a certain way in the present, or how a client's past actions have contributed to a present situation.[4]

None of this is true in coaching. In coaching, a coach does not know what the client needs—only the client knows what he/she needs. The client comes to the coach for help in making clear choices and be supported in making positive changes. And in coaching, it is always assumed (unless proven otherwise) that the client is mentally healthy and is capable of making responsible, reasonable choices. If a potential client presents with a diagnosed mental health disorder, psychological counseling may be more appropriate than coaching, and a professional referral should be made. It's best to have at least one referral source in your address file before you begin offering coaching services, just in case.[4]

Finally, coaching is focused on the present and the future. We don't want to help clients relive the past—we want to help them see a different, healthier future! Instead of helping clients explain their past or current behaviors, we help them create and practice new behaviors that lead to new outcomes. For example, if a client were overweight, a therapist might delve into the client's past relationship with an abusive lover, which led the client to eat as a source of comfort. Whereas in coaching, a coach would not get into these reasons for overeating, but would instead encourage the client to be aware of eating patterns and help him/her start to add small, healthier changes in eating habits, one step at a time, until they become a normal part of the client's routine—no matter what the previous reasons for overeating were. Thus, therapy focuses on understanding habits, while coaching works to actively change them![4]

Coaching is also a successful means for achieving wellness goals because coaches assume their clients are mentally healthy and actually able to change themselves. Unlike a therapist, who assumes a client is flawed and needs fixing, a coach believes wholeheartedly in the power the client has within to make choices that can be benefit her for the rest of her life.[4]

And one of the most important ways coaches help clients access this skill is by asking meaningful questions. Coaching is ALL about asking questions—until the client comes up with her own, individually appropriate answers. By doing so, the coach is handing over the responsibility for the client's actions to the CLIENT. And this leads us to probably the most crucial feature of coaching—clients are responsible for the actions they perform while involved in a coaching program. The coach is supportive and informative, but only the client can be held accountable for reaching weekly, monthly, and long-term goals because the client actually decides on these goals herself. No one is telling her what to do or how to do it. This is where most wellness professionals find a bit of resistance and confusion from their clients—and even amongst themselves! After years of always taking control of a client's well-being and making all the choices, and sometimes taking the blame, for a client's success or failure, this time it is up to the client to make her program successful. The coach is there to ask questions so the client becomes very clear on the path that will work.[4]

And in order to help the client on this likely totally new path, the coach must listen and truly hear the client, and totally support the client as he/she tries new paths to obtain the desired outcomes.

Listening is an "art". First, you must not think, plan, or wonder while the client is speaking—your job is just to listen. Turn off the expert in your brain, and focus on what's being said by the client. Remember, you have only known your client for a short period of time. You don't have the answers - the client does! So when listening, first, connect fully with the client. This is easy if you have the proper mindset. Your client is a human being with dreams and goals, and you must believe in his/her ability to effect change. Next, you must be "present". It's amazing what you can hear people say when you—your history, your knowledge, your assumptions—don't exist. Keep in mind that silence is your best friend in many coaching moments. From silence, come answers. What kind of answers come from silence? The client's answers! In successful coaching the client has the answers. The coach is simply a partner that supports a willing client through desired lifestyle changes.[4]

IDENTIFYING CLIENTS

So why is coaching so effective in helping people make healthy life changes? First and foremost, coaches (or smart coaches) only choose to work with clients who are ready to change. In the initial client screening process, you will want to be diligent about weeding out those clients who really are not ready to take responsibility for their choices and actions.[4]

If you want to run a successful coaching business, built around successful and enthusiastic clients, you need to make one major judgment when first meeting a potential client: Is this person ready to change or not? It's very likely that 90% of the people that come to you will be ready to change something—that's why they made the choice to call you in the first place! But some people might not understand that coaching actually requires them to act—not just sit idly by while you spew information at them and allow them to blame other people for their unhealthy condition.[4]

Stages of Readiness to Change

The Stages of Readiness to Change, made famous by Dr. James Prochaska, is a useful tool to see if this person has what it takes to be your client.[4]

Precontemplation Stage

The precontemplation stage is the stage in which the client is not yet ready to change. The client may deny that there is a problem (Yes, I'm overweight and my doctor wants me to lose weight, but we all need to die from something); blame someone else for the problem (It's my spouse's fault that I can't stick to a healthy regimen); or blame themselves (I can't make any positive changes in my life). Most often, the problem is identified by a doctor, family member or friend. Offering a fitness prescription at this stage is contraindicated. It will merely frustrate you and place you into a no-win situation.

It's actually pretty easy to identify clients who are not ready to change. When you begin communicating with the potential client, you will hear excuses, usually lots of excuses, when you ask "What seems to be the matter that you'd like to change?" Keep your ears open for the blame in their responses: Who is responsible for their condition? Is it time, or lack of time, that's to blame? Their job? Their boss? Husband? Kids? Who or what is the reason they use to take the responsibility for their condition off of their own shoulders? If you hear the blame game from the beginning, the potential client is probably not a potential client at all. You can feel comfortable saying to this person, "I hear you are frustrated with your situation, but unless you can take the responsibility for your current habits and situation, I can't help you. Can you tell me what you can do to change your current situation to make it better for your health?" And then let them think about it. If they come up with some solid answers that reveal that they, themselves, need to change some things, then there is a glimmer of hope.

Contemplation Stage

The contemplation stage is characterized by ambivalence. One easy way to tell if a client is ready to

---

STAGES OF READINESS TO CHANGE[7]

1. Precontemplation
    Client is not ready to change
    May deny or blame someone else for their problem

2. Contemplation
    Thinking about change
    Ambivalence is the key here

3. Preparation
    Getting ready to change
    Developing the fitness prescription with the client

4. Action
    Ready to make changes
    Putting the fitness prescription into actual behaviors

5. Maintenance
    Maintain behavior changes
    Ways to support the behavior

6. Relapse and Recycling
    Slipping into old behavior patterns and trying to
    resume fitness prescription
    Ways to rebuild motivation and support

---

change a behavior is to listen to him/her speaking about the behavior.   For example, if you hear a client say that he/she has tried a certain diet plan, but it's not working and would like some other ideas, then that client is actively seeking solutions to the problem and is in the preparation phase. If, however, the client is not interested in changing his/ her high-fat diet and blames the parents for too many desserts, that client is precontemplative and is not able to be helped with that habit. If the client is not sure—expressing desire to change, accompanied by fear and doubt that changes will actually work—then this client is a contemplator. This client can be educated about the potential for change, the causes of the fear, and the concept of practicing until something fits. This client may well be a great client after a bit more understanding about the process of change.[4]

Preparation Stage

This stage is characterized by the client's asking for advise on what to do in order to make healthy lifestyle changes. This is the window of opportunity. The client becomes less defensive and more willing to discuss modification of current behavior. He or she will begin to make self-motivational statements such as "I need to do something".   This is where a fitness prescription devised with the help of the client becomes beneficial. This is the stage that feels rewarding because clients are beginning to take charge of their health. It is not to say that all will run smoothly, but there is a definite feeling of motivation.

Action Stage

The action stage is that wonderful stage where we see behaviors that indicate positive lifestyle changes. If the client has been a partner in developing the plan, he or she is more likely to buy into the plan and make it work. Our role in this stage is to reinforce and affirm the client's commitment to change. We may need to modify the fitness prescription if the client has areas of difficulty.

Maintenance Stage

Maintenance is helping the client to maintain positive lifestyle changes. This may include the need to vary the fitness prescription. Strategies in this stage may require different strategies than those used in the Action Stage. Ambivalence may reappear at this stage. I've had clients who have had to work through the loss of old bad habits. They are aware of the old habits as being unhealthy (the midnight refrigerator raids), but there is still a need to mourn the loss. Support and reaffirmation at this time is critical.

Relapse and Recycling

Any change in behavior takes with it the possibility of relapsing into old, established behaviors. The key to success is helping the client to understand that relapse is a part of developing permanent behavior changes. It is important that we don't add to the client's guilt over relapsing into old behaviors. Our role is to help them analyze stumbling blocks and reframe the experience as a learning tool. Helping the client navigate through this stage requires that we assist them in coping with feelings of failure. We go back to the preparation stage with them and renegotiate a plan. What was it that worked for them in the past and what didn't? What small changes can be made to reinforce self-efficacy?

One way to test what stage a client is at is by questioning. 1. Are you able to make changes? 2. Why is now the time to change? 3. Is it possible to try new habits? 4. Is it impossible or just difficult to change? 5. What will changing do for you? 6. What will happen if you don't change? The first answer must contain a personally relevant reason, something that is emotionally meaningful to the client. They may give you an external reason at first (such as "My doctor told me to"). But keep asking the question, stressing "Why do YOU feel it's time to change?" Your goal is to see if they have a real, internal reason for changing. The second answer must be YES, or some indication of willingness to try. The third answer must be YES.[4]

The fourth answer must be "just difficult!" If she says "impossible," she's not ready to change! The fifth answer must usually be reality-checked by the coach. We must listen for any grandiose ideas of major life improvements coming from small body-centered changes. Listen to what the client says, and decide if this is the kind of client you can work with or not. If the expected outcomes seem far-fetched to you, ask if the results expected are realistic. Challenge the client until expectations be-come more realistic.[4] The sixth answer must be free of all-or-nothing thoughts, like suicide. In such cases, referral to a psychologist may be recommended. Listen for emotionally charged answers, such as "I will hate myself," or "I might not live to see my granddaughter graduate high school, and I don't want that!" If an emotion is driving the decision, the client can likely do the work that a coaching relationship involves. But again, reasons must be personally powerful and relevant.[4]

It should be obvious at this point that the client is part of the reason coaching works, too! In a successful coaching relationship, the client: Truly wants to make life changes; accepts responsibility for choices, actions, and consequences; is not afraid to try; understands that failure is not a personal flaw; learns to change thinking patterns and habits.[4]

When a potential client comes to you and says "I really want to change—what do I need to do?" Then you have the makings for a beautiful coaching relationship. The desire to change is the first key to making changes that stick![4]

The next major key to success is a willingness on the client's part to take responsibility for actions. And in so doing, can't be afraid to try new methods. The client can't continue to believe—as most people do, especially those who try diet plans—that a failed plan is an indication of failure as a person. Nothing could be further from the truth. The successful coaching client must understand that trying and failing are part of making life changes—and the client must be willing to keep at it![4] Finally, in order to make lasting changes in a client's life, both the coach and client must understand that a complete change in the way the client thinks must occur. Coaching works because a coach reinforces healthy and effective ways of thinking and acting. And a client feels the ramifications of acting and thinking in unhealthy, unproductive ways. For example, if a client believes he/she is a failure and that nothing will ever work, he/she is right! But if the client believes he/she can try anything, and that is bound to succeed at some point, he/she is also right! As coaches, it's our job to make it very clear that what the client thinks will truly shape reality. It's the client's job to then believe in their own capacity to succeed in healthy changes.[4]

Understanding the change process

We, like all animals, learn how to act by imitating our parents and those people we are exposed to in our early years. Unlike animals, who act clearly on the instinct that will keep them alive, we humans can choose actions at any time that clearly act against our own survival! People eat too much, drink too much, and let their bodies go to waste—which animals would never do because they are hardwired to act only for survival. So as a baby human, we can be exposed to habits and actions from our parents that are NOT healthy, and not conducive to our wellbeing. Unfortunately, as babies and small children, we don't know enough to differentiate between healthy and unhealthy habits. So we take everything we are shown, and we adopt it as our own. And only later, as thinking adults, can we choose healthier habits based on what we want our lives, bodies, and futures to be like.[4]

So we have to remind—and usually convince—our clients that they CAN and should choose habits and outcomes that work for them. If something isn't working in a client's life, the client must be able to see that it is a choice to change the actions that lead to that outcome. For example, if the client's family overate and the client learned poor eating habits that lead to excess weight gain, he/she needs to see that he/she can choose to learn better eating habits that will lead to weight loss—IF that truly is the goal. Clients must see that, as an adult, they have every possibility to change any habit they have ever learned—it just takes work and time. And the coaching relationship is a safe, effective place to undertake such work.[4]

As humans, we are mammals with survival instincts. Our instinct, genes, physical makeup—whatever you want to call it—is set to keep us alive. And one of the keys to staying alive in any environment is knowing what's coming. If you can predict what will happen when certain actions take place, you can control the outcome of such actions in your favor. For example, if you know that when you are really stressed out and you eat ice cream, you feel sedated and full, you will eat ice cream. If you have never just taken a walk or written in your journal when you feel stressed, you will have no idea how you will feel afterward and you will be wary and even fearful of trying these alternatives: What will I feel like after I walk or write in my journal? Will I still be hungry for ice cream? Will I feel even more stressed out? You don't know the outcome, so you feel afraid to try the new action.[4]

Therefore when our clients are starting the change process, we have to help them control their environment as much as possible so they can feel safe in making healthy changes. So if stress triggers a desire to eat ice cream, and the habit we'd like to form is that stress triggers a desire to go for a walk, we must either remove the habitual outcome (ie, the ice cream) or reduce/eliminate the habitual stimulus for eating ice cream: the stress. Now obviously not all stress can be eliminated from anyone's life, but some types of stress can be reduced—and those are the ones we can help the client work to reduce. So our job as coaches is to help the client see what is causing the unhealthy habits, and what stimuli and/or outcomes can be removed from his/her daily environment. Then the client can actively choose new outcomes related to those prior, unhealthy stimuli.[4]

The great thing about coaching is, you understand the change process and can help the client explain to her loved ones the type of support she needs: unconditional belief in her ability to change, and undying enthusiasm for her intended success. With a coach who demonstrates this type of support, clients usually can recruit effective helpers outside of the coaching relationship after just a few weeks of coaching. Thus, as your clients work with you, their circle of support will likely grow—making the change process that much easier, their potential for lasting change that much greater, and the likeli-hood of them pushing your personal boundaries that much lower.[4]

A client's reason for going through this difficult process must have some sort of emotionally-charged reward attached to it. Did you know that people make a majority of their choices based on their feelings, not based on fact or rational arguments? It's true in advertising, and it's true in life! For example, what do Goodyear tires have to do with cute babies and little puppies? Nothing, but the advertising geniuses that Goodyear hired knew that people make decisions based on emotions, and babies and puppies elicit warm and fuzzy emotions in most of us—they represent things that we feel a need to protect. So when we see their brand at the mechanics garage, we will remember the pleasing feelings we felt while viewing Goodyear commercials, and we'll feel good about buying their tires. "They've got babies and puppies riding in their tires," we think, "They must be safe!" And we plunk down our money—even though Firestone tires might be exactly as safe, or even safer! The process of change plays on the same emotional response that advertising does. Facts, or logic, don't necessarily matter—it's emotion that counts! A client must have that emotionally-charged reason to change or they will not make it through the change process. It's that strong feeling that will carry them through the tough times when relapse is a real danger. Because, as we know, it is always easier NOT to change! We know the outcomes of the habits we've been practicing for years and years—even if they are totally unhealthy and have gotten us into a mess, they are safe and predict-able and easy for us to do.[4]

Related to that is the client's perception of the costs and benefits of making the change. The perceived or projected benefits of making the change must be greater than the perceived or projected costs of making the change. For example, the desire to feel happy in a skimpy swimsuit on the beach, and the projected positive outcomes attached to that image, must far outweigh the perceived difficulties or costs in actually making the changes necessary to achieve that desired goal. If eating smaller portions, limiting alcohol consumption, and greatly increasing exercise are deemed to be more costly for the client than the perceived joy of achieving the swimsuit dream, the client will not put the effort forth to achieve the goal. In the process of change, the benefits of change must always outweigh the perceived cost of making the change.[4]

If change is so difficult, How can we convince our clients that they can change? The answer to this dilemma. is practice! The more you do something, the better or more efficient you get at doing it. So if you want to eat better, or exercise more, or drink more water, all you have to do is start doing it— once—and then repeat it—again and again and again until it becomes as natural as brushing your teeth or answering the phone when it rings.   Hence, coaching focuses on present and future actions. It's a way for clients to feel safe and supported as they try new habits on for size, and then modify their new habits according to what works for them?[4]

Smart Rule

Modifying habits requires an understanding of the parameters involved in goal setting. We need to help clients set goals and objectives that are reasonable and not overwhelming. And they must follow the SMART Rule.

S stands for specific—the goal must be specific. If the goal is too broad it will be beyond achievement.

M stands for measurable—the goal must be measurable. One can set goals, but if they are not measurable there is no way of knowing if that goal has been achieved.

A value—the goal must be important and of value to the client. If not important, then it will not be accomplished. For example, a client losing weight for a spouse will not work. The client must set a goal that is important to him or her.

Realistic—the goal must be realistic. For a person who is 50% body fat, achieving 20% body fat in 6 months is unrealistic and will only frustrate the client.

Time frame—all goals must have a deadline. If no deadline exists, then there is no incentive to achieve the goal.

Before setting effective goals we need to understand the concerns of our clients/students, i.e. "I want to lose 15 pounds in 6 months because I have to get into a bathing suit". It is important to discuss with them the reasonableness or unreasonableness of their concerns/goals. At this point, it is critical to discuss the futility of dieting and the importance of focusing on health (which is a much greater motivator) rather than focusing on "how they will look in spandex".

We need to educate clients/students to the difference between losing weight as measured by a scale and losing body fat as measured by body fat analysis. A better way to phrase the goal is to reduce body fat by 1% per month for a year. Losing one to three percent fat per month is the standard or average fat loss. This goal is reasonable, measurable, specific, and has a time frame. The only issue is the importance to the client. This is where applying all of the educational tools at our disposal becomes critical.

The first step in goal setting is to set long term goals, i.e. achieve a healthy body in one or two years. When long term goals have been agreed upon, the next step is to set short range goals which are still reasonable and measurable, i.e. one month, three months.

Once the short term goals are set, the next step is to create a calendar that specifically identifies the daily tasks required to accomplish the short term goal. On the calendar, the client can summarize daily exercise, and daily food totals. At the end of the time period, the fitness professional can review the calendar with the client. While this task is arduous, and time consuming it produces the wanted results; i.e. the client didn't lose any weight and the reason is discovered by analyzing his/her calendar which shows that exercise was sparse (only once a week) and extra calories were consumed every day (ice cream).

SUMMARY

Forty-one states have laws that regulate the profession of dietetics and nutrition. Implementation of any nutrition program by professions other than dietetics requires a thorough understanding of these laws. However, the laws governing nutrition education are skewed and politically motivated. While most states have licensure laws providing details about qualifications required for individuals providing nutrition education, these same legal requirements provide clauses that allow individuals in health food stores to provide nutrition education with absolutely no qualifications. Also, there are no limitations on writing nutrition and diet books. So anyone can write a book dealing with nutrition with absolutely no nutrition background whatsoever.

The American Academy of Sports Dietitians and Nutritionists (AASDN) is a non-profit organization dedicated to providing fitness professionals with a scope of practice for implementing nutrition programs. The goal of this *National Nutrition Scope of Practice for Health and Fitness Professionals* is to eliminate confusion as to the scope and depth of nutrition information that can be administered legally, safely, ethically, and professionally by all health and fitness professionals nationwide.[6]

Why a specific scope of practice for health and fitness professionals? Frustration and confusion exists in the health and fitness profession when it comes to nutrition education, advice, and services that can be provided, not only legally, but professionally as well. Some fitness professionals provide nutrition education based solely on "anecdotal data", while other more qualified professionals are afraid to provide information because they have been told it is beyond their scope of practice.

Choosing a qualified professional to oversee fitness programs is of utmost importance. It must not be assumed that all dietitians have the appropriate background to institute a wellness program, or have the appropriate background to oversee health and fitness programs. Dietitians are allowed to advertise a wellness "specialty" on the ADA website but are not required to indicate any experience or education. Hence, it should not be assumed that a dietitian has knowledge or experience in wellness or fitness. Dietitians wishing to work in a wellness venue must obtain further education upon graduation. It is also recommended that dietitians obtain a fitness certification. Visit www.aasdn.org for more details.

Working with clients requires a working knowledge of coaching skills. You've obviously heard about coaching by this point in your career. There are business coaches, career coaches, relationship coaches—you name the field, there seems to be a coach for it. But what IS it? The definition on your screen is a concisely worded description of this powerful concept: Coaching is a co-creative partnership between a qualified coach and a willing client that supports the client through desired life changes.[4]

Coaching is different from psychological counseling or "therapy" in three very important ways. One, in counseling or therapy it is assumed that something is "wrong" with the client. Two, a counselor or therapist is assumed to "know what's wrong and how to fix it" based on a body of knowledge that the client can be compared against. And three, counseling and therapy look to the PAST to try to help explain WHY a client acts a certain way in the present, or how a client's past actions have contributed to a present situation.[4]

If you want to run a successful coaching business, built around successful and enthusiastic clients, you need to make one major judgment when first meeting a potential client: Is this person ready to change or not? It's very likely that 90% of the people that come to you will be ready to change something—that's why they made the choice to call you in the first place! But some people might not understand that coaching actually requires them to act—not just sit idly by while you spew information at them and allow them to blame other people for their unhealthy condition.[4]

CHAPTER 11 - SAMPLE TEST

1. Why is it important to understand state licensure laws?

2. How can fitness professionals incorporate nutrition programs while still adhering to state licensure laws?

3. What is coaching?

4. Describe the difference between coaching and counseling.

5. List the states of readiness to change and provide details of each stage.

REFERENCES

1. http://www.eatright.org/cps/rde/xchg/ada/hs.xsl/career_2192_ENU_HTML.htm.

2. http://www.time.com/time/magazine/article/0,9171,1018093,00.html.

3. Hauber, S. *Essentials of Coaching for Wellness Professionals*/www.lifestylemanagement.com. 2006.

4. http://lifestylemanagement.com/state_law_pages/laws_illinois.htm.

5. http://lifestylemanagement.com/state_law_pages/laws_connecticut.htm

6. http://aasdn.org/

7.http://topics.nytimes.com/top/reference/timestopics/subjects/e/exercise/ index.html?query=CAPATI,%20ANNE%20MARIE&field=per&match=exact.

8. Prochaska,JO. CC DiClimente. *The transtheoretical approach: Crossing traditional boundaries of therapy.* Homewood, IL:Dow Jones/Irwin, 1984.

Chapter 12
Implementing Programs

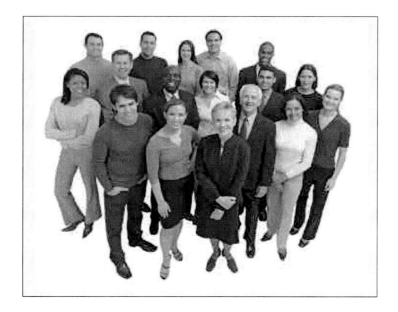

This chapter will focus on the details of implementing a nutrition program. Details will be provided on how to implement an individual program, a group program, a youth program, and other services.

Objectives

After reading and studying this chapter, you should:

1. Be able to implement a one-on-one nutrition program.

2. Be able to implement a group program.

3. Be able to implement a youth program.

4. Be able to implement programs for obese individuals, seniors, and athletes.

INTRODUCTION

The challenge facing professionals today is one of "moderation" and lifestyle changes, not dieting. We must convince the population that fitness can NOT be accomplished through dieting; nor does fitness require 3 hours a day in the gym and never eating ice cream again. We need to renew the belief that fitness isn't that difficult and can even be fun and rewarding. Slow, small, acceptable and palatable changes are the secret. The changes must be ones that the client can live with without feeling deprived. For example, going from whole milk to 2% milk is a much easier transition that trying to go from whole milk to skim milk. As professionals, dedicated to teaching healthy lifestyles, we need to develop patience and not try to bring individuals to our level of fitness overnight.

While exercise is not a major component of this textbook, it is assumed that you are familiar with exercise prescription and recommendations. Building muscle and burning fat must include aerobic exercise, muscle strengthening exercise (assuming flexibility as well) and proper nutrition to fuel the body. The statement "a calorie is a calorie, etc." may be true in dieting but not in body composition change. In muscle building and fat burning it's not only calories, but the type of calories and when those calories are eaten (in conjunction with exercise). The information contained in this chapter will produce muscle building and fat burning only if a program includes aerobic exercise, muscle strengthening exercise, proper eating and control of catabolic factors (caffeine, stress, etc.).

The following program outlines are suggestions. There are many possible variations and the following is simply one option. There are also many qualified professionals with materials available to provide nutrition services. Be sure to choose a program that fits your business model.

Before attempting to implement any of the suggested programs in this chapter, be sure that you have studied previous chapters in this textbook. It is assumed that you understand the biochemistry of the energy nutrients, energy production, supplements, nutrition research and the prerequisites involved before implementing a program.

Information in this chapter should not be used to alter a medically prescribed regimen or as a form of self treatment. Implementing any of the programs in this chapter requires working directly with a qualified professional.

INDIVIDUAL PROGRAM

The first step in instituting an individual program is to set up a preliminary interview (15 minutes) with all potential clients. This interview is designed to determine the client's stage of readiness to change.

Interview

The goal as a coach is to work with clients in the preparation and action phases, support clients in maintenance, and help clients through any times of relapse. The fitness professional has a good understanding of the coaching process if he/she can convince a contemplator to start the change process.

The section on coaching described methods to determine the stage of readiness to change. One way to test what stage a client is at is by questioning. Examples of questions to ask include: Are you able to make changes; why is now the time to change; is it possible to try new habits; is it impossible or just difficult to change; what will changing do for you; what will happen if you don't change. The first answer must contain a personally relevant reason, something that is emotionally meaningful to the client. They may give you an external reason at first (such as "My doctor told me to"). But keep asking the question, stressing "Why do YOU feel it's time to change?" Your goal is to see if they have a real, internal reason for changing. The second answer must be YES, or some indication of willing-ness to try. The third answer must be YES.[4] The fourth answer must be "just difficult!" If the client says "impossible," then he/she is not ready to change!

Trying to work with clients in the precontemplative stage will only cause frustration, and can actually induce failure on the part of the client. It's important to understand that some individuals are not ready to make lifestyle changes. As much as we wish we could "save everyone", we can not. Your role during the interview is to identify which clients are ready and which clients are not ready to enter your program.

Watch for the excuses. Potential clients in the precontemplation stage do not take responsibility, but rather provide lots of excuses concerning their lack of success. If you hear the blame game from the beginning, this potential client is not a good candidate. You can feel comfortable saying to this person, "I hear you are frustrated with your situation, but unless you can take the responsibility for your current habits and situation, I can't help you. Can you tell me what you can do to change your current situation to make it better for your health?" And then let them think about it. If they come up with some solid answers that reveal that they, themselves, need to change some things, then there is a glimmer of hope.

If a potential client is in the precontemplation stage your next course of action is to explain that your program is not the best program for him/her and, as stated above, explain that you can't help him/her. If the individual is thinking about making changes, or is ready to make changes, the interview then becomes your chance to convince him/her that nutrition is a large component to success in body composition change.

It is important to note here that many individuals believe they know what to eat. They are convinced that they are not successful because they do not have the willpower to follow through. However, the truth of the matter is most individuals do not know what to eat. Quizzing the individual on his or her knowledge of nutrition (on such topics as protein needs, caloric needs, why diets fail, etc.) will quickly make the individual aware that he/she does not know how to fuel the body properly to optimize muscle building and fat burning.

Depending on how and where you conduct business, you can perform an initial client interview in person or over the phone. The process is nearly identical. The first priority of this interview is to ascertain whether you are speaking to a person who is, indeed, ready to change their lifestyle habits.

Nutrition Knowledge Quiz[1]

1. After the age of thirty, adults lose approximately 1/2 pound of muscle per year. Five pounds of muscle can burn 6 pounds of fat in one year (and that's without exercise). Do you know how much protein you should have in your diet daily to maintain muscle?

2. Can you list dietary sources of protein?

3. Do you know what types of fat in your diet are stored as fat in your fat cells?

4. Do you know how much fat you should have in your diet daily to maintain vital immune and cell functions?

5. Carbohydrates are the primary source of energy for the body. If carbohydrates (in the form of glucose) are not available, your body will have to use the proteins in your diet to make glucose (rather than use them for muscle building). Do you know how many grams of carbohydrates you should have daily?

6. Vitamins do not provide calories, but are required for muscle building and energy. Do you know how many servings of fruits and veggies you should have every day?

7. Without adequate water intake your body can not eliminate the by products of fat burning. Do you know how much water you should drink daily?

Once you're certain that the person is ready to make changes, the next component of the interview is to describe your services in detail. What can the client expect from you, and what will his/her responsibilities be? You will want to provide details concerning your program such as the length of the program, services you will provide, etc.

This is the time to have the individual sign up for your program (more on pricing, selling etc., in chapter on Making it a Business). Most of us in the fitness profession do not perceive ourselves as sales people; but in a very real sense we are. We are selling the most valuable commodity there is - health.

Once the individual signs up for your program, the rest of the interview consists of receiving payment, having the new client sign a legal agreement, a responsibility clause, and discussing preparations for the first appointment.

Receiving payment is absolutely essential. You must have payment before the first appointment. Many fitness professionals have a difficult time asking for payment. A believe has been fostered that because fitness professionals care and are passionate about what they do (selling health), payment somehow diminishes their dedication. This is absolutely false. There are several important reasons to never work for "free". First, a financial commitment on the part of the client produces accountability. So fitness professionals must charge to insure client success. Second, if fitness professionals do not charge (and charge a substantial amount) for this service they will not be perceived as professional. It is a known fact in business that the higher the cost for a product/service the greater the perceived value. To be perceived as an expert, fitness professionals must charge industry rates.

If a fitness professional has a hard time asking for money, the process can be scripted. Scripting will be discussed in Chapter 14 but in essence it simply means writing appropriate statements, memorizing these statements and having them available when difficult situations arise. An example of such a script might consist of the following: "Great – I believe we will work well together. So how would you like to pay for the program? We accept credit cards, cash, and check." If a potential client says he/she does not have the money, the script may continue: "Oh darn, that's too bad. I do believe this program would be a great fit for you. As soon as you do have the money, let me know and we will set up an appointment". Or you can go through the questioning process and point out that your it may not be a matter of finances, but a matter of priorities. In either case, professionals need to write their own "script".

By the end of the interview (or before the first appointment) you should have obtained a clearance form to exercise, a physician's approval if necessary, and a legal agreement.

The client must also sign a "responsibility" agreement. At this point in the interview, the client should be aware that responsibility for success rests with him/her. This must be emphasized and clearly stated at the beginning of the program. The client should read the agreement out loud then sign the agreement. The fitness professional must then sign the agreement as well. Keep in mind that the fitness professionals are not responsible for success or failure. They are simply educators.

Be sure to have the client sign a comprehensive legal agreement that includes both exercise and nutrition.

The final component of the interview is to be provide the client with details concerning the first appointment: completion of a comprehensive client profile sheet, goal setting, and baseline body composition measurements. You'll want to describe the body composition measures, reasons for taking the measurements, and details of how to dress, etc. See the discussion on body composition measures in Chapter 5.

Responsibility Agreement[2]

Welcome to _____.   The next ____ weeks are crucial to ensuring your success in lifelong weight management. Please make this program your top priority. Many obstacles to your success will undoubtedly crop up in the next few weeks. Don't let these obstacles stand in your way. Be aware that you will probably go through several psychological stages during your program. We will ask you to determine what causes you to overeat and/or what prevents you from exercising.   In some cases, eating issues are a cover up for other more deep rooted problems. During your program you must continuously ask yourself if the changes you are making are lifestyle changes - changes you can live with the rest of your life without feeling deprived or stressed. If these changes are difficult and "unpleasant", then we must "talk". We will work with you to make this program the "beginning of the rest of your life". We will also be asking you to periodically keep a food log of everything you eat. A food log can actually decrease your obsession with food. Remember, the only way we can help you is if we have all the facts. We are your educators, motivators, and your confidants - not your judges.

We, the staff of _____ are at your disposal to help ease you into lifestyle transitions. However, you must do all the work. Therefore, we ask that you read the agreement below carefully, and   sign only if you are in complete agreement:

I _____ agree to follow the exercise program as prescribed in our sessions;

I _____ also agree to make changes in my eating patterns as agreed upon.

Signed: _____   Date: _____

Witness: _____   Date: _____

First Appointment

In this first appointment, the fitness professional will need to complete a client profile, perform body composition measurements and instruct the client on how to keep a "food log".

Client Profile

It is essential to collect accurate and complete health and lifestyle data for each client. Data can be classified into the following categories: demographics, health history, physical activity history, weight history, eating patterns/eating issues, stress levels, goals and objectives. Demographics refer to information such as name, address, telephone number, age, gender, etc. A health history form should contain questions concerning past and present health issues. There are many forms and variations of health history questionnaires. The most commonly used form is known as the Par-Q. Refer to your exercise manuals for a copy of a health history questionnaire, or combine the best features of a few forms to create your own. Also see "Client Profile" in the case studies at the end of this chapter.

A physical activity questionnaire should provide all the information necessary to prescribe a safe and effective exercise program. It should provide detailed information concerning past exercise, any injuries due to exercise, and current exercise habits. Information concerning weight history is valuable in providing you with information concerning large weight fluctuations and any possible eating disorders. Clients with large weight fluctuations – also known as yo-yo dieters— will have a much harder time with body composition change. Yo-yo dieting leads to loss of muscle mass and the addition of fat stores. These individuals have low metabolism due to this muscle loss and even their organs may become smaller. Metabolism must be improved through fueling the body during exercise. It may be months before actual body composition measures will indicate change, since internal organs must first be brought back to original health. It's best not to make comments on any of the information your client gives you at this time. Ask questions, yes, but don't give any opinions or make judgments. Remember, this is a delicate issue for MOST people. Let your clients fill out the form honestly in a non-judgmental atmosphere. You will approach each "red flag" in a very supportive manner in future appointments.

Another important question concerning weight history is addressing whether or not the individual believes he or she has, or has ever had, an eating disorder. If a possible eating disorder is present, you must refer this individual to your licensed dietitian. You also want to address eating patterns and food issues. You will obtain detailed information when performing a diet analysis after your second appointment together, but it is helpful to obtain general information here. It is also important to learn whether your client eats when depressed or stressed. Experts agree that identifying these issues can actually help to resolve them. If a client admits that she eats when depressed, you can advise her to keep track of this in her food log journal and you will discuss possible solutions during the course of her program.

As previously discussed, stress is catabolic, and in order to maintain health, stress must be controlled. Hence, it is critical to obtain information concerning the client's perceived stress levels. On a scale of 1 to 10, with 10 being high, ask the client what his/her stress levels are at home and at work. Stress levels 7 or above indicate a catabolic response is occurring in the body. While we are

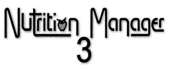

Lifestyle Management Associates
Dr. Jane Pentz
800-617-4615

Client Profile

Client Name:	Address:
Mr. Johnny Sample	5555 Apple Lane

City: Hometown	State or Province: MA	Zipcode: 55555

Phone Day	Ext.	Phone Night	Phone Cell	Height	Weight	Stress Level 1-10
800-800-8000				Feet 6'	Pounds:	Home 2 / Work 4
Date of Birth: 04/17/1977	Gender: Male	Occupation: Software programmer		Inches 4"	220 lbs	

Emergency Contact Name (First / Last)	Blood Type A+	Weight@Heaviest / Age 260 lbs 22 yrs
Phone Day	Extension	Phone Night	Weight@Lightest / Age 195 lbs 18 yrs

Personal History

Do you have any limitations to exercise? No

If so what are these limitations?

What is your exercise program now? Nothing

How long have you been following this regimen?

Have you had any injuries due to exercise? No

Medical History

Are you seeing a physician for any reason? No

Are you taking any medications? No

Are you allergic to any medications? No

Do you smoke? No

Did you ever smoke? Yes

If you did smoke when did you quit? 04/17/2003

How long did you smoke? 10 years

Eating Patterns

What is your largest meal? Dinner

Do you snack during the day? Yes

What types of snacks? Candy Chips

Do you snack after dinner? Yes

What size do you consider your portions? Large

Do you eat when depressed? No

Do you eat when stressed? No

Do you feel you have any eating disorders? No

Have you ever had any eating disorders? No

Comments

I want to lose weight/body fat and eat healthier.

Disease History

Medications Currently Using

Allergy History

not experts on stress reduction, we can provide clients details concerning stress.

Setting Effective Goals

Be sure to review the section in Chapter 11 on setting effective goals and objectives. Discuss goals and objectives with the client to be sure they follow the SMART rule.

Body Composition

Three important measures of body composition are Body Mass Index, percent body fat, and waist-to-hip ratio. See Chapter 5 for details. In order to get an accurate picture of your client's disease risk, you will want to perform all three body composition measures during your first appointment. You may choose NOT to provide all three results to the client after you calculate the results, but they are nonetheless important for your records. You will need to have written instructions on how you will perform body composition measures so that you and the client are properly prepared during this first appointment. For more details on body composition see Chapter 5.

Food Intake Record

Fitness professionals must be working directly with a qualified/licensed professional before complet-ing a diet analysis or providing a menu plans. As discussed in detail in Chapter 11, it is illegal in most states to provide these individualized services without the direct guidance of a qualified professional.

A diet history is created when someone recalls what they ate in the past; this method is not very accurate since it is easy for people to forget what they ate.
Food frequency is determined by providing a person a list of foods and asking them how often they eat the particular food. This form of food intake is typically used when conducting research. Indi-viduals were asked questions such as how often do you eat strawberries in season: daily weekly, monthly, or never. As you can see, this method is not very accurate, but in research if you see a statistically significant difference in responses then you know you truly have a difference.
A diet record (or food log) is a record of what is eaten throughout the day. This can also be inaccu-rate, but is the most accurate method we have thus far. You should be aware that not all persons will be completely honest. It is vital that you educate your client to the importance of providing you with accurate information. You are the professional trying to help them make healthy lifestyle changes. You can't help them if they do not provide you with an accurate picture of what they are doing.   A food log should contain types of foods eaten, quantities eaten, time of day, and mood when eaten. These last points will be especially important when trying to identify patterns of eating that must be altered. The food log also allows the fitness professional to prescribe a program that incorporates the clients food preferences. This is a major component to lifelong success. Food preferences must be incorporated into the clients menu planning.

A one or two day food log may not be truly representative of the client's intake. A five to seven day food log that is then averaged is a much truer picture of the client's typical eating pattern. Be sure to include weekdays and weekend days since weekends may be very different. A sample diet analysis of a food log can be found in chapter 5 and   a portion size chart in this section can be used to instruct the client on estimating portion sizes.

Example of Lifestyle Journal[4]

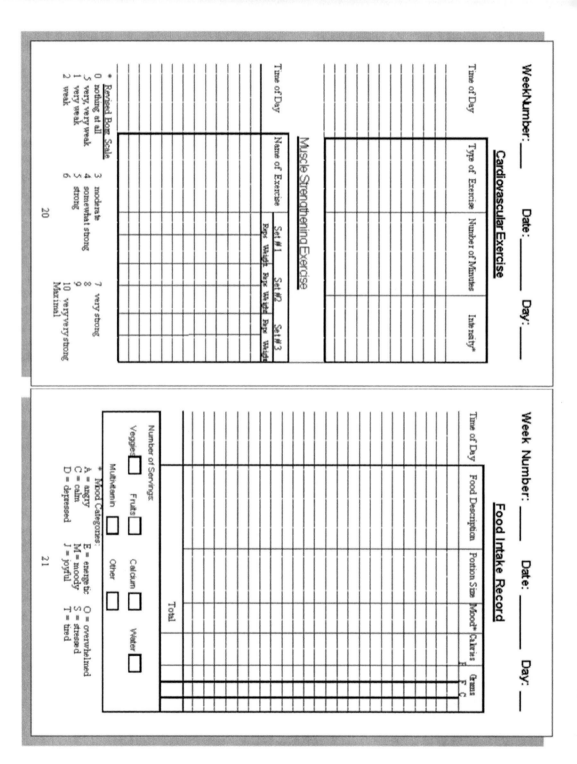

A food log should contain types of foods eaten, quantities eaten, time of day eaten, and the person's mood when foods are eaten. These last points will be especially important when trying to identify patterns of eating that must be altered. The food log also allows the fitness professional to prescribe a program that incorporates the clients food preferences. This is a major component to lifelong success. Food preferences must be incorporated into the client's menu planning, or the client will never adhere to the program. A one or two day food log may not be truly representative of the client's intake. A five to seven day food log that is then averaged is a much truer picture of the client's typical eating pattern. Be sure to include weekdays and weekend days since weekends may consist of different eating patterns (see example on next page).

To analyze an individual's diet you can use a food counts book, obtain the information from labels, and perform the calculations manually as in this slide. Calculation of energy nutrients can be taxing, but calculations of all the micronutrients (vitamins and minerals) by hand, is literally impossible. To truly analyze an individual's diet you will require diet analysis software. There are many software packages available – from very inexpensive to very expensive. If you do purchase software be sure you can add foods to the data base because no data base will have all foods listed. Other components to look for are: does the software list all micronutrients; and does the software provide details concerning protein quality.

Food Log Instruction

Instruct the client on how to keep a food log using the lifestyle journal on the previous page and the food chart on the next page. The food chart is for estimating portion sizes. Remember, the goal is not to measure all foods with a scale and a ruler, but to simply have the client become aware of estimates of portion sizes so that you can enter correct information into your computer software, or find accurate nutrient content in your food counts book.

Be sure to reiterate that these measurements are to help the client estimate what they are eating - and not to be viewed as "what they should be eating". For example, ½ cup of cut up fruit or grapes is the size of a light bulb; one pancake is the size of a CD, 1 cup of salad (packed) is the size of a baseball; 1 cup of pasta, rice or potatoes is the size of a fist; 1 oz. of cubed cheese is the size of 4 small dice; 1 medium fruit is the size of a tennis ball; 1 teaspoon of oil is the size of a quarter; 3 oz. of meat or fish cooked is the size of a deck of cards; ¼ cup raisins is the size of a large egg; 1 medium potato is the size of a computer mouse; 1 slice of bread is (slightly larger) than an audio cassette; and 1 oz. nuts is the size of 2 shot glasses. Before you end the appointment, use the chart on the next page[5] with your clients to run through a few examples of how they would record their portions on their food log so they feel comfortable providing you with accurate estimates when exact measures are not available. And ask your client to be as detailed as possible when they record their foods: writing "Tropicana Calcium Plus OJ ½ cup", "Two 12-oz. cans of Diet Dr. Pepper," and "Fuji apple, extra large" is much more helpful to you and will yield a more accurate diet analysis than simply "glass of OJ, 2 cans of pop, and an apple."

First Appointment Wrap-up

You'll want to explain to your client at this time what it is you will be doing with the information that has been collecting. You can describe briefly the diet analysis process, and how you will be entering

You Are What You Eat . . .
Are Your Portion Sizes Too Much?

Living a healthy lifestyle involves making the right choices about food, exercise and other daily activities. Americans are waging a war against an epidemic of obesity, partly due to eating too much food. Over half of the adults in the United States are overweight or obese—and today, obesity in children is rapidly becoming a major health crisis. Heart disease, type 2 diabetes and some types of cancers are just a few of the health risks associated with being overweight. Choosing healthier foods in the right proportion and exercising regularly can make a difference in your quality of life. Here are some easy ways to help you understand serving sizes. ©Paulette Mason, 2003

SERVING SIZE SAME SIZE AS

1/2 cup of grapes = light bulb

SERVING SIZE SAME SIZE AS

1 pancake = compact disc

SERVING SIZE SAME SIZE AS

1 cup of green salad = baseball

SERVING SIZE SAME SIZE AS

1 cup of pasta, rice or potatoes = fist

SERVING SIZE SAME SIZE AS

1 oz. of cubed cheese = 4 dice

SERVING SIZE SAME SIZE AS

1 medium fruit = tennis ball

SERVING SIZE SAME SIZE AS

1 teaspoon of oil or mayo = quarter

SERVING SIZE SAME SIZE AS

3 oz. of cooked meat, fish, or poultry = deck of cards

SERVING SIZE SAME SIZE AS

1/4 cup of raisins = large egg

SERVING SIZE SAME SIZE AS

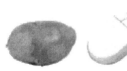

1 medium potato = computer mouse

SERVING SIZE SAME SIZE AS

1 slice of bread = audiocassette

SERVING SIZE SAME SIZE AS

1 oz. nuts = 2 shot glasses full

the information provided into high-tech software that will determine deficiencies or overdoses of various nutrients. It's important that the client understand that the accuracy of the food log is of the utmost importance. If the portions or the food content are not accurate the entire program could be a waste of time and money! You can also reveal that you will be doing your own homework before the next session. Using the body composition numbers you took, and the client's profile sheet, you will be determining a baseline Total Energy Expenditure for the client as described in chapter 5.   You will also come back to the second appointment armed with a pre-approved menu plan for someone in your client's particular caloric range as determined by your TEE calculations. You can reiterate that you are BOTH highly invested in your client's success, and that, while you understand that keeping a food log can be a daunting task, you are confident that it will be much easier and more interesting than your client imagines.

Behind the Scenes Calculations

With the information you collected in the first session, you'll want to determine the body composition measures described, then use the resulting body fat % to determine the client's total energy expenditure.   Once you've gotten the client's body composition measures, and have calculated their TEE, you are ready for appointment number 2. Take a few minutes to review the client's profile sheet, and make some notes regarding issues you think might deserve discussion.

Second Appointment

At the second appointment, you'll first want to collect your client's food log and give it a quick look. Do you see exact measures? Do you see details? If so, congratulations! You did your job and your client understands the value of an accurate food log. Thank the client and explain that you will have a thorough diet analysis at your next session. Ask the client how the process was for him/her, and if he/she has any specific questions about the food log.

So the second appointment arrives, and if you've both done your assigned homework, you will be armed with the client's body composition measures, a Total Energy Expenditure number, and a corresponding LMA Menu Plan. Your client will be handing you a 3- to 5-day food log, and some SMART goals she'd like to achieve. Let's take a look at what you'll do with this information, and the details of this second appointment. Next you will want to provide the client with at least one of the three body composition measures you calculated, the TEE calculation you arrived at, and the appropriate menu plan for the client's TEE. Take some time to go over these results, and perhaps draw on the food log your client has brought to the appointment. Are there a few small issues you see right away that deserve mention? Does the client relate your TEE results to her food log results? Any discussion here is good, as it gets the client thinking about making changes already. Just remember not to make value judgments, just listen and state facts. And remember, until your diet analysis is done, you can't offer "answers" for what your client needs to do.

What you can do, however, is ask the client about his/her SMART goals at this time, and help make sure they meet all the requirements: They must be Specific, Measurable, A value, Realistic, and Timed. If they don't meet the criteria, help the client figure out how to re-word them. Above all, make sure the goals are realistic. You'll need to use your fitness knowledge and give your client an honest appraisal of achievable goals. You know by this point where the client is starting. Are the chosen goals too far out of reach for the chosen time frame? Remember, it's better to start small and set longer-term, larger goals as you move along in the program.

Help your client set a couple of small SMART goals to achieve by your next appointment. He/she will not need to keep a food log this time, but might tell you he/she wants to do it because it helped with eating healthy; or the client may want to set an activity goal. Whatever it is, it is important to keep your client involved in the program by setting SMART goals at every appointment. Maybe a goal is to have read your session handout on "Why Diets Don't Work" by the next time you meet. Something as simple as this will keep your client actively invested in the program. It's a good idea to explain that this process is time intensive. You have to enter each food item into your software (or look them up in a food counts book and add them by hand if you are not using software) to get useful numbers that will be your client's guide as he/she starts to add muscle and lose fat.

When you feel comfortable that the client has learned a thing or two in the second appointment, and is excited about achieving SMART goals for the next time you meet, it's time to set up the third appointment. Give yourself at least 5-7 days between appointments, as the food log analysis can't be rushed.

Behind The Scenes Analysis

Analyze the client food log using a computerized program. Take a long look at the energy nutrients first. What are the total calories eaten versus the recommended number of calories. Is the client eating too much or too little? Is the client eating enough protein or too much protein, etc? Next, look at the carbohydrate and fats and compare. Follow the same analysis for all the micronutrients. Make a list of possible changes that are required for a healthy eating plan. You will also want to provide your client with a list of nutrient content in foods (see Appendix). This list provides the names of foods high in certain nutrients. For example, if your client's analysis indicates that he/she is low in vitamin C you can point out foods that are high in vitamin C. You will want to present the results to your client in the next appointment.

See the diet analysis printouts in this chapter for examples of computerized printouts. Become familiar with the actual intake versus DRI (recommended). Nutrition Manager software includes analysis of water, fiber, and amino acids.

Third Appointment

In the next appointment you will want to present the results of the diet analysis. As you discuss the results with the client, start to point out areas that might require some work. "So, Mary, I see that you use whole milk in your coffee, and you drink 2 glasses at lunch as well. Would you be open to choosing low-fat milk with your coffee, and perhaps switching to 2% milk in the afternoon? This would be better for your cholesterol, which we can see is quite high from my software analysis."

This comment will help your client get started thinking about do-able changes. Remember that ALL changes must be palatable for the client. Asking Mary to stop drinking milk or to go directly from whole milk to skim would be a big jump. If she suggests it and she really believes it is not sacrifice,do it! But it must be her idea. She must be committed to every goal that she chooses.

And that is a crucial point. When you begin coaching nutrition clients, their actions MUST be their choice, not YOURS! You can make recommendations, of course, but no goal will be achieved unless it is the client's chosen goal. Even if you want your client to stop drinking a 6-pack of beer a night, if he/she says "I guess I could drink light beer instead this week." Go with it! The client is changing, and will change at a pace that is right for him/her. You made a recommendation to "Look at alcohol content, because it was adding to the dangerous fat stores around the waist, and that is a major indicator of higher risk for heart disease and stroke." The client grasped the severity of that comment, and chose the goal. THAT is the art of coaching.

Review the goals your client set in the last appointment. How did they go? If your client raises an issue that corresponds to any of session handouts (see outline in Appendix), you'll want to give provide a copy of the handout to take home, and spend a couple of minutes talking about the issue together. And you always want to end a session with a fresh set of SMART goals to be achieved by your next appointment date.

Follow-up Appointments

Your follow-up appointments are much less structured than the first 3 because all of your calculations are done. Each session from here on out will include a discussion of the goals set at the previous appointment, and how the client fared. You can introduce other topics that you feel the client might be ready to tackle, and you can use the approved session handouts (see appendix) and appropriate handouts from other organizations and from other qualified licensed individuals. Your main goal with each session is to ensure that the client understands that she is making progress every week, and that lifestyle change is a SLOW process. You'll have to use every ounce of compassion and every bit of knowledge to help the client understand that he/she can't lose 6 sizes in 4 weeks. Always focus on the positive changes the client IS making, and reflect on how far he/she has come already, just by signing up for a program such as yours.

Ending a Program

Once your client is satisfied with his/her own efficacy in regard to lifestyle change, begins to set SMART goals, and understands the steps needed to continue, it's your job to ask if the client is ready to move on without your help. If the client no longer needs your guidance and is ready to go it alone, you've done your job! Ask the client for feedback about the program. Sending clients a pre-written questionnaire is always a great idea. Use open-ended questions, such as "What parts of your program did you find the most helpful?" and "Was there anything you had hoped to learn during your program that you did not get to explore? If so, what?" This way, the client provides invaluable help as you fine-tune your programs and services.

Note that the first 3 sessions include a LOT of background work. It's very important to spend those first 3 sessions really getting into the nitty gritty of a client's history, specific measurements, and goals, so that your program will be built on a strong foundation. You've got to spend those first 3 sessions really figuring out what that client has come to you for, and how your work together can help change his/her life. The rest of your sessions from then on can be a joy.

GROUP PROGRAMS

Group programs offer an added benefit of interaction with other individuals with similar goals. This can be seen from the success of groups such as Weight Watchers. Fitness professionals can build on this concept by providing exercise prescription and more detailed information at each meeting. It is important to structure a group program that includes a "curriculum". A curriculum ensures that participants will complete the program with a new level of acquired information. See the Appendix for the curriculum outline used in a pilot program presented by Lifestyle Management Associates.[3]

Informational Meeting[6]

Informational meetings should be open to the public and free. This is a great opportunity to draw new members to your facility. Everyone must exercise and non exercising individuals will need a place to exercise. Below are several examples of how to include a temporary membership while participating in the program:

- provide a 3 month membership at a reduced rate
- provide a 3 month membership and if they join after the three months you will eliminate the joining fees
- provide a partial refund if they attend all classes.

Begin the informational meeting by introducing yourself (see Keys to A Successful Class on the next page) and describing the program. Include the date and time of the weekly sessions, the cost, and the commitment that they attend all meetings. Also explain the commitment to exercise, small changes in eating patterns, and a willingness to look at their stress levels.

Include the information on why diets don't work. Display a hard ball and beach ball and explain that both balls weigh the same. Provide details on why dieting doesn't work and has never worked (see section on diets). Describe the skills required to complete the program - willingness to change; diet analysis software to be loaded onto their own computers; completing the Informational Meeting Questionnaire.

Allow time for questions and answers. Don't worry if you don't know all the answers. Let individuals know that your work directly with a qualified/licensed professional that can answer all their questions (through you).

Explain that only ten individuals can be chosen for the program but all attendees will receive a follow up phone call. This is a critical component. All attendees MUST BE CONTACTED. It is just as important to call individuals not chosen for the program as it is to call individuals that are chosen. For those individuals not chosen explain the reason for their non-acceptance (not willing to exercise, not willing to remove problem foods from the home, etc.) Also critical is to offer non chosen attendees with other options. For example: discounted membership to your facility; possibly one-on-one pro-gram; discounted personal training session; refer them to a sports dietitian, etc.

Groups should be formed with common goals. For example, everyone in the group does the cooking, or grocery shopping, or wants to lose weight, etc. Once your chosen group is established, the group program should include some one-on-one time with each participant. During the one-on-one consultation you can discuss goals and objectives, exercise regimen, and how to keep a food log.

Group meetings should contain similar topics as individual programs. In a pilot program, completed by Lifestyle Management Associates, the group program consisted of 8 sessions. Results of the pilot are included in the Appendix. At the end of the 8 week program, participants were invited to return in 4 weeks for a free body composition. During these follow up appointments participants were offered options for continued support: individual consultations, another group program, weekly meetings, etc. The program was very successful in that all participants indicated that they had learned everything they needed to know about designing a healthy eating program centered on their food preferences. Topics for each session ranged from discussion of energy nutrients, reading labels, fiber, stress, alcohol, and of course exercise. See Appendix for copies of the session handouts.

It's impossible to address each participant's individual concerns during a group program, so it works best to choose a topic based on participant interest or need. Group programs do not necessarily need to last 8 weeks. Successful programs can include as many sessions as needed to for participants to become successful in make lifestyle changes.

Group programs can follow a similar pattern to individual programs. However, analyzing food intakes for 10 participants is too time consuming and will result in your losing money rather than making money. In the pilot program mentioned above, participants were give a copy of the Nutrition Manger software and entered their own food data. Participants learned to enter their own food data but were not able to analyze the results. The results were brought to class and participants formulated their own lifestyle changes. Participants were then provided with menu plans from Dr. Pentz's book.[4] Participants used the menu plans to help develop their own healthy eating plan.

Keys to a Successful Class[6]

Keys to implementing a successful class include:
1. Non-threatening environment: It takes great courage to attend an informational meeting. Many individuals, if not most, have failed many times at weight management. Be sure your meetings are situated in a non-threatening environment. Having a meeting in the middle of a workout area, with lots of "thin" people in skimpy outfits is very threatening to overweight and inactive people.
2. Take Charge: Help make individuals comfortable by introducing yourself. Humor is always a great way to make people feel comfortable. Be sure your comments are humorous to everyone. Ask questions. People like to talk about themselves. Keep the questions light: so what do you do; do you live close by; are you a member here, etc.
3. Positive Attitude: One of the greatest assets you can bring to the group is a positive attitude. Always maximize the positive and "eliminate the negative".
4. Welcome: It is important to be sure that you specifically welcome everyone to the informational meeting. Introduce yourself and let them know that you appreciate their taking time from their busy schedules to attend. Have each individual introduce themselves. This is also a great time to ask light questions about themselves.
5. Remember names: I always feel special when someone remembers my name when first meeting me. As people introduce themselves, jot down notes to help you remember their

names. Along with remembering names, it is also important to jot down something that the person has said about themselves. This is also a great way to remember names.

Working with individuals: Even though you are facilitating a group program, the program is made up of individuals with very different reasons for attending and very different needs.

6. Learn to Listen: We so often feel like we have to do all the talking. After all, we're the teachers. But listening is even more important. Through careful listening, you can learn and understand each person's needs.

7. Empathy: Empathy is defined as "understanding of another's feelings. While you may not have the same experiences as participants, there is always "commonality" of experiences. I was an obese child, so I can certainly empathize with anyone that has been or is obese. While I never had an eating disorder, I can certainly empathize about poor body image, etc.

8. Coaching: Your role in this program is that of educator and coach. Coaching is a co-creative partnership between a qualified coach and a willing client that supports the client through desired life changes. In other words, you don't tell people what needs to be changed, you help them discover themselves what needs to be changed. See section on coaching for further details.

Follow Up

Upon completion of the program it's important to provide follow up options for participants. The 8 week pilot program established a follow up visit at 12 weeks (4 weeks after completion of the program). Participants were given a free body composition analysis and a 15 minute meeting with the fitness professional. Follow up options were itemized: one-one-one consultations; another group program; weekly meeting with other program graduates, personal training, etc.

Group programs are very cost effective and a great opportunity for people to meet each other and provide support. It's also a great opportunity to have volunteers help you with future programs. The pilot program completed by Lifestyle Management Associates produced volunteers to help train new program participants on how to use the diet analysis software.

YOUTH PROGRAM

Guidelines listed on mypyramid.gov state that healthy eating is an important life skill. It helps children grow, develop, and do well in school. It prevents childhood and adolescent health problems such as obesity, dental caries, and iron deficiency anemia. It lowers the risk of future chronic disease such as heart disease, stroke, diabetes, and cancer and reduces potential health care costs. Healthy eating is defined as following the *Dietary Guidelines for Americans* recommended by the Department of Agriculture and the Department of Health and Human Services. The guidelines recommend that children aim for a healthy weight; be physically active each day; use the Pyramid guide your food choices; choose a variety of grains daily, especially whole grains; choose a variety of fruits and vegetables daily; choose a diet that is low in saturated fat and cholesterol and moderate in total fat; choose beverages and foods to moderate your intake of sugars; choose and prepare foods with less salt.[3]

Many children are flunking healthy eating. Only 2 percent meet all the recommendations of the Food Guide Pyramid; 16 percent do not meet any of the recommendations; less than 15 percent of school children eat the recommended servings of fruit; less than 20 percent eat the recommended servings of vegetables; about 25 percent eat the recommended servings of grains; only 30 percent consume the recommended milk group servings; only 19 percent of girls ages 9 to 19 meet the recommended intakes for calcium; only 16 percent of school children meet the guidelines for saturated fat. The consequences are troubling. Childhood obesity is a national epidemic, likely to result in earlier onset and increased prevalence of disease. The percentage of young people who are overweight has more than doubled in the past 30 years. Unhealthy eating and physical inactivity are causes of obesity and chronic disease, resulting in at least 300,000 deaths each year. Poor nutrition associated with heart disease, stroke, cancer, and diabetes, alone, now costs $71 billion a year.[3]

Fitness professionals, again, are an ideal profession to take on the challenge of reducing childhood obesity rates. Free materials to educate children on healthy lifestyles abound. Materials are available free of charge from mypyramid.gov (click on resource library).[7]

      Available Resources for K-12 Schools include:

            Changing the Scene: Improving the School Nutrition Environment
            Community Nutrition Action Kit
            Connections, Volume 9
            Getting It Started and Keeping It Going, Team Nutrition
            Making It Happen! School Nutrition Success Stories
            MyPyramid Anatomy
            MyPyramid Mini Poster
            MyPyramid Poster
            Sense-ational Food poster (Spanish)
            Serving Up Success
      Available Resources for Elementary Schools include:
            Eat Smart. Play Hard. Table Tents
            Enjoy Moving Flyer
            Enjoy Moving Poster

MyPyramid for Kids: A Close Look
MyPyramid for Kids Blast Off
MyPyramid for Kids Classroom Materials
MyPyramid for Kids Coloring Page
MyPyramid for Kids Poster
MyPyramid for Kids Tips for Families
MyPyramid for Kids Worksheet
Team Up at Home: Team Nutrition Activity Booklet
Available Resources for Middle and High Schools
Empowering Youth
Food for A Day Available Resources for Middle and High Schools
Empowering Youth
Food for A Day
How Much Do You Eat poster
Move It! poster
Nutrition Essentials
The Power of Choice: Helping Youth Make Healthy Eating and Fitness Decisions
Read It Before You Eat It poster
yourSELF Middle School Nutrition Education Kit

Kids Health (www.kidshealth.org) is another nutrition site proving materials for children. They provide materials aimed at helping parents incorporate healthy lifestyles. They provide hints on how to have regular family meals, eat a variety of foods, avoid battles over food and involving kids in the process.

Another site that provides free materials is Learn to Be Healthy (www.learntobehealthy.org). This site offers materials for children, parents, and educators.

Googling" children's nutrition materials will bring up dozens of other sites providing free materials.

While these sites are informative and provide a plethora of free materials, there are several problems associates with using these materials and initiating a youth program. One problem is that free materials do not provide a curriculum. It is up to the instructor to decide on available topics and develop a curriculum - a time consuming project. Another problem is that exercise is typically not included in combination with the nutrition component. So fitness professionals would need to invest a considerable amount of time to construct a program. Visit www.lifestylemanagement.com for details on an established program that incorporates exercise and nutrition - *Healthy Kids & Families*.

WORKING WITH SPECIAL POPULATIONS

Working with the obese population, seniors and athletes is very similar to the programs already mentioned.

Obese Clients

The simplistic definition of obesity is excess body fat that accumulates when people take in more food energy than they expend. Many factors are involved in this simplistic definition. Obesity has many interrelated causes and is not simply a matter of what one eats. Obesity is a combination of behavioral, psychological, biological, genetic, metabolic, and dietary components.

Several studies have concluded that genetics is one of the determining factors in obesity.[5] When both parents are obese the chances that their offspring will be obese can be as high as 80%. When neither parent is obese, the chances fall to about 10%. Differences in BMR between individuals are greater than can be explained by age, sex, and body composition, hence metabolism may also be involved in obesity.[6] The enzyme lipoprotein lipase functions in promoting fat storage. This enzyme is partially regulated by estrogen and testosterone. Obese persons have higher levels of this enzyme. In obese persons who have lost weight, lipoprotein lipase levels are increased.

Physiological variables such as blood glucose, blood pH, and body temperature remain stable even under a variety of conditions. This fact led to the "set point theory". This theory proposes that the body tends to maintain a certain weight by means of its own internal controls. This theory is controversial and unproven. However, many researchers seem to agree that the body somehow regulates its weight. Other factors involved in obesity, such as environmental and behavioral, have received much attention over the past years. Many people assume that every overweight person can achieve weight loss through control. There are innumerable prejudices involved with this assumption. Suffice is to say that obese persons can be compared to persons with high blood pressure, diabetes, etc. Obesity is a serious health problem and obese persons are a subpopulation that require health care. Obese persons die younger from a host of causes, including heart attacks, strokes, certain types of cancer, and complications of diabetes.

Working with obese clients requires patience, understanding, and constant reinforcement. Losing weight the right way is slow and arduous. It is the responsibility of the fitness professional to offer constant positive reinforcement. Goal setting must be reasonable and the client needs to understand that the process is slow.

The steps in working with obese clients are similar to working with non-obese populations. The first step is to obtain a client profile, then a food diary. Analysis of the food diary will determine the client's likes, dislikes, overeating patterns, etc. The calculations and the recommendations will be the same as for a normal population. You will determine total energy expenditure—being sure to adjust for percent body fat. You then reduce or increase calories slightly, being sure to help the client achieve the proper protein, carbohydrate, and fat ratio. Your exercise program should contain all the components of a program designed for obese persons as recommended by the American College of Sports Medicine.

Aging Population

Working with seniors can be a very rewarding experience. Seniors don't care about how they look in "spandex" and don't (typically) bombard you with questions about the latest supplements.

There is not denying it. We are all aging daily. We look in the mirror and wonder who is that aging person looking back at me. For most of us the aging process is unwanted and dreaded. Our only option is age as gracefully as possible. Aging is one of those vague terms that we use constantly but can't define with precision. We can point to friends and relatives who are old, but a specific definition eludes us. We are born, we grow from childhood to adulthood, and then we grow old and die. An English gerontologist defined aging as an increased liability to die.[8]

Have you noticed that 70 and 80 year olds do not look as old as 70 and 80 year olds a decade ago. Is there an explanation for this? Researchers at the USDA Human Nutrition Research Center on Aging at Tufts University tell us "yes".[9] Many persons today are doing their part in slowing the aging process. While genetics plays a role in how well we age, there are many factors that we have control over that can slow the process; and in some cases even reverse it.

Researchers at Tufts have discarded the chronological approach to aging. Biologically as people age they become more diverse than the younger population; i.e., younger people are much more similar physiologically than are older persons. As people age the diversity in physiological parameters increases immensely. Some eighty year olds look more like thirty year olds when measuring certain physiological parameters; similarly, some twenty five year olds physiologically look more like fifty year olds. Researchers at Tufts have focused on a more positive definition of aging. They resurrected a concept that the medical research community has used for years. The term "biomarkers" is used to refer to biological markers of aging. Researchers at Tufts have narrowed the definition to include only the physiological functions that can be altered for the better by changes in a person's lifestyle.

Aging Successfully

What does it take to age successfully? Some of the critical factors involved in maximizing health throughout life include the role of exercise and nutrition, smoking, sleep, stress, personal relationships and heredity.[10] Before examining the major role of exercise and nutrition it is important to understand the aging process and eliminate any prejudices we may have toward this diverse group of people that span more than five decades.

Ageism

When you see an older, frail woman do you automatically think "little old lady" and assume that she is slow, incompetent, or senile? This is a form of prejudice called ageism.[11] Ageism can be defined as any attitude, action, or institutional structure which subordinates a person or group because of age, or any assignment of roles in society purely on the basis of age. Our language and our humor toward the aging reflect this prejudice in terms such as over the hill, fuddy-duddy, little old lady, old hag, old coot, dirty old man.

Our own individual ageist attitudes can be identified and eliminated through continuous exposure to and working with older adults. When working with the older population, it soon became apparent to me that the majority are not senile, are not set in their ways, and are certainly capable of learning new information. After my first presentation to older adults (all were over the age of 90) I had one lovely woman take the time to explain to me: "Dear, please understand that for many of us our hearing is fine, we are not senile, and we are very bright. It simply takes a few seconds longer for the words to go from our ears to our brains; so, please speak more slowly and we will understand every word you say".

Genetics Versus Lifestyle

A common belief that aging is mostly inherited is unfounded.[9] Genetics accounts for less than 30 percent of all aging effects and becomes less important as a person ages so that by the age of eighty, lifestyle choices account for almost 100% of a person's overall health and longevity. Even if sedentary individuals begin at 50 years old to implement exercise and healthy eating they can regain 90 percent of the health benefits of their younger counterparts by age 70.

While we have very little control over the outward signs of aging, we do have tremendous control over the physiological aspects of aging. In essence, everything we do either contributes to or prevents aging and many of the choices that prevent aging are easy and simple to do.

People age at a similar rate until they reach their late twenties or mid thirties.[8] Then between the ages of 28 and 36 most individuals reach a transition point from growing to aging. As people age chronologically variability among individuals becomes great; so much so that averages become meaningless. Certain functions, such as mental activity and IQ, in some individuals show almost no decline and even improve from chronological age 35 to 75.

The challenges facing this diverse group of older adults who span more than five decades are also varied. As individuals approach their seventies and eighties many of the challenges they face are actually a reversal of the challenges they faced in their younger years.

The 50 to 70 Year Old Adult

The 50 to 70 year old must still face the battle of added weight gain and increased risk of chronic diseases associated with weight gain (diabetes, heart disease, hypertension, etc.). Also many adults in this age range are still working and face similar challenges of a hectic, stressful lifestyle as their younger counterparts.[9]

No matter what physical limitations exist, everyone must exercise to remain physiologically young. Exercise is the closest thing we do have to a "magic pill". As previously mentioned, physiological variability in this group is great and heart rate varies widely among individuals. In determining exercise intensity, the BORG scale is recommended. The goal using the BORG scale is to reach an intensity of 15/16 on the original scale, or 7 on the new scale. If the older person has any trace of heart disease a cardiovascular event may occur. The problem is seriously compounded if the older person sits or lies down immediately, takes a hot shower or plunges into a hot tub or steam room. These situations should be avoided for at least 45 minutes to an hour.

Up until the mid-1980's it was assumed that muscle loss (sarcopenia) was age related and inevitable.[9]   However, in the mid-1980's, Walter Frontera, completed research at Tufts University that revised the way we look at exercise.[5] Dr. Frontera investigated the effects of resistance training in sixty and seventy old males.[6] They performed exercises at 80 percent of their one repetition maximum.   In just twelve weeks, muscle hypertrophy increased 10 to 12 percent and muscle strength increased 100 to 175%. The amount of hypertrophy was as much as was expected in young people doing the same amount of exercise. Hence, many of the factors once associated with aging are now known to be due to inactivity. (fat gain, muscle loss, diabetes, heart disease, etc.) Strength training can prevent sarcopenia. It can also improve balance, help prevent osteoporosis, and lessen arthritis pain through stronger muscles which can ease the strain.

A resistance training program for this population should concentrate on a minimum of exercises encompassing all large muscle groups. The participants in the above cited research performed 5 exercises to failure. It is not necessary to add several exercises per muscle group for this population. Maintaining flexibility is critical for this age group if they are to maintain their activities of daily living.[9]

Nutritional Requirements

The evidence is undisputed that diet and nutrition are directly linked to many of the chronic diseases afflicting older adults today. If one is to age successfully then healthy eating in conjunction with exercise is a must.

The single most important nutrition factor is aging successfully is the addition of 5 to 9 servings of fruits and vegetables.[9] Fruits and vegetables are nutrient dense foods that contain large amounts of micronutrients. They contain antioxidants, phytochemicals, fiber, and are low in calories. While all micronutrients – vitamin and minerals - are necessary for successful aging, several nutrients specific to this age group are vitamin D, folate, vitamin B12, vitamin B6, and calcium. Limiting alcohol intake is also a significant factor in aging successfully.

The Over 70 Year Old Adult

Many older adults are faced with very different challenges than their younger counterparts. If exercise has been lacking, this group is typified by decreased muscle mass (sarcopenia) and increased body fat. Rather than facing obesity, they face decreased caloric intake associated with sarcpenia and are therefore at increased risk for nutritional deficiencies.[9] Nutritional status surveys have indeed shown a marked increase in risk of malnutrition and subclinical deficiencies in this group. Dietary quality becomes difficult to ensure since overall energy intake becomes so low.

If successful aging is to continue in this age group, cardiovascular exercise is a must. In addition to the aerobic benefits, cardiovascular exercise increases appetite, which in turn can help ward off nutritional deficiencies typically seen in this group. Precautions for this group are similar to that for the 50 to 70 year old adult. However, this group is typified by more limitations to exercise and exercise prescription may have to be modified. Tufts University guidelines emphasize the use of the BORG scale for this population as well, and recommend a 10 minute warm up and cool down.[9]

Resistance training also becomes more critical in this group if successfully aging is to occur. Not only is it possible for individuals over 70 to increase muscle mass, but all individuals, even centurions, can build muscle. In 1990, Dr. Maria Fiatarone published her research in which men and women in their eighties and nineties increased muscle strength by 175% and muscle hypertrophy by 10% in 8 weeks.[12] Resistance training can prevent sarcopenia and hence prevent the nutritional deficiencies associated with it.

Resistance training programs, along with stretching programs for this population have been published in several books.[13]

Nutritional Requirements

Tufts University researchers have developed a separate pyramid to address the specific needs of this age group.[12] As previously mentioned this group faces the challenge of adequate caloric intake. The base of the "70+ Pyramid" is narrowed signifying the reduced energy intake of 1200 to 1600 calories per day for many adults in this age group. With advancing age nutrient intake typically becomes more and more decreased making prevention of deficiencies a prime factor. The trick to preventing deficiency is to eat as many nutrient dense foods as possible, while minimizing non nutritive foods.

Older people in this age group are more prone to constipation and other adverse gastrointestinal conditions. The base of the "70+ Pyramid" indicates that they should make a conscious effort to take in at least 8 glasses of water every day. A lack of fluid is a major contributor to constipation, and many elderly people do not get enough fluids. The thirst mechanism becomes blunted with age, hence this population can not depend on this mechanism to determine fluid intake.[12]

Because of the reduced energy intake in this group, emphasis is placed on obtaining nutrient dense foods in each category, such as whole grain foods, varied colored fruits and vegetables, low fat dairy products, and lean meats, fish, and poultry.[12]

Icons throughout the grains, fruits, and vegetable groups of the pyramid highlight the importance of fiber for this population. Fiber is emphasized to a greater extent in this population as a hedge against constipation which is a common and serious problem. Fiber also helps ward off diverticulitis which becomes more common in this population. Diverticulitis is an infection in the large intestine which causes acute abdominal pain, fever, and nausea and sometimes requires surgery. To obtain the recommended minimum 20 grams of fiber, whole grain breads, whole fruits over juices, and high-fiber cereals are again emphasized. Tufts researchers also recommend choosing beans over meat as a main dish several times a week. A half cup of beans contain between five to ten grams of fiber.[12]

To obtain adequate amounts of vitamin C, beta carotene, and folate deeply colored vegetables are recommended; dark green, orange, and yellow vegetables, whether fresh, frozen, or canned.

Another key difference in the 70+ pyramid is that it is topped with a flag that represents the possible need for dietary supplements. As mentioned previously, both calcium and vitamin D absorption decrease with age; this has adverse effects on bone health and increases the risk of fractures. The ability to absorb vitamin B12 needed for normal nerve function also decreases with age, making this another nutrient that may need to be supplemented. All individuals in this age group should discuss supplementation with their health care provider.[12]

The Tufts researchers point out that these dietary recommendations are aimed at healthy, mobile seniors with the resources needed to prepare adequate meals. It is not designed to consider the special dietary needs of those with significant health problems, nor does it address socioeconomic factors, such as decreased income and mobility, that make it harder for many seniors to meet nutrient needs. But all seniors should still head the pyramid's main messages: people over 70 have specific needs and meeting these needs is critical in aging successfully.[12]

Obtaining all of the essential nutrients need not be a daunting task. Many of the added supplements previously discussed can be obtained in a multivitamin. Be sure to look for the recommended dosages. When looking for a multivitamin, remember that supplement companies buy their vitamins and minerals from the same small group of multinational manufacturers. Since there are no federal standards it is advised to look for USP on the label which indicates that the tablets have met the voluntary standards set by the U.S. Pharmacopoeia, and that they dissolve in a lab test designed to mimic what happens in the gut. Another way to make sure that the vitamin disintegrates is to buy chewable brands or large drug chains or retailers who are large enough to demand top quality from vitamin makers.

Most experts recommend taking the multivitamin with meals because some nutrients are better absorbed with food. As previously discussed, calcium may be an exception, depending on the type of supplement. Also calcium and iron should not be taken together. See section on "Choosing a Multivitamin".

Athletes

Working with athletes is very similar to working with other populations. Special considerations include the amounts of carbohydrates, water, fats, proteins, vitamins and minerals.

Carbohydrates

Athletes benefit the most from the amount of carbohydrates stored in the body. In the early stages of moderate exercise, carbohydrates provide 40 to 50 percent of the energy requirement. Carbohydrates yield more energy per unit of oxygen consumed than fats. Because oxygen often is the limiting factor in long duration events, it is beneficial for the athlete to use the energy source requiring the least amount of oxygen per kilocalorie produced. As work intensity increases, carbohydrate utilization increases.[14-17]

During exercise, the glycogen is converted back to glucose and is used for energy. The ability to sustain prolonged vigorous exercise is directly related to initial levels of muscle glycogen. The body stores a limited amount of carbohydrate in the muscles and liver. If the event lasts for less than 90 minutes, the glycogen stored in the muscle is enough to supply the needed energy. Extra carbohydrates will not help, any more than adding gas to a half-full tank will make the car go faster.[14-17]

For events that require heavy work for more than 90 minutes, a high-carbohydrate diet eaten for two to three days before the event allows glycogen storage spaces to be filled. Long distance runners, cyclists, cross-country skiers, canoe racers, swimmers and soccer players report benefits from a pre-competition diet where 70 percent of the calories comes from carbohydrates.[16]

According to the Olympic Training Center in Colorado Springs, endurance athletes on a high-carbohydrate diet can exercise longer than athletes eating a low-carbohydrate, high-fat diet. Eating a high-carbohydrate diet constantly is not advised. This conditions the body to use only carbohydrates for fuel and not the fatty acids derived from fats.[14-]

For continuous activities of three to four hours, make sure that glycogen stores in the muscles and liver are at a maximum. Consider taking carbohydrates during the event in the form of carbohydrate solutions. The current recommendation is a 6 to 8 percent glucose solution.[17]

You can make an excellent home-brewed 7.6 percent sports drink with reasonable sodium amounts. Add 6 tablespoons sugar and 1/3 teaspoon salt to each quart of water. Dissolve sugar and cool. The salt translates into a sodium concentration of 650 mg/liter. This small amount is good for marathon runners.[17]

Electrolyte beverages can be used if the athlete tolerates them, but other electrolytes are not essential until after the event. Experiment during training to find the best beverage for you.[14-17]

Eating sugar or honey just before an event does not provide any extra energy for the event. It takes about 30 minutes for the sugar to enter the blood stream. This practice may also lead to dehydration. Water is needed to absorb the sugar into the cells. Furthermore, sugar eaten before an event may hinder performance because it triggers a surge of insulin. The insulin causes a sharp drop in blood sugar level in about 30 minutes. Competing when the blood sugar level is low leads to fatigue, nausea and dehydration.[16]

A diet where 70 percent of calories comes from carbohydrates for three days prior to the event is sometimes helpful for endurance athletes. Water retention is often associated with carbohydrate loading. This may cause stiffness in the muscles and sluggishness early in the event. A three-day regimen minimizes this effect. The previously suggested seven days of deprivation/repletion is not recommended due to increased risks of coronary heart disease. In addition, electrocardiograph abnormalities may occur and training during the deprivation phase may be difficult.

Water

Water is an important nutrient for the athlete. Athletes should start any event hydrated and replace as much lost fluid as possible by drinking chilled liquids at frequent intervals during the event. Chilled fluids are absorbed faster and help lower body temperature.[14-17]

Fats

Fat also provides body fuel. For moderate exercise, about half of the total energy expenditure is derived from free fatty acid metabolism. If the event lasts more than an hour, the body may use mostly fats for energy. Using fat as fuel depends on the event's duration and the athlete's condition. Trained athletes use fat for energy more quickly than untrained athletes.[14-17]

Fat may contribute as much as 75 percent of the energy demand during prolonged aerobic work in the endurance-trained athlete. There is evidence that the rate of fat metabolism may be accelerated by ingesting caffeine prior to and during endurance performance. However, insomnia, restlessness and ringing of the ears can occur. Furthermore, caffeine acts as a diuretic and athletes want to avoid the need to urinate during competition.[16]

Protein

After carbohydrates and fats, protein provides energy for the body. Exercise may increase an athlete's need for protein, depending on the type and frequency of exercise. Extra protein is stored as fat. In the fully grown athlete, it is training that builds muscle, not protein per se. The ADA reports that a protein intake of 10 to 12 percent of total calories is sufficient. Most authorities recommend that endurance athletes eat between 1.2-1.4 grams protein per kg of body weight per day; resistance and strength-trained athletes may need as much as 1.6-1.7 grams protein per kg of body weight. (A kilogram equals 2.2 pounds.)

Japanese researchers demonstrated that "sports anemia" may appear in the early stages of training with intakes of less than 1 gram/kg of body weight per day of high quality protein. To calculate your protein needs, divide your ideal weight by 2.2 pounds to obtain your weight in kilograms. Then multiply kilograms by the grams of protein recommended.[14-17]

A varied diet will provide more than enough protein as caloric intake increases. Furthermore, Americans tend to eat more than the recommended amounts of protein. Excess protein can deprive the athlete of more efficient fuel and can lead to dehydration. High-protein diets increase the water requirement necessary to eliminate the nitrogen through the urine. Also, an increase in metabolic rate can occur and, therefore, increased oxygen consumption. Protein supplements are unnecessary and not recommended. Increased caloric intake through a varied diet ensures a sufficient amount of vitamins and minerals for the athlete. There is no evidence that taking more vitamins than is obtained by eating a variety of foods will improve performance. Thiamin, riboflavin and niacin (B vitamins) are needed to produce energy from the fuel sources in the diet. However, more than enough of these vitamins will be obtained from the foods eaten. Carbohydrate and protein foods are excellent sources of these vitamins. Furthermore, the B vitamins are water soluble and are not stored in the body. Some female athletes may lack riboflavin. Milk products not only increase the riboflavin level but also provide protein and calcium. The body stores excess fat-soluble vitamins A, D, E and K. Excessive amounts of fat-soluble vitamins may have toxic effects.[14-17]

Vitamins and Minerals

Minerals play an important role in performance. Heavy exercise affects the body's supply of sodium, potassium, iron and calcium. To replenish sodium lost through sweating, eat normally following the competition. Avoid excessive amounts of sodium. Eating potassium-rich foods such as oranges, bananas and potatoes supplies necessary potassium. Salt tablets are not recommended.[17]

Sweating naturally increases the concentration of salt in the body. Salt tablets take water from the cells, causing weak muscles. They also increase potassium losses. Potassium is important to help regulate muscle activity. Salt added to beverages during endurance events may be helpful.

Iron carries oxygen and is another important mineral for athletes. Female athletes and athletes between 13 and 19 years old may have inadequate supplies of iron. Female athletes who train heavily have a high incidence of amenorrhea and thus conserve iron stores. Amenorrhea is the absence of regular, monthly periods. Iron supplements may be prescribed by a physician if laboratory tests indicate an iron deficiency. Excess iron can cause constipation. To avoid this problem, eat fruits, vegetables, whole grain breads and cereals.[17]

Calcium is an important nutrient for everyone. Female athletes should have an adequate supply of calcium to avoid calcium loss from bones. Calcium loss may lead to osteoporosis later in life. Dairy products, especially low-fat choices, are the best source of calcium.[17]

Pre-Game Meal

A pre-game meal three to four hours before the event allows for optimal digestion and energy supply. Most authorities recommend small pre-game meals that provide 500 to 1,000 calories.[17]

The meal should be high in starch, which breaks down more easily than protein and fats. The starch should be in the form of complex carbohydrates (breads, cold cereal, pasta, fruits and vegetables). They are digested at a rate that provides consistent energy to the body and are emptied from the stomach in two to three hours.[17]

High-sugar foods lead to a rapid rise in blood sugar, followed by a decline in blood sugar and less energy. In addition, concentrated sweets can draw fluid into the gastrointestinal tract and contribute to dehydration, cramping, nausea and diarrhea. Don't consume any carbohydrates one and a half to two hours before an event. This may lead to premature exhaustion of glycogen stores in endurance events.

Avoid a meal high in fats. Fat takes longer to digest. Fiber has a similar effect, as well.

Take in adequate fluids during this pre-game time. Caffeine (cola, coffee, tea) may lead to dehydration by increasing urine production.

Don't ignore the psychological aspect of eating foods you enjoy and tolerate well before an event. However, choose wisely — bake meat instead of frying it, for example.

Some athletes may prefer a liquid pre-game meal, especially if the event begins within two or three hours. A liquid meal will move out of the stomach by the time a meet or match begins. Remember, include water with this meal.

Regardless of age, gender or sport, the pre-game meal recommendations are the same. Following a training session or competition, a small meal eaten within thirty minutes is very beneficial. The meal should be mixed, meaning it contains carbohydrate, protein, and fat. Protein synthesis is greatest during the window of time immediately following a workout and carbohydrates will help replete diminished glycogen stores.

Maintain nutritional conditioning not only for athletic events, but all the time. A pre-game meal or special diet for several days prior to competition cannot make up for an inadequate daily food intake in previous months or years.[18]

Lifelong good nutrition habits must be emphasized. Combine good eating practices with a good training and conditioning program plus good genes, and a winning athlete can result!

Vegetarians

People who exclude animal products from their diets do so for many varied reasons. Some people exclude red meat only while others exclude chicken, fish, eggs and dairy products. Lactovegetarians omit meats, eggs, fish and poultry but include dairy products. Lacto-ovo-vegetarians include milk products and eggs, but exclude meat, poultry, fish and seafood. Vegans exclude all animal products including meat, poultry, fish, eggs, and dairy products.[18]

Research on the health benefits of vegetarian diets is complex since this population differs in other respects as well. Vegetarians are typically active, use little alcohol and refrain from smoking. Available research does point to health benefits of vegetarian diets. In general, vegetarians maintain a lower and healthier body weight than nonvegetarians.[5] Vegetarians tend to have lower pressure and lower rates of hypertension than nonvegetarians and the incidence of heart disease is much lower. Vegetarians have a significantly lower rate of cancer than the general population.[18]

Vegetarians can easily obtain large quantities of most nutrients with a few exceptions. Protein from vegetable products has a lower digestibility rating and contains lower amounts of protein. Many vegetarians supplement their protein intake with textured vegetable proteins. These foods are formulated to look like animal products and are often fortified with vitamins and minerals.

Vegetarians must also pay attention to iron intake. The iron in plant foods is poorly absorbed. However, iron absorption is enhanced by vitamin C (chili has iron in the beans and the tomatoes have lots of vitamin C) hence vegetarians are not any more likely to be iron deficient than the general public.[18]

Zinc is similar to iron in that meat provides the richest sources of iron and plant sources are not well absorbed. Also, soy, a staple in most vegetarian diets, interferes with zinc absorption. Vegetarians are advised to include lots of whole grains, nuts, and legumes.[18]

Vegetarians who consume no dairy products risk becoming deficient in calcium. These vegetarians must pay special attention to selecting foods such as fortified juices, soy milk and breakfast cereals.

Vitamin B12 is found in animal products. Small amounts are found in tempeh, seaweed, and chlorella but the amounts are insignificant. Vegetarians must rely on fortified sources or supplements to obtain enough B12. Without adequate amounts of B12 nerve damage can occur.[18]

Vegans that do not eat fish may become deficient in omega-3-fatty acids. To obtain sufficient amounts of B12 vegetarians need to consume flaxseed, walnuts, soybeans and their oils.[18]

SUMMARY

Before attempting to implement any of the suggested programs in this chapter, be sure that you have studied previous chapters in this manual. It is assumed that you understand the biochemistry of the energy nutrients, energy production, supplements, nutrition research and the prerequisites involved before implementing a program.

Information in this chapter should not be used to alter a medically prescribed regimen or as a form of self treatment. Implementing any of the programs in this chapter requires working directly with a qualified professional.

The first step in instituting an individual program is to set up a preliminary interview (15 minutes) with all potential clients. This interview is designed to determine the client's stage of readiness to change. Trying to work with clients in the precontemplative stage will only cause frustration and can actually induce failure on the part of the client. It's important to understand that some individuals are not ready to make lifestyle changes. As much as we wish we could "save everyone", we can not. Your role during the interview is to identify which clients are ready and which clients are not ready to enter your program. If a potential client is in the precontemplation stage your next course of action is to explain that your program is not the best program for him/her and, as stated above, explain that you can't help him/her. If the individual is thinking about making changes, or is ready to make changes, the interview then becomes your chance to convince him/her that nutrition is a large component to success in body composition change. Once you're certain that the person is ready to make changes, the next component of the interview is to describe your services in detail. What can the client expect from you, and what will his/her responsibilities be? You will want to provide details concerning your program such as the length of the program, services you will provide, etc. This is the time to have the individual sign up for your program (more on pricing, selling etc., in chapter on "Making it a Business"). Most of us in the fitness profession do not perceive ourselves as sales people; but in a very real sense we are. We are selling the most valuable commodity there is - health. Once the individual signs up for your program, the rest of the interview consists of receiving payment, having the new client sign a legal agreement, a responsibility clause, and discussing preparations for the first appointment.

In this first appointment, the fitness professional will need to complete a client profile, perform body composition measurements and instruct the client on how to keep a "food log". With the information you collected in the first session, the next stop is to determine the body composition measures described, then use the resulting body fat % to determine the client's total energy expenditure. See Appendix for TEE calculation worksheet. Once the client's body comp measures are completed, TEE can be calculated. The second appointment consists of collecting the client's food log and providing the client with at least one of the three body composition measures you calculated, the TEE calculation you arrived at, and the appropriate menu plan for the client's TEE. Review client goals at this point to be sure they meet the criteria for SMART goals. If they don't meet the criteria, help the client figure out how to re-word them. After the second appointment, analyze the client food log using a computerized program. Make a list of possible changes that are required for a healthy eating plan. You will also want to provide your client with a list of nutrient content in foods (see Appendix).

In the third appointment you will want to present the results of the diet analysis. Once your client is satisfied with his/her own efficacy in regard to lifestyle change, begins to set SMART goals and understands the steps needed to continue, it's your job to ask if the client is ready to move on without your help. If the client no longer needs your guidance and is ready to go it alone, you've done your job!

Group programs offer an added benefit of interaction with other individuals with similar goals. This can be seen from the success of groups such as Weight Watchers. Fitness professionals can build on this concept by providing exercise prescription and more detailed information at each meeting. It is important to structure a group program that includes a "curriculum". A curriculum ensures that participants will complete the program with a new level of acquired information.

Fitness professionals, again, are an ideal profession to take on the challenge of reducing childhood obesity rates. Free materials to educate children on healthy lifestyles abound. Materials are available free of charge from mypyramid.gov (click on resource library).[4]   While these sites are informative and provide a plethora of free materials, there are several problems associates with using these materials and initiating a youth program. One problem is that free materials do not provide a curriculum. It is up to the instructor to decide on available topics and develop a curriculum - a time consuming project.   Another problem is that exercise is typically not included in combination with the nutrition component. So fitness professionals would need to invest a considerable amount of time to construct a program.

The steps in working with obese clients are similar to working with non-obse populations. The first step is to obtain a client profile, then a food diary. Analysis of the food diary will determine the clients likes, dislikes, overeating patterns, etc. The calculations and the recommendations will be the same as for a healthy population. You will determine total energy expenditure—being sure to adjust for percent body fat. You then reduce or increase calories slightly, being sure to help the client achieve the proper protein, carbohydrate, and fat ratio. Your exercise program should contain all the components of a program designed for obese persons as recommended by the American College of Sports Medicine.

Working with seniors can be a very rewarding experience. Seniors don't care about how they look in "spandex" and don't (typically) bombard you with questions about the latest supplements. There is no denying it. We are all aging daily. We look in the mirror and wonder who is that aging person looking back at me. For most of us the aging process is unwanted and dreaded. Our only option is age as gracefully as possible.

Working with athletes is very similar to working with other populations. Special considerations include the amounts of carbohydrates, water, fats, proteins, vitamins and minerals.

Vegetarian diets offer many healthy benefits but can also lead to possible deficiencies in protein, iron, zinc, calcium, and vitamin B12. Strict vegetarians need to be aware of the possibility of deficiencies and guard against them by eating a variety of foods, along with enriched foods and possibly a supplement.

CHAPTER 12 - SAMPLE TEST

1. Describe the steps in instituting an individual nutrition program.

2. Describe the differences between instituting a group nutrition program versus an individual nutrition program.

3. Describe the difficulties with instituting a youth program.

4. Describe how to implement a program for obese individuals, seniors, and athletes.

5. Complete the case studies at the end of this chapter.

REFERENCES

1. Pentz, J. Nutrition Specialist Manual,7th ed. *Nutrition Knowledge Quiz*, LMA Publishing: MA. 2005.

2. Pentz, J. Nutrition Specialist Manual, 7th ed. *Responsibility Agreement*. LMA Publishing: MA.,2005.

3. Pentz, J. Nutrition Manager Pro Series Software, 2003.

4. Pentz, J. *Lifestyle Journal.* LMA Publishing: MA. 2003.

5. Pentz, J. You Are What You Eat. Nutrition Specialist Manual,7th ed. *Nutrition Knowledge Quiz*, LMA Publishing: MA. 2005.

6. Pentz, J. Healthy Balance Instructor Manual. LMA Publishing: MA. 2003.

7. http://kidshealth.org/parent/nutrition_fit/nutrition/habits.html

8. Comfort, A. The biology of senescence, 3rde. NY: Elsever, 1979.

9. Evans, W, IH Rosenberg. *Biomarkers.* NY: Simon & Schuster, 1991.

10. Napier, K. Cancer fighting foods. webmd.com, February 21, 2000.

11. Ageism; www.webster.edu/woolflm/ageismintro.html.

12. Fiatarone, MA, et al. High intensity strength training in nonagenarians: Effects on skeletal muscle, *Journal of the American Medical Association,* 263:3029-3034, 1990.

13. Nelson, M. Strong Women Stay Young: Bantan Doubleday Dell, 1997.

14. Advances in Sports Medicine and Fitness, Volume 2, 1989.

15. Nutrition for Fitness and Sports, Melvin Williams; Brown, Benchmark, 1995.

16. Nutrition for the Recreational Athlete, Catherine Jackson, editor; CRC Press, 1995

17. http://www.ext.colostate.edu/PUBS/foodnut/09362.html.

18. P.K.Newby, K.L. Tucker, et al. Rish of overweight and obesity among semivegetarian, lactovegetarian, and vegan women. Amer J of Clinical Nutrition. 81: 1267-1274. 2005.

Case Study 1 - Sally Stressed

Sally is a 28 year old single RN who cannot ever remember being anything but overweight. During High School and College she was "big" but during a relationship of several years which recently ended, she ended up "bigger than ever". She has been working with a trainer for approximately 6 months and has managed to lose about 20 pounds but she has plateaued at just over 200 lbs. She is now 208 at 5'10". Her trainer is asking her to eat more often and eat more calories but Sally is afraid she is going to gain back the weight she has lost already. She is strength training with her trainer 3 days per week and doing cardio for at least 3 days per week, 30 minutes per day. She does not want working out to consume her entire life and is reaching out for a solution that does not involve 3 hours per day at the gym.

See client profile on next page for more details.

1. Determine Sally's body mass index and waist to hip ratio.
2. Determine Sally's estimated total energy expenditure.
3. Analyze the following computerized analysis. Compare the actual intake with the DRI for all nutrients.
4. Based on all the information, what recommendations would you make to help Sally achieve her goals.

Results:

BMI _____

Waist to Hip _____

Percent Body Fat _____

Recommendation _____

_____

_____

_____

_____

_____

_____

_____

Sally Stressed

Phone Day	Ext.	Phone Night	Phone Cell	Height		Weight	Stress Level 1-10	
				Feet 5'		Pounds:	Home	Work
Date of Birth: 09/15/1980	**Gender:** Female	**Occupation:** RN		Inches 10"		208 lbs	3	6

Emergency Contact Name (First / Last)	Blood Type	Weight@Heaviest / Age
		230 lbs 26 yrs
Phone Day Extension **Phone Night**		Weight@Lightest / Age
		185 lbs 18 yrs

Personal History

Do you have any limitations to exercise? No

If so what are these limitations?

What is your exercise program now? 3x strength with trainer, 2 - 3x cardio 30 -60 minutes

How long have you been following this regimen? 6 monthe

Have you had any injuries due to exercise? no

Medical History

Are you seeing a physician for any reason? No

Are you taking any medications? No

Are you allergic to any medications? No

Do you smoke? No

Did you ever smoke? No

If you did smoke when did you quit? n0

How long did you smoke? n/a

Disease History

Medications Currently Using

Eating Patterns

What is your largest meal?   Lunch

Do you snack during the day?   No

What types of snacks?

Do you snack after dinner?   Sometimes

What size do you consider your portions?   Large

Do you eat when depressed? Yes

Do you eat when stressed? Yes

Do you feel you have any eating disorders?   No

Have you ever had any eating disorders?   No

Comments

Allergy History

Medical Evaluation

1/15/2008 ~ Diet Analysis Summary

Sally Stressed

Blood Test Results
Glucose
Hematocrit
Hemoglobin
MCH
Serum Iron
GIBC
Ferritin

Date	01/15/2008

Circulatory
R.H.R.
BP Systolic
BP Diastolic

Serum Lipids
HDL
LDL
Cholesterol
Triglycerides

Body Composition	
Body Weight	208 lbs
Height	5' 10"
BMI	29.93
Body Fat	34.0 %
Waist to hip Ratio	

Energy Nutrient Evaluation
Tuesday, January 15, 2008

Sally Stressed

Date	01/15/2008	

Macronutrient Ratio		
	Protein	Carbs	Lipids

	Protein	Carbs	Lipids
Calories	400	926	584
Ratio	21%	49%	31%

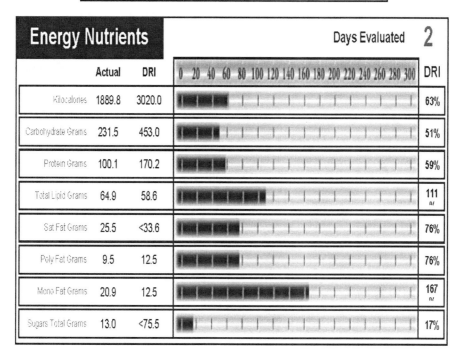

Energy Nutrients
Days Evaluated 2

	Actual	DRI	0 20 40 60 80 100 120 140 160 180 200 220 240 260 280 300	DRI
Kilocalories	1889.8	3020.0		63%
Carbohydrate Grams	231.5	453.0		51%
Protein Grams	100.1	170.2		59%
Total Lipid Grams	64.9	58.6		111
Sat Fat Grams	25.5	<33.6		76%
Poly Fat Grams	9.5	12.5		76%
Mono Fat Grams	20.9	12.5		167
Sugars Total Grams	13.0	<75.5		17%

Micronutrient Evaluation
Tuesday, January 15, 2008

Sally Stressed

	Actual	DRI	0 20 40 60 80 100 120 140 160 180 200 220 240 260 280 300	DRI
Vitamin A IU	23232.2	2333.8		995%
Thiamin B1 mg	0.9	1.1		84%
Riboflavin B2 mg	1.7	1.1		157%
Vitamin B6 mg	2.4	1.3		182%
Vitamin B12 mcg	4.5	2.4		186%
Pant. Acid mg	4.6	5.0		93%
Folate mcg	315.8	400.0		79%
Niacin mg	15.9	14.0		114%
Biotin mcg	45.0	30.0		150%
Vitamin C mg	173.4	75.0		231%
Vitamin D IU	5.0	200.0		3%
Vitamin E mg	12.9	15.0		86%
Vitamin K mcg	0.0	90.0		0%
Sodium mg	2088.8	<1500.0		139%
Calcium mg	1063.0	1000.0		106%
Potassium mg	3214.5	4700.0		68%
Phosphorus mg	1300.9	700.0		186%
Copper mg	1.8	9.0		20%
Magnesium mg	310.2	310.0		100%
Iron mg	14.7	18.0		81%
Zinc mg	13.2	8.0		166%
Selenium mcg	41.1	55.0		75%
Manganese mg	2.2	1.8		125%
Molybdenum mcg	0.0	45.0		0%
Iodine mcg	22.5	150.0		15%
Chloride mg	0.0	2300.0		0%
Chromium mcg	0.0	25.0		0%

Sally Stressed

Essential Amino Acids

	Actual	DRI	0 20 40 60 80 100 120 140 160 180 200 220 240 260 280 300	DRI
Histidine g	1.8	1.1		154%
Isoleucine g	2.6	2.8		93%
Leucine g	4.5	4.5		99%
Lysine g	4.2	3.5		118%
Methionine g	1.3	1.8		70%
Cystine g	0.6	1.8		32%
Phenylalanine g	2.4	4.5		54%
Tyrosine g	2.1	4.5		46%
Throenine g	2.2	1.8		122%
Tryptophan g	0.7	0.7		99%
Valine g	2.9	2.5		115%

Other

	Actual	DRI	0 20 40 60 80 100 120 140 160 180 200 220 240 260 280 300	DRI
Cholesterol mg	142.9	<300.0		48%
Fiber Total g	19.9	25.0		80%
Choline mg	0.0	425.0		0%
Water oz	105.6	134.2		79%
Alcohol g	0.0			
Caffeine	274.9			

Sally Stressed - One Day Food Log

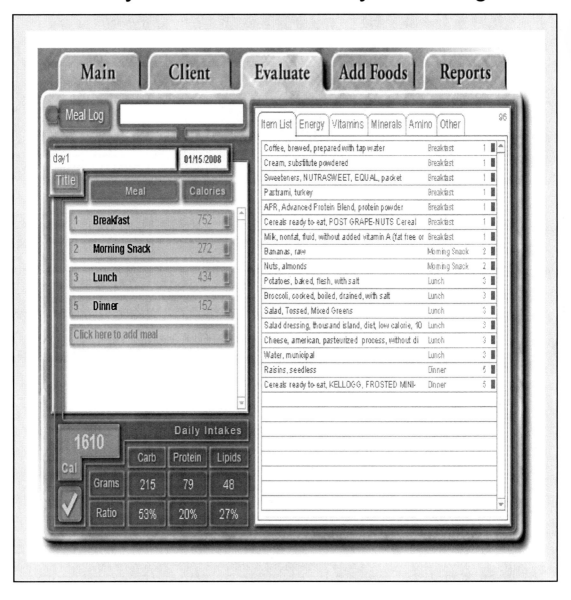

355

Case Study 2 – Derrick Dunn

Derrick is a 53 year old CIO and Internet consultant. He has a home gym and is extremely regimented about his eating and about his workout program. He lifts weights 5 days per week and runs a few miles 2 or 3 days per week, sprinting the last several yards back to his home. He filters his water, avoids certain foods such as bottom feeding fish for their lack of dietary cleanliness, avoids all sugars, HFCS, trans fats and food additives. He rarely eats out and he measures everything that he eats to exact quantities. He eats very small portions of food, despite the variety. Derrick is pleased with his lean look but would like to add muscle to his structure, without adding any fat. He is 5'9", weighs 143 pounds and his body fat is 10%. He likes a wide variety of fruits and vegetables, (organic) prefers vegetarian protein sources but will eat chicken and white fillet type fish, though it is not his favorite, and eats only organic grains and organic eggs.

See client profile on next page for more details.

1. Determine Derrick's body mass index and waist to hip ratio.
2. Determine Derrick's estimated total energy expenditure.
3. Analyze the following computerized analysis. Compare the actual intake with the DRI for all nutrients.
4. Based on all the information, what recommendations would you make to help Derrick achieve his goals.

```
Results:

BMI               _____

Waist to Hip      _____

Percent Body Fat  _____

Recommendation    _____

_____
_____
_____
_____
_____
_____
_____
_____
```

Derrick Dunn

Phone Day	Ext.	Phone Night	Phone Cell	Height	Weight	Stress Level 1-10

						Home	Work

Height — Feet 5' Inches 9"

Weight — Pounds: 138 lbs

Stress Level — Home 3 Work 6

Date of Birth: 12/20/1953	Gender: Male	Occupation: CIO

Emergency Contact Name (First / Last)	Blood Type	Weight@Heaviest / Age
		145 lbs 45 yrs

Phone Day	Extension	Phone Night	Weight@Lightest / Age
			140 lbs 45 yrs

Personal History

Do you have any limitations to exercise? No

If so what are these limitations?

What is your exercise program now? run 3 x per week, lift 5x per week

How long have you been following this regimen? years

Have you had any injuries due to exercise? no

Medical History

Are you seeing a physician for any reason? No

Are you taking any medications? No

Are you allergic to any medications? No

Do you smoke? No

Did you ever smoke? No

If you did smoke when did you quit?

How long did you smoke?

Eating Patterns

What is your largest meal?   Lunch

Do you snack during the day? Yes

What types of snacks?   Nuts Fruits

Do you snack after dinner?

What size do you consider your portions? Small

Do you eat when depressed? No

Do you eat when stressed? No

Do you feel you have any eating disorders? No

Have you ever had any eating disorders? No

Comments

Disease History

Medications Currently Using

Allergy History

Medical Evaluation
12/6/2007 ~ Diet Analysis Summary

Derrick Dunn

Blood Test Results

Glucose
Hematocrit
Hemoglobin
MCH
Serum Iron
GIBC
Ferritin

Serum Lipids

HDL
LDL
Cholesterol
Triglycerides

Date

12/06/2007

Circulatory

R.H.R.
BP Systolic
BP Diastolic

Body Composition

Body Weight	138 lbs
Height	5' 9"
BMI	20.43
Body Fat	10.0 %
Waist to hip Ratio	

Energy Nutrient Evaluation
Thursday, December 6, 2007

Derrick Dunn

Date	12/06/2007	

Macronutrient Ratio

	Protein	Carbs	Lipids
Calories	372	1133	567
Ratio	18%	56%	28%

Energy Nutrients — Days Evaluated 1

	Actual	DRI	0 20 40 60 80 100 120 140 160 180 200 220 240 260 280 300	DRI
Kilocalories	2022.2	2951.0		69%
Carbohydrate Grams	283.2	442.7		64%
Protein Grams	92.9	94.1		99%
Total Lipid Grams	63.1	89.3		71%
Sat Fat Grams	9.1	<32.8		28%
Poly Fat Grams	15.7	28.3		55%
Mono Fat Grams	29.2	28.3		103%
Sugars Total Grams	20.7	<73.8		28%

Micronutrient Evaluation
Thursday, December 6, 2007

Derrick Dunn

	Actual	DRI	0 20 40 60 80 100 120 140 160 180 200 220 240 260 280 300	DRI
Vitamin A IU	9101.1	3000.6		303%
Thiamin B1 mg	1.7	1.2		142%
Riboflavin B2 mg	2.0	1.3		153%
Vitamin B6 mg	1.9	1.7		115%
Vitamin B12 mcg	4.0	2.4		165%
Pant. Acid mg	4.7	5.0		93%
Folate mcg	182.5	400.0		46%
Niacin mg	17.5	16.0		109%
Biotin mcg	0.0	30.0		0%
Vitamin C mg	103.1	90.0		115%
Vitamin D IU	0.0	400.0		0%
Vitamin E mg	10.5	15.0		70%
Vitamin K mcg	0.0	120.0		0%
Sodium mg	2723.9	<1300.0		210%
Calcium mg	647.1	1200.0		54%
Potassium mg	3430.0	4700.0		73%
Phosphorus mg	1185.2	700.0		169%
Copper mg	1.5	9.0		17%
Magnesium mg	409.3	420.0		97%
Iron mg	11.6	8.0		145%
Zinc mg	6.4	11.0		58%
Selenium mcg	129.4	55.0		235%
Manganese mg	6.3	2.3		274%
Molybdenum mcg	0.0	45.0		0%
Iodine mcg	0.0	150.0		0%
Chloride mg	0.0	2000.0		0%
Chromium mcg	0.0	30.0		0%

Derrick Dunn

Essential Amino Acids

	Actual	DRI	0 20 40 60 80 100 120 140 160 180 200 220 240 260 280 300	DRI
Histidine g	2.0	0.8		265%
Isoleucine g	3.5	1.8		191%
Leucine g	6.0	3.0		199%
Lysine g	4.8	2.4		205%
Methionine g	1.8	1.2		151%
Cystine g	1.3	1.2		105%
Phenylalanine g	3.7	3.0		122%
Tyrosine g	2.6	3.0		86%
Throenine g	3.0	1.2		247%
Tryptophan g	0.9	0.4		200%
Valine g	4.0	1.7		237%

Other

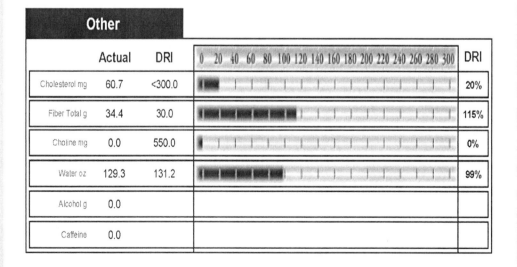

	Actual	DRI	0 20 40 60 80 100 120 140 160 180 200 220 240 260 280 300	DRI
Cholesterol mg	60.7	<300.0		20%
Fiber Total g	34.4	30.0		115%
Choline mg	0.0	550.0		0%
Water oz	129.3	131.2		99%
Alcohol g	0.0			
Caffeine	0.0			

One Day Food Log – Derrick Dunn

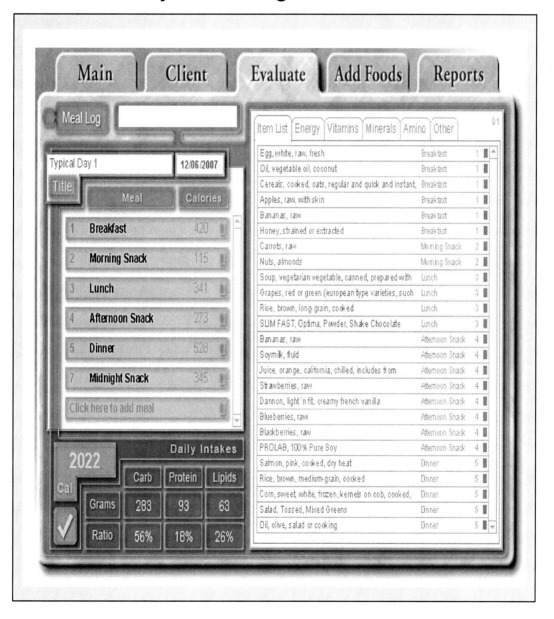

Case Study 3 – Emily Energetic

Emily is a very active, very energetic 74 year old. She grows many of her own fruits and vegetables, does a home strength training program daily, gulfs at least 4 or 5 times per week and walks with her lab mix dog daily. Emily has had some problems with acid reflux recently and bouts of diarrhea. She would like to lose 8 or 10 pounds and feels like she cannot control her snacking during the evening hours. Her husband has no interest in eating "healthfully" – he enjoys his meats, salty snacks and desserts, but she is concerned for both of their health as they are seniors. She was raised in the generation where you eat large portions, clean your plate, and never snack before a meal, because it spoils your appetite. Emily is 5'1" tall, weighs 145 pounds and measures 35% body fat.

See client profile on next page for more details.

1. Determine Emily's body mass index and waist to hip ratio.
2. Determine Emily's estimated total energy expenditure.
3. Analyze the following computerized analysis. Compare the actual intake with the DRI for all nutrients.
4. Based on all the information, what recommendations would you make to help Emily achieve her goals.

Results:

BMI _____

Waist to Hip _____

Percent Body Fat _____

Recommendation _____

_____

_____

_____

_____

_____

_____

_____

_____

Emily Energetic

Phone Day	Ext.	Phone Night	Phone Cell	Height	Weight	Stress Level 1-10

Feet 5'

Inches 1"

Pounds: 145 lbs

| Home | Work |

| Date of Birth: 01/01/1933 | Gender: Female | Occupation: retiree |

| Emergency Contact Name (First / Last) | Blood Type | Weight@Heaviest / Age 152 lbs 70 yrs |
| Phone Day | Extension | Phone Night | Weight@Lightest / Age 130 lbs 30 yrs |

Personal History

Do you have any limitations to exercise? No

If so what are these limitations?

What is your exercise program now? golf 5 days per week, lift weights at home 3 -4 x per

How long have you been following this regimen? 10 years

Have you had any injuries due to exercise? no

Medical History

Are you seeing a physician for any reason? Yes

Are you taking any medications? Yes

Are you allergic to any medications? No

Do you smoke? No

Did you ever smoke? No

If you did smoke when did you quit?

How long did you smoke?

Eating Patterns

What is your largest meal? Dinner

Do you snack during the day? Yes

What types of snacks? Chips Fruits Cookies

Do you snack after dinner? Yes

What size do you consider your portions? Large

Do you eat when depressed? No

Do you eat when stressed? Yes

Do you feel you have any eating disorders? No

Have you ever had any eating disorders? No

Comments

lately bouts of diarehea seem to be related to milk/dairy intake

acid reflux type feeling after eating certain foods, usually at night

Disease History

Medications Currently Using

Allergy History

Medical Evaluation
5/2/2007 ~ Diet Analysis Summary
Emily Energetic

Blood Test Results

Glucose	
Hematocrit	
Hemoglobin	
MCH	
Serum Iron	
GIBC	
Ferritin	

Serum Lipids

HDL	
LDL	
Cholesterol	
Triglycerides	

Date	05/02/2007

Circulatory

R.H.R.	
BP Systolic	
BP Diastolic	

Body Composition

Body Weight	145 lbs
Height	5' 1"
BMI	27.47
Body Fat	35.0 %
Waist to hip Ratio	

Energy Nutrient Evaluation
Wednesday, May 2, 2007

Emily Energetic

Date	05/02/2007	

Macronutrient Ratio

	Protein	Carbs	Lipids
Calories	183	364	244
Ratio	23%	47%	31%

Energy Nutrients

Days Evaluated **5**

	Actual	DRI	0 20 40 60 80 100 120 140 160 180 200 220 240 260 280 300	DRI
Kilocalories	778.6	2082.0		37%
Carbohydrate Grams	91.1	312.3		29%
Protein Grams	45.7	79.1		58%
Total Lipid Grams	27.2	57.4		47%
Sat Fat Grams	9.1	<23.1		39%
Poly Fat Grams	3.6	17.1		21%
Mono Fat Grams	9.8	17.1		57%
Sugars Total Grams	23.8	<52.1		46%

Micronutrient Evaluation
Wednesday, May 2, 2007

Emily Energetic

	Actual	DRI	0 20 40 60 80 100 120 140 160 180 200 220 240 260 280 300	DRI
Vitamin A IU	7092.3	2333.8		304%
Thiamin B1 mg	0.6	1.1		53%
Riboflavin B2 mg	0.6	1.1		55%
Vitamin B6 mg	0.5	1.5		30%
Vitamin B12 mcg	2.0	2.4		85%
Pant Acid mg	1.0	5.0		21%
Folate mcg	125.2	400.0		31%
Niacin mg	7.2	14.0		51%
Biotin mcg	0.0	30.0		0%
Vitamin C mg	23.2	75.0		31%
Vitamin D IU	29.0	600.0		5%
Vitamin E mg	1.1	15.0		7%
Vitamin K mcg	0.0	90.0		0%
Sodium mg	1741.8	<1200.0		145%
Calcium mg	341.7	1200.0		28%
Potassium mg	1075.8	4700.0		23%
Phosphorus mg	445.0	700.0		64%
Copper mg	0.5	9.0		6%
Magnesium mg	101.6	320.0		32%
Iron mg	4.6	8.0		58%
Zinc mg	5.3	8.0		66%
Selenium mcg	49.0	55.0		89%
Manganese mg	1.0	1.8		56%
Molybdenum mcg	0.0	45.0		0%
Iodine mcg	0.0	150.0		0%
Chloride mg	0.0	1800.0		0%
Chromium mcg	0.0	20.0		0%

Emily Energetic

Essential Amino Acids

	Actual	DRI	0 20 40 60 80 100 120 140 160 180 200 220 240 260 280 300	DRI
Histidine g	1.1	0.8		145%
Isoleucine g	1.7	1.9		86%
Leucine g	2.8	3.2		90%
Lysine g	2.8	2.5		113%
Methionine g	0.9	1.3		70%
Cystine g	0.5	1.3		37%
Phenylalanine g	1.5	3.2		49%
Tyrosine g	1.3	3.2		41%
Threonine g	1.5	1.3		114%
Tryptophan g	0.4	0.5		93%
Valine g	1.9	1.8		107%

Other

	Actual	DRI	0 20 40 60 80 100 120 140 160 180 200 220 240 260 280 300	DRI
Cholesterol mg	96.4	<300.0		32%
Fiber Total g	10.1	21.0		48%
Choline mg	0.0	425.0		0%
Water oz	38.3	92.5		41%
Alcohol g	0.0			
Caffeine	274.9			

One Day Food Log - Emily Energetic

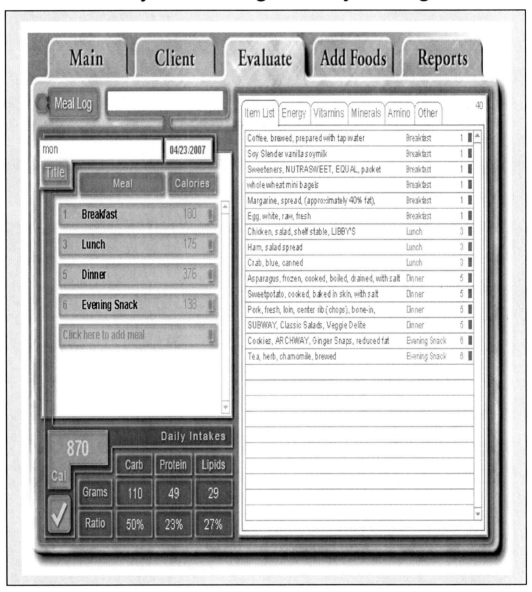

Case Study 4 - Linda Lucky

Linda is a very successful, 53 year old veterinarian. She has been working with a trainer for over 7 years, 2 or 3 days per week. Additionally she does some kind of cardio work 7 days per week for at least 30 minutes, sometimes 60 minutes each day. In her late 20's Linda was hospitalized for bulimia. She has weighed as much as 140 at 5'7" while working with her trainer, but now weighs around 128 pounds. At 140 lbs, her body fat reading was 22%; since she has lost weight, her body fat reading is at 23%. In the last year, which is when her weight loss occurred, her strength has decreased on pull-ups, chest presses, dips and bicep curls. Additionally, she reports constant fatigue and continuous joint pain. Her low back has always been a problem, and now she reports pain in her shoulders, elbows, wrists and knees almost daily. She is about to run a marathon but is not sure her knees and feet are going to cooperate through the entire run. She believes that all carbohydrates except non-starchy vegetables are off limits. She believes that fruit, grains, dairy.... are all foods that are very bad for the body. She will eat most meat, chicken, fish, drink alcohol occasionally, but not as much as she used to, and lives almost entirely on food bars and supplements created by a company claiming to have "real food" supplements.

See client profile on next page for more details.

1. Determine Linda's body mass index and waist to hip ratio.
2. Determine Linda's estimated total energy expenditure.
3. Analyze the following computerized analysis. Compare the actual intake with the DRI for all nutrients.
4. Based on all the information, what recommendations would you make to help Linda achieve her goals.

Results:

BMI   _____

Waist to Hip   _____

Percent Body Fat   _____

Recommendation _____

_____

_____

_____

_____

_____

_____

_____

Linda Lucky

Phone Day	Ext.	Phone Night	Phone Cell	Height	Weight	Stress Level 1-10	
				Feet 5'	Pounds:	Home	Work
Date of Birth: 07/01/1955	Gender: Female	Occupation: veternarian		Inches 7"	128 lbs	4	7

Emergency Contact Name (First / Last)	Blood Type	Weight@Heaviest / Age
		145 lbs 50 yrs
Phone Day Extension Phone Night		Weight@Lightest / Age
		115 lbs 28 yrs

Personal History

Do you have any limitations to exercise? No

If so what are these limitations?

What is your exercise program now? 7 days per week cardio 30 minutes or more, 3x per

How long have you been following this regimen? 7 years

Have you had any injuries due to exercise? nothing bad - a little joint pain, constant low back

Medical History

Are you seeing a physician for any reason? No

Are you taking any medications? No

Are you allergic to any medications? No

Do you smoke? No

Did you ever smoke? No

If you did smoke when did you quit? n/a

How long did you smoke? n/a

Eating Patterns

What is your largest meal?   Dinner

Do you snack during the day?   No

What types of snacks?

Do you snack after dinner?

What size do you consider your portions?   Large

Do you eat when depressed?   No

Do you eat when stressed?   No

Do you feel you have any eating disorders?   No

Have you ever had any eating disorders?   Yes

Comments

Bullemic in 20's when had 3 young kids, was going to vet school and married to a relatively unsupportive man who did not help much with the kids.

Disease History

Medications Currently Using

Allergy History

Medical Evaluation
2/13/2008 ~ Diet Analysis Summary
Linda Lucky

Blood Test Results
Glucose
Hematocrit
Hemoglobin
MCH
Serum Iron
GIBC
Ferritin

Serum Lipids
HDL
LDL
Cholesterol
Triglycerides

Date	02/13/2008

Circulatory
R.H.R.
BP Systolic
BP Diastolic

Body Composition		
Body Weight	128 lbs	
Height	5'	7"
BMI	20.1	
Body Fat	23.0 %	
Waist to hip Ratio		

Energy Nutrient Evaluation
Wednesday, February 13, 2008

Linda Lucky

Date	02/13/2008	

Macronutrient Ratio

	Protein	Carbs	Lipids
Calories	322	433	288
Ratio	31%	42%	28%

Energy Nutrients

Days Evaluated 1

	Actual	DRI	0 20 40 60 80 100 120 140 160 180 200 220 240 260 280 300	DRI
Kilocalories	1030.6	2300.0		45%
Carbohydrate Grams	108.1	345.0		31%
Protein Grams	80.5	87.3		92%
Total Lipid Grams	32.0	63.4		50%
Sat Fat Grams	13.3	<25.6		52%
Poly Fat Grams	4.2	18.9		22%
Mono Fat Grams	2.4	18.9		13%
Sugars Total Grams	2.0	<57.5		3%

Micronutrient Evaluation
Wednesday, February 13, 2008

Linda Lucky

	Actual	DRI	0 20 40 60 80 100 120 140 160 180 200 220 240 260 280 300	DRI
Vitamin A IU	14405.0	2333.8		617%
Thiamin B1 mg	3.7	1.1		333%
Riboflavin B2 mg	4.3	1.1		389%
Vitamin B6 mg	16.2	1.5		1081%
Vitamin B12 mcg	47.7	2.4		1989%
Pant. Acid mg	53.6	5.0		1071%
Folate mcg	179.1	400.0		45%
Niacin mg	71.6	14.0		511%
Biotin mcg	90.0	30.0		300%
Vitamin C mg	209.4	75.0		279%
Vitamin D IU	0.0	400.0		0%
Vitamin E mg	18.9	15.0		126%
Vitamin K mcg	0.0	90.0		0%
Sodium mg	2033.3	<1200.0		169%
Calcium mg	500.0	1200.0		42%
Potassium mg	962.8	4700.0		20%
Phosphorus mg	539.9	700.0		77%
Copper mg	0.9	9.0		10%
Magnesium mg	219.8	320.0		69%
Iron mg	10.8	8.0		134%
Zinc mg	8.9	8.0		111%
Selenium mcg	43.2	55.0		79%
Manganese mg	1.1	1.8		61%
Molybdenum mcg	0.0	45.0		0%
Iodine mcg	37.5	150.0		25%
Chloride mg	0.0	2000.0		0%
Chromium mcg	24.0	20.0		120%

Essential Amino Acids — Linda Lucky

Essential Amino Acids	Actual	DRI	0 20 40 60 80 100 120 140 160 180 200 220 240 260 280 300	DRI
Histidine g	0.8	0.7		116%
Isoleucine g	1.3	1.7		78%
Leucine g	2.2	2.8		79%
Lysine g	2.4	2.2		108%
Methionine g	0.7	1.1		63%
Cystine g	0.3	1.1		26%
Phenylalanine g	1.1	2.8		41%
Tyrosine g	0.9	2.8		32%
Throenine g	1.2	1.1		108%
Tryptophan g	0.3	0.4		76%
Valine g	1.5	1.6		94%

Other

Other	Actual	DRI	0 20 40 60 80 100 120 140 160 180 200 220 240 260 280 300	DRI
Cholesterol mg	70.3	<300.0		23%
Fiber Total g	20.8	21.0		99%
Choline mg	0.0	425.0		0%
Water oz	52.4	102.2		51%
Alcohol g	19.0			
Caffeine	0.0			

One Day Food Log – Linda Lucky

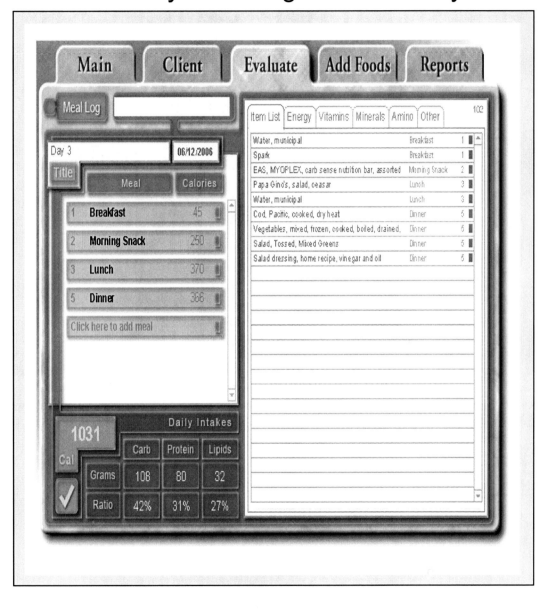

Chapter 13
Promoting Success

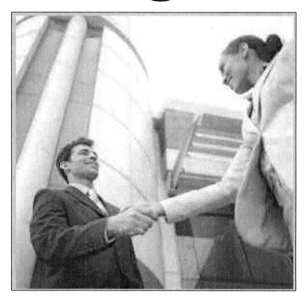

This chapter focuses on ensuring success in health and life long weight management through exercise and healthy eating - not dieting. We will initially investigate many of the pitfalls associated with dieting. We will then take a look at the steps to success in health and long term weight management.

Objectives

After reading and studying this chapter, you should:

1. Be able to describe the history of dieting and debunk some of the latest fad diets.

2. Be able to describe why dieting doesn't work in long term weight management.

3. Be able to provide details concerning labeling regulations by the FDA and USDA.

4. Be able to provide details concerning healthy choices when eating out.

INTRODUCTION

Success in maintaining life long health requires acquiring important skills. This chapter will focus on some of the pitfalls that sabotage people from being successful.

Discussion will center on obstacles to success. An entire section is dedicated to diets. We are a nation addicted to dieting. Diets don't work; they have never worked. So why are we still addicted to a process that simply doesn't work? The history of dieting sheds light on how we became a nation addicted to dieting.

This chapter will then look at labeling laws. Many of your well intentioned clients, athletes, and patients are making what they believe to be healthy choices at the grocery store, but they are instead being sabotaged by inconsistencies and often ambiguous labeling regulations. Deciphering food labels and health claims is not for amateurs anymore. It has become an exercise in under-standing legal rhetoric. "Whole grain" doesn't mean whole grain; "93% lean ground beef" isn't 93% lean by calories, and the definition of "free-range" is far from what you may envision.

Next the discussion will focus on eating out. Most people are totally unaware of what they are eating when they eat out.

The final discussion in this chapter will center on sabotaging practices such as eating too many calories in the evening, dealing with problem foods in the home, deprivation of favorite foods, eating too fast, shopping when hungry, not planning, eating by the numbers, friendly saboteurs and stress eating. This section will look at difficult situations and provide possible solution to traveling, eating out, business meetings and holidays.

DIET - A FOUR LETTER WORD

Diets - Big Fat Lies

Diets do not work; diets never work! The diet industry is a $54 billion industry with a 95% fail rate. Despite all our "diet foods" we are still getting fatter.[1] Despite all the money spent yearly on dieting, 66 percent of Americans are overweight today compared to 58 percent in 1983. If this weight increase were considered a disease, it would be an epidemic.

History of Dieting[2]

Dieting has been around for thousands of years, although not in any structured way like we see all around us today. It wasn't very common until the 1800's simply because people who were over-weight were not very common; only the rich and well to do were overweight. So being fat was not a problem for most Americans. So any diet at the time involved reducing calories.

As time progressed, many more people became wealthy and thus had much greater access to the same foods as the wealthy. Eating and drinking too much became a sign of affluence.

But strangely enough it wasn't entirely the health factors of being overweight that first got the modern diet off the starting blocks, as well as health concerns, it was the war against sin! Yea, the immorality of excess from the glutton will cause a more sinful world. And we all know what the punishment of sin is.

A world entirely full of thin sticks of people would doubtlessly be just as sinful, but not to the Ameri-can Presbyterian minister Sylvester Graham, who after being ordained in 1826, began to preach in the 1830's that the ills of health; physical, moral, and spiritual, could all be remedied by a basic vegetarian diet. He also encouraged such behavior as; sleeping on hard and unyielding mattresses, the opening of bedroom windows (whatever the weather), regular cold showers, brisk hearty exer-cise, clothing to include only loose garments, learning about the benefits of drinking pure water (fair enough), and of course chastity!

So as you can imagine, this luminary of the temperance movement in the city of Philadelphia was not entirely popular in some quarters, and he was referred to as 'Dr. Sawdust' by his detractors; though he did attract a number a followers who obediently did as they were told and became known as 'the Grahamites'. They, after being converted to the ways of the diet, further spread his word, and thousands would attend his lectures. Those not able to could read of his theories in the Graham Journal of Health and Longevity. The originator of graham flour and the flat bread known as graham crackers, he stated that the vitality, strength and all-round health of the orangutan proved that vegetarianism was the way forward, and tirelessly campaigned against all alcohol and also coffee, tea and tobacco as stimulants.

Because of his regaling against the bakers of the day, who used refined flour where the wheat had been stripped of most of its' nutritional goodness to facilitate a faster baked loaf, he sometimes needed bodyguards at his meetings. Milk producers also suffered his wrath. They fed their cows on swill leftover from the distilleries, and had to add the likes of chalk and molasses to their sold milk, to neutralize the taste of the alcoholic content and make it presentable to the public.

England, and the Banting Plan

In 1850's England, a man called William Banting was in a seriously obese state of affairs, and he had had enough of it. This unfortunate fellow was so fat that he supposedly could not tie his own shoes, and it is said that he had to go downstairs backwards. Despairing at the inability of the doctors to help him, their advice on exercise, steam baths, temporary starvations and chemical purges had all come to naught, he at last found something that worked.

One medical practitioner, a Doctor Harvey, had suggested that he might find the answer by not eating any more than a minimum of sugars and starches. Low carbohydrate diets had been born.

William Banting followed this advice, and lost fifty pounds in a year. So delighted at his success, he wrote a book, which was the world's first diet book, to tell of his experience, the splendidly titled: "Letter on Corpulence Addressed to the Public," that was published in 1862.

His obesity had been cured but the British Medical Association immediately attacked this approach, and because Banting was not a scientist, claimed that it had no scientific value and would not work for others. The public however was impressed, and people all over the English speaking world read of his plan and lost weight themselves, not caring about the doubters. It proved so popular, that it was translated into other languages and thus spread even wider.

'The Great Masticator'

One way of success had been found, but many approaches can work. Another was to involve the mechanism of chewing, or masticating, as it is properly known. Around the end of the nineteenth century; William Ewart Gladstone, the four times British Prime Minister, had apparently advised that a person should always masticate thirty two times before swallowing (why thirty two? - The same number as the total of teeth in the mouth). This would inevitably lead to a lessening of the appetite and subsequent weight loss for better health.

Powerful world leaders usually have their opinions listened to with respect, but one American considered this with more than a passing interest. He was to come to believe that it was the perfect answer to the fat problem. This man was Horace Fletcher, who would become better known to the citizenry in the United States by the nicknames of 'The Chew-Chew Man' and `The Great Masticator.'

Horace Fletcher might have been himself inspired by Gladstone, but he was to take this enthusiasm for chewing to heights surely undreamt of, even by that worthy. The chewing should continue, he proclaimed, until the food becomes a liquid in the mouth. And any food that does not (like fiber) should therefore not be chewed in the first place.

Leaving fiber out of a diet leads to constipation, as those caught up in the frenzy of mastication were to painfully discover, but Fletcher persisted that this was right and a small price to pay, and lost over sixty pounds in weight by this approach.

In an unlikely parallel with Rev. Sylvester Graham, that earlier notable of American dieting, the Great Masticator held that all meat should be avoided, as well as coffee, tea and alcohol. He also wrote in his book, The A-Z of our own Nutrition, that no-one should eat until they were hungry, and that they should try to be happy at mealtimes. Most important though, they should chew until "the food swallowed itself."

A side note here is that a Dr. John Kellogg thought that the advice from Fletcher to avoid fiber was so wrong that he founded his famous cereal company to make sure Americans were getting plenty of fiber in their diets.

Calories Arrive on the Scene

The theory of the calorific value of foodstuffs, which is how much thermal energy they give off when burned, was started by a chemist called Wilbur Atwater. But it was around two decades later, in 1918 before the calorie left the world of academia and hit the mainstream.

Lulu Hunt Peters, a Californian doctor, introduced the concept of counting calories in a diet to aid weight loss in her bestseller book Diet and Health with a Key to the Calories. This scientific way of looking at things was a big hit with the public, and despite her honest message that dieting could be a tough road to follow at times, with an emphasis on self-discipline and willpower to win the war against fat, her work is influential to this day.

She also showed that a lot of money could be made by anyone coming up with new ideas to help overweight people. More of whom were now around in society than ever before, and combined with the phenomenon of movie theaters and subsequent beginnings of the hero worship of the stars of the silver screen, almost all of whom were good looking of course, the public's obsession with fat was off to a running start. This was noted by both genuine writers on the subject of dieting advice, and complete cranks.

Some came up with variations of the idea (and still do) that how much food is eaten is almost an irrelevance; the only thing that matters is what combinations of foods are consumed at the same time.

The first of these was William H. Hay, who recommended that proteins, starches and sugars should be eaten completely separately to avoid the putting on of excess fat. He also advised that having an enema each and every day was a key to proper health.

Others took this up and altered it slightly, claiming that some food could change the fatty properties of other foods, if digested together. This was apparently the miracle cure for obesity. But despite the validity of this theory never being even partly proven by proper research, it has been still loudly proclaimed by many that their particular method of matching foodstuffs will guarantee that fat is burned quicker, or otherwise dispensed with.

Diets, More Diets, and More Diets

And people are still eating more, weighing more, and dieting more. There have been far too many diets set upon the public to discuss in one article, but let's have a look at a timeline and include a few notable points in dieting history.

☐   1930's - The Hollywood Diet (soon to be better known as the Grapefruit Diet) is introduced. Seaweeds such as kelp and bladderwrack are promoted as the food of choice to end weight   problems.

☐   'Diet Guru' Victor Lindlahr, regularly broadcasts on the nations' radios to spread news of `reverse calorie foods.' This is a catabolic system of weight loss he has discovered where some foods use up more calories to be digested, than they give out to the body; like celery and apples.

☐   1940's and 1950's - "Ideal Weight" charts are invented by matching a weight with gender, height and frame.

☐   Diet pills are introduced that are based on Amphetamine derivatives. It is soon realized that they are dangerous.

☐   1960's - A woman named Jean Nidetch and friends hold a meeting in her apartment to share support and advice on dieting. It is the beginning of Weight Watchers.

☐   Dr. Atkins releases his plan for weight loss, the high protein, high fat and low carbohydrate diet causes a storm of controversy that still rages today as multiple health fears are voiced by critics.

☐   1970's - The Food & Drug Administration (FDA) calls for a ban on saccharin in the United States. Because of voter fury, the US Congress does not heed this advice.

☐   The Pritikin Diet Program with low fat and high fiber is introduced for those with heart complaints, but quickly is taken up by others for weight loss.

☐   The eating disorder anorexia nervosa is described for the first time by Psychiatrists as many continual dieters are becoming underweight.

☐   A new diet drug called fenfluramine is introduced which makes the brain think the stomach is full.

☐   Dr. Robert Linn invents a protein drink called Prolinn, which is made up of slaughterhouse byproducts like crushed horns and hooves and hides, which are treated with artificial flavorings and enzymes. He urges for all looking to lose weight, to completely omit food and break the fast only by the use of his product in The Last Chance Diet. Somewhere around 3 million weight worriers give it a go.

☐   The book entitled Fit for Life is written by Harvey and Marilyn Diamond. In it are claims that the human body has changing physiological needs for certain foodstuffs depending on the time of the day.

☐   1980's - The Beverly Hills Diet becomes the latest dieting craze. It holds that only fruit should be eaten for the first ten days of the plan.

☐   An anti-diabetes system called The Glycemic Index is developed by Dr. David Jenkins and a team of scientists at the University of Toronto. To help simplify the problems suffered by diabetics, this index charts how quickly a range of diverse foodstuffs affects blood sugar levels. This research is also often misappropriated by authors of fad diets to back up their weight loss claims.

☐   TV personality Oprah Winfrey loses almost 70 pounds on a liquid diet.

☐   Health writer Susan Powter advises her female readers to diet less and exercise more.

☐   1990's - The FDA demands that food labeling should include more detailed information about calories and fat content to assist dieting consumers, and for better general public health.

☐   A shocking report indicates that 40% of nine and ten year old children in the United States are dieting for weight loss reasons.

☐   The diet pills containing fenfluramine and the related dexfenfluramine are withdrawn by their manufacturers as the FDA reports on them being a cause of heart valve disease.

☐   2000's - Some researchers claim that for the first time in recorded human history, the number of underfed people in the world has been equaled by those overweight.

How to Write Your Own Diet Book[3]

Bonnie Liebman, in "How to Write a Diet Book (Nutrition Action Healthletter, July, 2006)" provides details on how to create a diet book. "After all," she says, "You've been eating all your life haven't you? Don't worry about having any expertise or degree."

In Step 1, Bonnie says to name your book after a trendy place (South Beach, Beverly Hills, Scarsdale, etc.). Next make up a diet that will banish unwanted fat forever. It doesn't matter what it is people

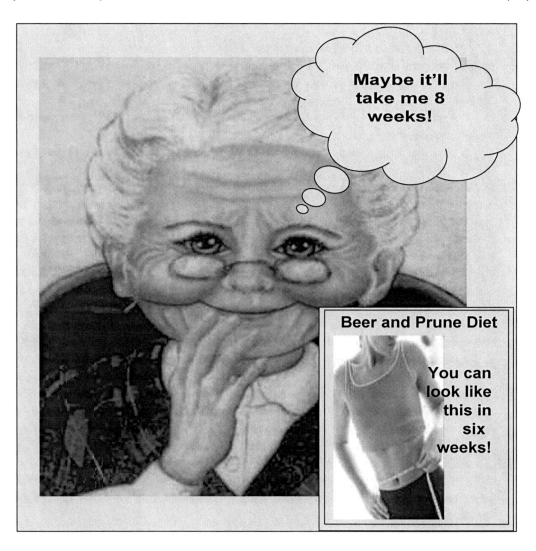

will believe it. Then personalize it by tailoring it to the masses (Eat Right 4 Your Type, Carbohydrate Addict's Diet, The Zone, etc.). Zero in on a body part (Abs Diet, Cellulite Breakthrough, The Butt Book, etc.) Single out a food that currently isn't in vogue (Grapefruit Diet, Cabbage Soup Diet) and single out a nutrient (low carb, low-fat, etc.).

In Step 2, tell people they won't be hungry on your diet; people on your diet will lose weight even when all other diets failed; tell people they will not only lose weight, but they will have more energy, be healthier and will show no signs of aging. Also tell people that they don't have to give up their favorite foods, don't have to count calories, will lose weight fast and will detox their body. Be sure to tell people that your diet is backed by scientific research and to boost sales tell people that the scientific community has completely ignored your research.

Step 3 - Keep it complicated (or simple). For people who don't like to read fill chapters with foods to avoid, recipes, blank pages that people can write on and lots of charts listing fiber, calories, etc. For science lovers, deluge people with scientific evidence, especially if it has been ignored. Use scientific names (lippprotein lipase, cortisol, leptin, resistin, etc.) and be sure to explain how your diet will prevent diseases. Be sure to have at least 50 references and a list of supplements to take. You can even create your own supplements.

Step 4 - Think outside the box. Go beyond what's been done. How about a beer and prune diet; or a wine and cheese diet? What about a diet for postmenopausal women? "You can think of it as a creative writing course," says Bonnie.

And on and on we go, most still worrying about our weight as the wealth of society increases; it seems there will always be self-made problems for humanity to deal with. Bountiful advances on some fields are inevitably the harbingers of coming trouble elsewhere. As a last word for now on this topic, that well loved bear Winnie the Pooh, once asked how long it took to get thin. The answer, it appears, is still not fully available.

Diets and Muscle Loss

Dieting doesn't work for many reasons. First, no one can sacrifice forever. Caloric restriction, in and of itself, can lead to binge-eating episodes. Second, low calorie diets produce tired, cranky people. Third, low calorie diets utilize lean muscle as an energy source—hence fat burning machinery is lost. The scale goes down but is destined to go right back up. When the weight is gained back it's all fat. The only known method of permanent weight loss is exercise and healthy eating.[4,]

Similar to low calorie diets, fasting (twelve to sixteen hours without eating) forces the body to switch to a wasting metabolism; i.e., exhausting carbohydrate reserves, and drawing on vital protein tissues.[5] In the first few days of a fast or a low calorie diet, body protein provides about 90 percent of the needed glucose. If body proteins were to continue to be utilized at this rate, death would ensue within three weeks. However, as the low calorie diet or fast continues, the body finds a way to use fat by-products as a fuel source for some brain cells. Fats are broken down to produce by-products that look similar to glucose—ketones. Ketones can be used by some brain cells, but others still rely on glucose, hence body protein continues to be broken down. This is a dangerous process, since ketones can cause a disease known as acidosis—changes in pH which can eventually cause death. Fasting reduces energy output and the body conserves both its fat and lean tissue. As the lean organ tissues shrink, they perform less metabolic work and so demand less energy.[5]

Consider the following example. The beach ball and baseball in this picture weigh the same. The scale provides no information about size, only weight. Most Americans use the scale as a measure of determining size and health status. However, body composition is the more important measure.[6]

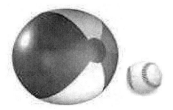

Consider another example.[6] Mike is a 55-year-old executive trying desperately to win the battle of the bulge. He steps on the scale every morning to monitor his weight. At six foot, two inches and 200 pounds, he doesn't look "overweight." But Mike is frustrated. He eats less (by skipping lunch) and exercises more in order to keep his weight from creeping up, but he now buys clothes a size larger. He is always tired and hungry, and often cranky. The scale is deceiving Mike. The scale only measures his total mass - 200 pounds. The question the scale answers for Mike is, "How much do I weigh?" It cannot answer the more important question, "How much of those 200 pounds is calorie-burning muscle versus metabolically inactive fat?" Therefore, the scale provides an unreliable "picture" of Mike's true condition.

Mike, like millions of Americans, believes his body is burning fat when he does not eat, but the truth of the matter is that by following his low-calorie regimen, he is actually losing muscle at a rate equal to or greater than his loss of fat.

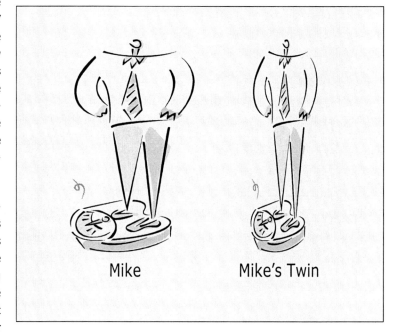

Mike   Mike's Twin

To end this vicious cycle of eating less and increasing his body fat, Mike must fuel his muscles with adequate amounts of carbohydrates every day. He must be sure to limit the fat in his diet and incorporate adequate amounts of protein. So where does Mike start? How can he, and millions of Americans like him, break the cycle? Menu planning discussed later in this session is the answer - not dieting.

Eating Enough and On Time[7]

Changing body composition (building muscle and utilizing fat stores for energy) requires fueling the body, not dieting. The July/August, 1999 issue of ACSM Health & Fitness Journal provides an in depth discussion of the necessity to fuel the body in exercise, and the consequences of not doing so (reiterating all of the information in this chapter).[21] While this summary report may seem outdated, the information still holds true and is very helpful when trying to convince clients about the futility of dieting.

According to the authors, when healthy people exercise during a time of severe energy deprivation, the potential benefits of exercise can be lost. Also, energy inadequacies may be the reason that people turn to performance enhancing ergogenic aids. They can be fooled into thinking that ergogenic aids are conferring performance enhancing qualities when, in reality, they may simply be filling an energy or nutrient void that could more effectively be met by eating sufficient energy with a good distribution of nutrients.

Aging (muscle loss is the biggest factor) and dieting force the resting metabolic rate to make adjustments. These and other factors influence a person's total energy requirement and, to achieve energy balance, require an appropriate adjustment on the consumption side of the energy equation; i.e., decreased metabolic rate must be accompanied by decreased caloric intake or weight gain will occur.

Adaptations that occur from energy imbalance have been known for some time. For example, it's been shown that runners clearly expend more energy than nonrunners, yet they can maintain weight despite energy intakes equivalent to that of the nonrunners. In one study, the runners ran approximately 54 kilometers per week but maintained weight on an energy intake that was calculated to be about 645 calories below the predicted energy requirement.[2]

A person who has restricted his or her energy intake develops an associated lower rate of resting energy expenditure. On the other hand, overeating does not result in an equivalent increase in resting energy expenditure. Studies support the notion that energy restrictive diets often fail because they induce a lower resting energy expenditure that ultimately impedes weight loss. While this is particularly a problem for people who are disposed to gaining weight, it is also likely to be a problem in others because the compensatory reduction in resting energy expenditure is greater than would be expected by the weight loss induced from inadequate energy intake.[3] The human adaptive response to inadequate energy intake could be viewed as a means of preservation during a time of famine. In human history famine is likely to have been a more frequent and formidable problem in maintaining a population's viability than overabundance. Perhaps this explains why we are able to increase metabolic efficiency (burn fewer calories doing the same work) with inadequate energy intake, but are less capable of reducing metabolic efficiency (burn more calories doing the same work) in an environment of excess energy.

The impact of a caloric deficit may interfere with the capacity to increase muscle mass because of a lower production of insulin-like growth factor, and a reduced power production.[4] There is evidence that muscle mass may actually be reduced when exercise occurs in an energy-deficient environment. This may be associated with the long-understood tenet in nutrition that carbohydrates have a protein-sparing effect; that is, proteins are used as a source of energy when there is inadequate carbohydrate energy. A low energy intake (likely to be low in carbohydrates) would require that protein be used as a fuel rather than be spared for anabolic (muscle building) purposes. A low carbohydrate diet should be a red flag for exercisers who are trying to improve the conditioning and fitness level of their muscles. It would be hard to imagine anything more counterproductive than utilizing the very tissue you're trying to improve because of an insufficient level of appropriate energy from carbohydrates.

A person may consume sufficient energy to satisfy the general daily need for energy. If however, these energy providing foods are consumed at the wrong time or are not of the right type, the energy requirement may not be satisfied. A person who has an estimated daily energy requirement of 2,000 kilocalories can expect clearly different outcomes if the required energy is consumed in one meal at the end of the day or broken up into several meals spread throughout the day. Since exercise produces an insulin response more glucose and amino acids enter cells after exercising. There is a two hour window of increased ability for muscles to take up more of these nutrients after an exercise session. It is important, when possible, to take advantage of this effect. The determinant of how soon after exercise to eat depends on how long it takes for the individual to cool down so that blood flow can be diverted from working muscles to the gastrointestinal tract for absorption of nutrients.

The person who misses breakfast and lunch is likely to experience low blood sugar. For a variety of reasons, infrequent eating patterns are common among the general public, especially among people who are trying to induce weight loss through severe dietary restrictions. It is even common among elite athletes to complete an early morning exercise session before any source of energy is consumed. People commonly exercise in an energy-deficient state because the assumption is (albeit an incorrect one) that the body will run without fuel or will easily burn undesirable fat for fuel. Not true!

In summary, heavy physical exercise during an energy-deficit state may be counterproductive in producing the desired conditioning improvements. The energy deficit may be caused by inadequate caloric intake or poor distribution of caloric intake throughout the day. Since many people are wedded to a level of physical activity they are unlikely to reduce to achieve energy balance, a more realistic approach is needed to assure an adequate energy intake that creates an energy balance. Normal post meal blood glucose fluctuations suggest that some energy from food is needed approximately every three hours. An eating pattern that provides small amounts of energy throughout the day meets this recommendation. In the context of the problems associated with energy deficits, it makes sense for people to eat breakfast, mid-morning snack, lunch, mid-afternoon snack, dinner, and an evening snack. Focusing on obtaining an adequate total energy intake and avoiding within-day energy deficits is a good strategy for maintaining energy metabolism, getting more out of training, reducing injuries, improving nutrient intake, and maintaining a desired body composition.

LABELING

Many of well intentioned clients, athletes, and patients are making what they believe to be healthy choices at the grocery store, but they are instead being sabotaged by inconsistencies and often ambiguous labeling regulations. Deciphering food labels and health has become an exercise in understanding legal rhetoric. "Whole grain" doesn't mean whole grain; "93% lean ground beef" isn't 93% lean by calories, and the definition of "free-range" is far from what you may envision. The goal of this section is **NOT** to have your clients, patients and athletes throw away their can of Pam spray, or to totally eliminate beef from their diets. The goal is to educate them so that they can make healthier, more informed choices. Personally, I like to think of it as a "budget"—for calories. To be healthy your clients need to know how much they should eat, and how much of each nutrient they should eat. Understanding labeling regulations will help protect them from fraudulently being "cheated" out of their hard earned calories.

Food Labeling Regulations

In 1989 the FDA and USDA commissioned the National Academy of Sciences-Institute of Medicine (NAS-IOM) to write a background report on the current state of food labeling and make recommendations for revising them. However, the NAS-IOM's recommended revised labeling regulations did **not** withstand the scrutiny of industry lobbying groups. According to Jeff Nadelman, a former lobbyist for the very powerful Grocery Manufactures of America Association, "the goal of every food-industry association is to maintain the status quo, to delay, to fight, to lobby, and to obscure the facts so that manufacturers can reposition their products to compete for consumer demand" (www.menshealth.com, April 20, 2005). Present day food labeling regulations are a composite of these opposing forces: NAS-IOM and the food industry.

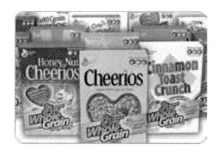

The Food and Drug Administration (FDA) is responsible for regulating most food products, while the United States Department of Agriculture (USDA) is responsible for regulating meat and poultry products. Each organization developed labeling requirements that are unique to their respective products and requirements. The National Labeling and Education Act (NLEA) passed by Congress in 1990 required mandatory nutrition labeling to appear on most packaged foods regulated by the FDA. No such regulations have been passed requiring the USDA to make meat labels comparable to the packaged food labels. This makes it very difficult for consumers to compare products. Prepackaged pizza with meat topping falls under USDA rules, while cheese pizza is labeled according to FDA rules. Let's look at some results of these convoluted laws.[8,9,13]

Whole Grain

The definition "made with whole grain" does not specify an amount of whole grain the product must contain:

o "Made with whole grain" means a product may contain either a little or a lot of whole grain – a specified amount is not required.

o "An excellent source of whole grain" means a product must contain at least 16 grams per serving or approximately nearly half of what most serving sizes are (30 to 55 grams).

o "A good source of whole grain" means there can be as little as 8 grams per serving. Is this truly a good source when the product may be less than 50% whole grain?

o "Multigrain" is a mixture of grains that can be mostly refined with minimal nutritional value.

General Mills claims their new whole grain cereals are "made with whole grains." So how do the newer cereals stack up against their older counterparts? By comparing older ingredient labels with the new ones it is clear the only thing that changed is the label.   You can Visit www.wholegrainscouncil.org for more information about whole grains, and where to find them in foods.

Fat free / Calorie Free

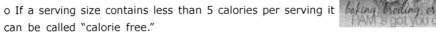

Are those products that claim to be calorie- and fat-free truly free of calories and fat? Not exactly!

o If a serving size contains less than 5 calories per serving it can be called "calorie free."

o If a serving size contains 1/2 gram of fat or less the product can be called "non-fat."

o The nutrition label on a can of Pam fat free cooking spray reads: serving size 1/3 second, calories 0, calories from fat 0. A side panel compares the fat in the Pam spray to the fat in butter. In a one second spray, Pam has 7 calories while a tablespoon of butter has 104 calories. A low fat alternative to be sure, but 7 calories per second does not mean calorie free. The can contains 702 (1/3 second) servings, in other words, 234 seconds, hence the can contains 1638 calories (234 seconds x 7calories/second). The labeling law states that if the serving size contains 1/2 gram of fat or less it can be called non fat, and if the serving size contains less than 5 calories per serving it can be called calorie free. So the 1/3 second serving size fulfills the legal requirements.

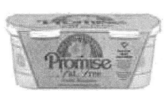

o Promise Ultra Fat-Free is 100% fat.

o This same regulation holds true for "trans-fats." Many new products are not truly free of trans-fats.

For definitions of terms such as low, lite, lean, extra lean, high, good source, and reduced, visit http://www.fda.gov/fdac/special/foodlabel/lite.html for a little "lite" reading.

Meat Industry Labeling

The USDA labeling guidelines allow meat and poultry products to label fat content by volume or weight rather than by calories as does the FDA labeling regulations.[8,]

· 93% lean ground beef (7% fat by weight) is actually 45% fat by calories.

· 97% lean pre-packaged meat is actually 18% fat by calories.

A label of ground beef that states it is 85% lean does not mean that the product is 15% fat by calories. The 85% lean refers to fat content by weight (not by calories). Beef that is 85% lean can be 45 to 50% fat by calories. For further details visit www.cspinet.net/nah/junebeef.htm.

Dairy Industry Labeling

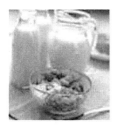

The dairy industry is also regulated by the USDA and falls under the same category as meat and poultry products.[8,]

o Milk labeled 1% fat is 18% fat by calories.

o Milk labeled 2% fat is 36% fat by calories.

o Whole milk is almost 50% fat by calories.

By definition, the FDA's guideline of low-fat is "a product containing three grams of fat or less". Therefore, under the USDA labeling guidelines, milk labeled 2% (containing 5 grams of fat) could make the low-fat claim. However, in 1998 the FDA disallowed the use of low-fat for 2% milk. The new term that is now used to replace low-fat is reduced-fat. Confusing? Yes! And there's more.

Net Carbs

The FDA does not evaluate or regulate terms placed on labels outside of the nutrition facts panel. The terms "net carbs," "impact carbs" and "non-impact carbs" have no legal or scientific definition. "These terms have been made up by food companies," says Wahida Karmally, PhD, RD, director of nutrition at the Irving Center for Clinical Research at Columbia University. So why doesn't the FDA step in if there isn't any science behind these terms? Congress chartered the FDA to regulate the nutrition facts panel only. These new terms are outside of this boundary and do not violate any laws. The FDA can only take action if such terms can be shown to be harmful. For more details on these marketing terms, visit http://www.webmd.com/content/article/92/101603.htm.

Nutrition Facts

Serving Size: 1 Bar (60g)
Servings Per Container: 1

Amount Per Serving	
Calories 220	Calories from Fat 80

	% Daily Value*
Total Fat 9g	14%
Saturated Fat 6g	30%
Trans Fat 0g	
Cholesterol 0mg	0%
Sodium 120mg	5%
Total Carbohydrate 27g	9%
Dietary Fiber 11g	44%
Sugar 1g	
Sugar Alcohol 4g	
Protein 17g	34%

• Vitamin A 25%		• Vitamin C 25%
• Calcium 35%		• Iron 10%
• Vitamin E 15%		• Vitamin K 15%
• Thiamin 15%		• Riboflavin 15%
• Niacin 15%		• Vitamin B6 15%
• Folate 15%		• Vitamin B12 15%
• Biotin 25%		• Magnesium 15%
• Phosphorus 10%		• Pantothenic Acid 15%
• Zinc 15%		• Selenium 15%
• Chromium 10%		

*Percent Daily Values are based on a 2,000 calorie diet. Your daily values may be higher or lower depending on your calorie needs:

		Calories	2,000	2,500
Total Fat	Less Than		65g	80g
Sat Fat	Less Than		20g	25g
Cholesterol	Less Than		300mg	300mg
Sodium	Less Than		2400mg	2400mg
Total Carbohydrate			300g	375g
Dietary Fiber			25g	30g
Protein			50g	65g

Organic[10]

The USDA is responsible for managing the National Organic Program, implemented in October 2002. By definition, organic farming avoids the use of most artificial inputs, such as synthetic pesticides and fertilizers. Also banned are the use of animal by-products, antibiotics and sewage sludge, among other practices. Any food product (except fish) using the word "organic" must be certified by an official USDA accredited certifier. Definitions are as follows:

o "Organic" must contain at least 95% organically produced ingredients.

o A "made with organic" label means a product must contain at least 70% organic ingredients. Products that contain fewer than 70% organic ingredients cannot bear the USDA Organic seal or display the word "organic" on the front of the package. However there are exceptions to these rules.

o Farms and handling operations that sell less than $5000 a year are exempt from certification and can label their products organic but can not use the USDA Organic seal.

o Grocery stores or restaurants do not have to be certified.

Items labeled "certified organic" must pass a clearly defined certificating process by federal agents. Items labeled "certified organic" can not be genetically modified or irradiated; produce cannot be farmed with most synthetic pesticides or fertilizers; organic dairy, poultry, meat and eggs are produced without growth hormones and antibiotics.[11]

When should you buy Organic? Consumers Union and other independent researchers indicate it may be worth the extra cost to buy organic but at other times is simply be a "waste of money".[11] The best bets to buy organic according to Consumers Union include: apples, bell peppers, celery, cherries, imported grapes, nectarines, peaches, pear, potatoes, red raspberries, spinach and strawberries. These foods known as the "dirty dozen" carry much higher levels of pesticide residue. Consumers Union also says it's worth the extra money to buy organic beef, poultry, eggs and dairy in order to avoid ingesting supplemental hormones and antibiotics. Marginally beneficial to buy organic is: asparagus, avocados, bananas, broccoli, cauliflower, sweet corn, kiwi, mangos, onions, papaya, pineapples, and sweet potatoes because multiple pesticides residues are rarely found on these foods. Again, according to Consumers Union, buying organic foods that aren't good for you doesn't make them healthy and don't bother buying organic seafood. The USDA has not developed organic certification standards for seafood. Wild or farmed fish can be labeled "organic" despite the presence of mercury, PCBs and other contaminants.

Non-government Logos[12]

Many different non-government logos, labeling and certification schemes now appear on products. Their abundance can be confusing and the criteria and assessment standards not always clear. It's easy to imagine free range chickens running free in a beautiful field. Think again.

o The definition of "free range" is regulated by the USDA and applies only to chickens.

o The use of "free range" on beef is unregulated and there is no standard definition of this term.

o "Free range" requires that birds be given access to the outdoors but what is not defined is the length of time per day. In other words, five minutes a day of open-air access could be adequate for manufacturers to use the "free range" claim on a poultry product.

o The term "free range" used on eggs is not regulated.

o The USDA considers the term "antibiotic-free" on dairy and meat "un-approvable" and has banned its use. Producers can only say "no antibiotics administered" or "raised without antibiotics."

o "Cruelty-free" on cleaning and personal hygiene products implies no animal testing was done. The ingredients may have once been tested on animals, or the company may have commissioned other labs to do the testing, but have themselves not tested the finished product.

o Other meaningless or unverified terms are "natural," "no chemical," "no hormones," "nonpolluting," "nontoxic," "ozone-friendly," or "sensitivity tested."

Visit www.eco-labels.org from Consumers Union Guide for more details.

General Terms[4]

The following is a summary on information that must be provided on labels.[4]

1. The common name of the product
2. Name and address of the manufacturer, packer, or distributor
3. Net contents
4. The ingredient list
5. The serving size and number of servings
6. The quantities of specified nutrients and food constituents

Ingredient List:

1. The FDA requires that all ingredients be listed in descending order of predominance by weight and to state on the label that they have done so.
2. When more than one sweetener is used, manufacturers must put them all together under the term "sweeteners" and list them in order of predominance. So if the label specifies sweeteners as the second ingredient then the total of sweeteners is the second largest component of the product.
3. Manufacturers are also required to list the specific fats and oils they have used. They can no longer use the terms and/or clause (soybeans and/or coconut).
4. Manufacturers must now also list all additives.

Serving Size:

1. Labels must identify the size of a serving and the number of servings.
2. The new standard serving size for beverages is 8 ounces.
3. Any package that contains less than 2 servings is considered a single serving item and the label must reflect the contents of the entire package.

Nutrition Information:

1. The label must show the quantities of certain nutrients, total calories, and calories from fat.
2. The label must indicate grams from total fat, saturated fat, cholesterol, and sodium.
3. The label must indicate total grams of carbohydrate, sugars, fiber, and protein.
4. Labels must present nutrient content information as compared with the percentage of recommended intakes: vitamin A, vitamin C, Iron, Calcium.

General Terms:

Free: nutritionally trivial and unlikely to have a physiological consequence: synonyms include without, no, and zero.

High: 20% or more of the Daily Value for a given nutrient per serving.

Less: at least 25% less of a given nutrient than the comparison food. Synonyms include fewer and reduced.

Light or lite: any use of the term, other than as defined below, must specify what it is referring to (for example, light in color, or light in texture).

Low: an amount that would allow frequent consumption of a food without exceeding the dietary guidelines. A food that is naturally low in a nutrient may make such a claim, but only as it applies to similar foods (for example, "fresh cauliflower, a low sodium food"); synonyms include little, few, and low source of.

More: at least 10% more of a given nutrient than the comparison food; synonyms include "added".

Good source of: Product provides between 10 and 19% of the Daily Value for a given nutrient per serving.

Cholesterol:

Foods containing more than 13 g total fat per serving or per 50 g must indicate those contents immediately after a cholesterol claim. As you will see, all cholesterol claims are prohibited when the food contains more than 2 g saturated fat/serving.

Cholesterol-free: less than 2 mg cholesterol per serving and 2 g or less saturated fat per serving.

Low in cholesterol: 20 mg or less per serving, and 2g or less of saturated fat per serving.

Less cholesterol: 25% or less cholesterol than the comparison food (reflecting a reduction of fat at least 20 mg per serving), and 2 g or less saturated fat per serving

Energy:

Kilocalorie-free: fewer than 5 kcal per serving.

Light: one-third fewer kilocalories than the comparison food.

Low kilocalorie: less than 40 kcal per serving.

Fat:

Extra lean: less than 5 g of fat, 2 g of saturated fat and 95 mg of cholesterol per serving and per 100 g of food.

Fat-free: less than 0.5 g of fat per serving (and no added fat or oil).

Lean: less than 10 g fat, 4 g saturated fat; 95 mg cholesterol per serving/per 100g of food.

Less fat: 25% or less fat than the comparison food.

Less saturated fat: 25% or less saturated fat than the comparison food.

Low fat: 3 g or less fat per serving.

Low saturated fat: 1 g or less saturated fat per serving.

Percent fat-free: may be used only if the product meets the definition of low fat or fat free and must reflect the amount of fat in 100 g.

Light: 50% or less of the fat than in the comparison food (for example, 50% less fat than our regular cookies).

Fiber:

High fiber: 20% or more of the Daily Value for fiber; a high-fiber claim made on a food that contains more than 3g of fat per serving and per 100g must also declare total fat.

Sodium:

Sodium-free and salt-free: less than 5 mg of sodium per serving.

Low sodium: less than 140 mg per serving.

Light: a low kilocalorie, low-fat food with a 50% reduction in sodium.

Light in sodium: no more than 50% of the sodium in the comparison food.

Very low sodium: less than 35 mg per serving.

Sugar-free: less than 0.5 g per serving.

Health Claims[19]

Unlike nutrition information, health messages on labels were strictly forbidden until 1987. Since 1987, some scientifically based health statements have been permitted on labels, subject to FDA approval. Healthy messages such as "Diets low in sodium may reduce the risk of high blood pressure," meant that the FDA had examined scientific evidence and reached the conclusion that here was a clear link between diet and health. Food manufacturers argued in court that they should be allowed to inform consumers about possible benefits based on less than clear and convincing evidence. The courts ruled in the favor of the food manufacturers and the FDA must now allow claims that are not backed by convincing scientific evidence. There are now several "grades" of health claims that manufacturers can use. See table below.[19]

Grade	Level of Confidence	Required Disclaimer
Grade A	High: Significant scientific agreement	Does not require a disclaimer.
Grade B	Moderate: Evidence is supportive but not conclusive	Disclaimer: "Although there is scientific evidence supporting this claim, the evidence is not conclusive"
Grade C	Low: Evidence is limited and not conclusive	Disclaimer: "Some scientific evidence suggests (health claim). However, FDA has determined that this evidence is limited and not conclusive."
Grade D	Very Low: Little scientific evidence supporting this claim.	Disclaimer: "Very limited and preliminary scientific evidence research suggests (health claim). FDA concludes that there is little scientific evidence supporting this claim."

Structure-Function Claims[19]

Unlike health claims, which require food manufacturers to collect scientific evidence and petition the FDA, structure-function claims can be made without any FDA approval. Manufacturers can add claims such as "improves bone health" or improves "cholesterol health" without any proof. However, manufacturers can not mention a disease or symptom. So claiming that a product "improves cholesterol levels" is illegal, but claiming that their product improves "cholesterol health" is legal. One can see how the public can be misled into believing product claims when no evidence exists.

EATING OUT

Eating out can produce panic in individuals beginning new lifestyle changes. Persons need to be educated in making wise choices when eating out. Yes, people can eat out and still maintain healthy habits. But, it's not easy; it can be a very confusing, difficult task.

Fast Food Restaurants

America has been called a 'fast food nation,' and for good reason. Everyday, one out of four Americans eats fast food. Most do it for the convenience – lack of time leads many people to the drive thru, and money plays a part as well. If you are eating out, fast food restaurants are often the cheapest option. Unfortunately, fast food restaurants are not the most nutritious option. Generally, fast food meals are higher in calories, sodium and fat, and often lacking in important vitamins and minerals. Until recently, french fries were the only vegetable option at many fast food restaurants. By most standards, it is a stretch to call fast food french fries a vegetable. Restaurant dining poses similar challenges. Restaurant meals also tend to include too much fat, salt, or sugar, and portions are almost always larger than normal.[14]

While fast food restaurants may not offer the healthiest options, most people find themselves eating fast food from time to time. How can you make the most of your fast food meal? For that matter, how can you make the most of any restaurant meal? The good news is that many restaurants, fast food and sit-down, are adding healthier menu options. It is now possible to eat a fairly nutritious meal on the go. Keep in mind portion control (no super sizing), high fat and calorie sauces and dressings (eliminate them or take them on the side and use sparingly), and sodas (drink water or low fat milk). Making good choices when you are eating out will help you maintain a healthy diet. Knowing what types of menu items are healthier than others can help limit temptation and will also help you encourage your children and grandchildren to make healthy choices as well.[14]

For a free PDF file of Fast Food 05 by Jayne Hurley and Bonnie Liebman visit http://www.cspinet.org/nah/03_05/fastfood.pdf.

Other Hints[14]

Studies show that people tend to consume more food when they are not eating at their own kitchen tables. When you take fast food home, you also have the option of providing a healthier side dish such as fruit or vegetables.

Avoid buffets – All-you-can-eat buffets promote overeating. If the temptation isn't in front of you, you are less likely to overindulge.

Stick to the light menu / Make careful menu selections – Many restaurants indicate healthy choices on their menus, and most sit-down places will modify menu items on your request. Additionally, fast food restaurants now offer a wider range of healthy choices and most will provide nutritional information on all of their offerings by request. Knowing how food is prepared can be a good indication of whether it will work with your diet or ruin it. Main courses which have been baked, broiled, roasted, poached or steamed will be more healthy than anything fried. Salads with plenty of fresh fruits and vegetables and lighter dressings will be better than salads with croutons, cheeses, meats and heavy dressings.

Don't be afraid to special order – Most restaurants have plenty of things that are good for you, but they are served in heavy sauces. Ask for your vegetables and main dishes to be served without the sauces. Ask if things are fried or cooked in oil or butter – if they are, see if you can order them in a more healthy way. Many restaurants, even fast food restaurants are happy to accommodate your requests.

Watch portion size – At a typical restaurant, a single serving provides enough calories for at least two meals. Portion sizes at restaurants are usually double or triple what a person would normally eat so it is important to keep that in mind when ordering and eating. If it is possible to order a smaller portion (often called 'half sizes'), that will help eliminate the temptation to overeat. If you can't order smaller portions, it is a good rule of thumb to leave at least one-third to one-half of the meal on your plate. Or, separate your meal before you start eating so that you create a distinction between what you are going to eat in the restaurant and what you want to take home. Ordering something that will reheat easily will provide you with a delicious lunch or dinner the next day.

Share – Sharing entrees, appetizers and desserts with dining partners is a great idea. It allows you to sample something that you really want to have while also helping you avoid the temptation to overindulge. If you are sharing with a friend or your partner, your portion size is automatically reduced and there is less available to eat. It is still important to make good menu choices, but sharing might make dessert (or something else indulgent) more of an option.

Order sauce and dressing on the side – If you ask for sauces and dressings on the side, you can control the amount that you eat. Often you can use less than is normally used and still enjoy the same taste.[16]

Remember the big picture – Think of eating out in the context of your whole diet. If it is a special occasion or a fun social occasion and you know you want to order your favorite meal at a nice restaurant, cut back on your earlier meals that day. Moderation is always key, but planning ahead can help you relax and enjoy your dining out experience without sacrificing good nutrition or diet control.

The most important thing to remember when eating out is to think of it as part of your overall healthy eating plan. Try to order wisely and if portions are big or the food is rich, consider taking some of it home for a meal the next day. Also, consider sharing entrees, appetizers or desserts with dining partners or friends. Everything in moderation is a wise guideline to follow when considering the menu at your favorite restaurant.[1]

When ordering grilled fish or vegetables, ask that the food either be grilled without butter or oil, or prepared "light," with little oil or butter.

When ordering pasta dishes look for tomato-based sauces rather than cream-based sauces. Tomato-based sauces are much lower in fat and calories. In addition, the tomato sauce (or marinara sauce) can count as a vegetable![16]

Drink water, diet soda, or unsweetened tea or coffee instead of regular soda or alcoholic beverages. This will save a lot of calories each day.

When choosing a soup, keep in mind that cream-based soups are higher in fat and calories than most other soups. Soup can serve as a great appetizer to a meal, or as an entree. Most soups are low in calories and will fill you up, so you eat less.

Other Restaurants

Chinese

For an excellent handout on eating out in Chinese restaurants From Nutrition Action visit www.cspinet.org/nah/chinese.html.[15] Two writers bought a total of fifteen Chinese take-out foods, from kung pao chicken to Moo Shu pork, and sent them off to the lab to be analyzed for fat, sodium content, etc. The authors include several tips on how to make your dining-out experience a little less hard on dieters.

Italian

According to the Nutrition Action Healthletter (Nov. 2007), there is nothing more American than Italian food. To get a handle on a typical menu, CAPQ analyzed popular dishes from the two most popular Italian food chains, Olive Garden and Romano's Macaroni Grill.[16] Best picks included Linguine alla Marinara and Capellini Pomodoro. Among the worst choices were Lasagna Classico which contains 28 grams of saturated fat. Fettuccine Alfredo has a whopping 1200 calories wtih 33 grams of saturated fat.

The Marcaroni Grill best pics included creating your own pasta and Chicken Florentine. Among the worst choices were Calamari Fritti which contains 1200 calories and 13 grams of saturated fat and Parmesan-Crusted Chicken with 1190 calories and 3230 mg of sodium. For the complete article visit www.cspinet.org and search their archives.[16]

Mall Food

Defensive eating - staying lean in a fattening world is another great article on calories and fat in typical mall foods. Visit http://findarticles.com/p/articles/mi_m0813/is_10_28/ai_80485397 to review the results.[17]

OTHER SABOTAGING PRACTICES

Advertisers and food distributors have truly distorted our view of serving sizes. How many times have you seen supersize, all you can eat, double or even triple burgers, big foot pizza, or 16 ounce sirloin? For years a soft drink was 8 ounces, now it is 4 times that size (an 8 ounce cola has 100 calories, vs the Big Gulp that has 800 calories).[15] In the January, 1995 issue of Times there was an article entitled Girth of a Nation. Scientists were stunned to find that during the 1980's the number of Americans considered obese went from 25% to 30%. The statistics today are even more staggering. Over half of Americans are overweight. A major factor in this disturbing weight increase is the amount of food we eat. Many people are unaware of just how much they are eating—they simply clean their plates.[18]

So how do we help clients deal with portion sizes? The food chart presented in chapter 12 is a very useful tool in helping clients understand how much they are eating.

Eating Too Many Calories in the evening

Too many calories at night forces the body to store more of the energy as fat. Someone consuming 1000 calories at night and not eating during the day will not be successful in weight management. Muscle will be utilized during the day for energy and the body will store many of the 1000 calories eaten at night as fat. Changing eating patterns is a very difficult obstacle to overcome. As already discussed, many people with stressful harried lifestyles associate eating in the evening with "unwinding" and "taking care of themselves". These individuals will need to find other alternatives to "fill in the gap". This is where a fun list is helpful. A fun list can help individuals replace the eating with a more positive activity. The client/student is asked to make a fun list consisting of at least five things that he or she enjoys. This fun list should be displayed in an area where it is readily seen (as on the refrigerator). When the problematic period approaches, the client then picks one of the fun activities instead of eating. While this sounds easy, in most cases it is not. Some persons may have a hard time coming up with a fun list, and then have tremendous difficulty implementing it. However, it's well worth the effort because it works.

Problem foods in the home

Temptation needs to be minimized, especially for beginners. Problem foods need to be removed from the home temporarily, if not permanently. Help your clients reach the understanding that this in no way means they are "failures", but is simply a part of human nature.

Deprivation of favorite foods

Deprivation produces binge-eating. Favorite foods can be eaten in moderation. Moderation is the key! Goals need to be set as to the timing of these favorite foods; i.e., "I'll have a piece of chocolate cake next weekend". To reiterate, these favorite foods should not be kept in the home, but should be bought in one serving sizes or eaten out.

Eating too fast

Many people "inhale" their food and have overeaten before their brains tell them that they are full. Eating slowly can be very helpful in preventing overeating.

Shopping when hungry

Never shop when hungry. Hungry people make lousy choices. The temptation is too great—no one should ever go food shopping when hungry. Have a healthy snack first, then attempt "entering the candy store without buying candy".

Not planning

Not planning is surely one of the biggest obstacles to overcome. For persons to be successful in long term weight management, planning must become part of their lifestyle. Planning does not take extra time—it requires thinking ahead of time. If healthy choices are not available, the hungry individual will undoubtedly make "lousy choices". This doesn't mean that the only choices are carrots and celery (rabbit food). Good choices can include yogurt, bagels, cereals, pretzels, fruits, milk, etc.

Eating by The Numbers

Prescribing a computerized list of foods that should be eaten does not produce success. Telling someone that they must eat cottage cheese every day when they hate cottage cheese will lead to failure. What will produce long term success is incorporating the individual's food preferences with changes centered on those preferences. For example, if your client loves cream cheese on his/her bagel for breakfast, switching to low fat cream cheese is an acceptable alternative. Eventually switching to nonfat cream cheese may also be an acceptable alternative. However, telling your client that cream cheese is a bad food and never to be eaten again may produce immediate results, but eventually will produce failure. Remember, no one can sacrifice forever. Also, it is important to work with clients/students to help come up with acceptable alternatives. If the same client as above hates low fat cream cheese, another alternative may be to put jelly on the bagel 6 out of 7 days, and on the seventh day indulge in the "real" thing.

Menu planning should also be easy. As professionals, we need to do the work of determining total caloric intake, adequate percentages of proteins, carbohydrates, and fats, which then needs to be transformed into easy to understand healthy alternatives.

Friendly Saboteurs

Saboteurs are essentially people who target behaviors for their own purposes. They offer food when it is not wanted, advice whether it is wise or not, and commentary not generally designed to facilitate attainment of goals. Saboteurs come in so many forms that it is often difficult to spot them until after the fact. Some mean well but produce harm through their ignorance, others are deliberately trying to sabotage, and yet others are simply selfish. The only commonality is, that regardless of their motives, saboteurs try to alter behavior from what should be done to what they want done. There are several steps in gaining the upper hand over people's efforts to control. The first is to really convince individuals that they have the right to say no. The second is to identify the principal saboteurs; they are not always obvious. The next step is to master strategies to produce assertiveness in your clients/students.

Stress Eating

Have ever had this experience? You come home from a long day feeling tired, down, and lonely. The day has been super-stressful and you have no one to greet you at the door. You look in the refrigerator for something to eat; you really do not feel like cooking dinner for yourself, so you have a snack of cheese and crackers. You have more cheese and crackers and decide that this was dinner. Then, since you have eaten a lousy dinner, dessert would fit right in. You open the freezer and have a few bites of ice cream. After thinking about your day and how you feel, you continue eating the ice cream until it's all gone.

Does this sound familiar? End of the day stress eating is very common. Strategies to deal with stress eating at night can include a fun list, healthy snacks available, etc.

People with hectic lifestyles often go long stretches without eating. Hungry, starving people make unhealthy choices. Here are some helpful hints and strategies: always be sure to eat breakfast; eat every 3 to 4 hours during the day; carry emergency food in the car or at the office; eat a snack before reaching home; on the drive home plan dinner.

Sometimes the thought of cooking dinner at the end of a long day is just overwhelming. This is an area where planning is key. Individuals should try to plan meals in advance of this "critical time period". If they are too tired to cook, options need to be determined. For example cottage cheese and fruit with a baked potato and salsa fulfills all of the nutritional requirements of a healthy meal (may not be a great sounding combination) and requires very little effort. Frozen vegetables added to soup with a large glass of milk and bread will also fulfill the requirements for a healthy meal. Of course, there is always the option of eating out, but beware; this is a time when it is easy to give in to all the temptations (I deserve it). If opting to eat out rules, the restaurant should be familiar and the choice made before entering the restaurant.

Traveling

Learning to eat healthy when traveling requires fortitude. Making healthy choices when traveling is a process of "trial and error". Carrying healthy snacks maybe the only alternative. Another pitfall is those "social" alcoholic drinks. See the next section on eating out for hints.

Business or Job Related Meetings

Many people feel compelled to eat at business meetings, while others eat because of boredom. Teach your clients to try to eat a healthy snack before meetings and to have water available to drink. If possible, they should bring their own healthy snacks. After the meeting, they should go back to their healthy eating program.

Holidays/Being a Guest

For some clients, holidays are terrifying; some people worry about holidays months ahead of time. They are afraid to say no to any food that their host presents (they do not want to be rude). This can be a very huge stumbling block for some clients. They will be dealing with psychological factors that have been ingrained for many years. The key to helping these clients is to emphasize the importance of becoming assertive enough to be able to say no (see the section on friendly saboteurs). Other strategies include filling up on vegetables and taking smaller portions of high fat alternatives— just enough to be polite. Offering to bring a low fat alternative can also be very helpful.

SUMMARY

As discussed in depth in the chapter on diets - diets do not work; diets never work! Again, the diet industry is a $54 billion industry with a 95% fail rate. Despite all our "diet foods" we are still getting fatter. Despite all the money spent yearly on dieting, 66 percent of Americans are overweight today compared to 58 percent in 1983. If this weight increase were considered a disease, it would be an epidemic.

Dieting has been around for thousands of years, although not in any structured way like we see all around us today. It wasn't very common until the 1800's simply because people who were over-weight were not very common; only the rich and well to do were overweight. So being fat was not a problem for most Americans. So any diet at the time involved reducing calories.

Bonnie Liebman, in "How to Write a Diet Book (Nutrition Action Healthletter, July, 2006)" provides details on how to create a diet book. "After all," she says, "You've been eating all your life haven't you? Don't worry about having any expertise or degree."

Dieting doesn't work for many reasons. First, no one can sacrifice forever. Caloric restriction, in and of itself, can lead to binge-eating episodes. Second, low calorie diets produce tired, cranky people. Third, low calorie diets utilize lean muscle as an energy source—hence fat burning machinery is lost. The scale goes down but is destined to go right back up. When the weight is gained back it's all fat. The only known method of permanent weight loss is exercise and healthy eating.[4,]

Changing body composition (building muscle and utilizing fat stores for energy) requires fueling the body, not dieting. The July/August, 1999 issue of ACSM Health & Fitness Journal provides an in depth discussion of the necessity to fuel the body in exercise, and the consequences of not doing so (reiterating all of the information in this chapter).[21] While this summary report may seem outdated, the information still holds true and is very helpful when trying to convince clients about the futility of dieting.

Many well intentioned clients, athletes, and patients are making what they believe to be healthy choices at the grocery store, but they are instead being sabotaged by inconsistencies and often ambiguous labeling regulations. Deciphering food labels and health has become an exercise in understanding legal rhetoric. Understanding labeling regulations will help protect them from fraudu-lently being "cheated" out of their hard earned calories.

Eating out can produce panic in individuals beginning new lifestyle changes. Persons need to be educated in making wise choices when eating out. Yes, people can eat out and still maintain healthy habits. But, it's not easy; it can be a very confusing, difficult task.

Other sabotaging effects include: eating too many calories in the evening; having problem foods in the home; telling people they can never eat their favorite foods; eating too fast; shopping when hungry; not planning; eating a computerized list of foods; friendly saboteurs; stress eating; travel-ing; meetings; holidays.

CHAPTER 13 - SAMPLE TEST

1. Describe the history of dieting and why diets don't work.

2. Provide details on how to write your own diet book.

3. Does a label stating 85% lean indicate that the contents are 15% fat by calories? Explain your answer.

4. Discuss the levels of "health claims" that manufacturers can use.

5. Describe the differences between the USDA labeling guidelines and the FDA guidelines.

6. Discuss ways of choosing healthier choices when eating out.

7. What would you say to a client who tells you that he or she does not have time to eat.

8. What are friendly saboteurs?

REFERENCES

1. http://www.campusrec.uci.edu/fitness/includes/healthywtloss.pdf.

2. http://www.thehistoryof.net/the-history-of-dieting.html.

3. Liebman, B. *How to Write A diet Book*. Nutrition Action Healthletter. July/August 2006.

4. Whitney, E. Rolfes, S. Understanding Nutrition. Thompson Wadsworth, US. 2008.

5. Pentz J. Nutrition Specialist Manual, 7th ed. LMA Publishing: MA. 2004.

6. Pentzj. If You Don't Take Care of Your Body Where Are You Going to Live. LMA Publishing; MA. 2004.

7. Bernardot, D and W. thompson. *Energy from food for Physical Activity, Enough and on Time*, ACSM's Health & Fitness Journal, July/August 1999.

8. http://www.fsis.usda.gov/about/labeling_&_consumer_protection/index.asp.

9. http://www.faqs.org/nutrition/Foo-Hea/Food-Labels.html.

10. http://www.organic.org/home/faq.

11. http://www.consumersunion.org/food/organicpr.htm.

12. http://www.consumersunion.org/pub/core_food_safety/000793.html

13. U.S. Food and Drug Administration Center for Food Safety & Applied Nutrition. A food labeling guide. May, 1997.

14. http://www.americanheart.org/presenter.jhtml?identifier=531

15. www.cspinet.org/nah/chinese.html.

16. Liebman, B, J Hurley. Belly-ssimo! Nutrition Action Healthletter. Nov 2007.

17. http://findarticles.com/p/articles/mi_m0813/is_10_28/ai_80485397.

18. http://www.time.com/time/covers/0,16641,19950116,00.html.

19. http://www.cfsan.fda.gov/~dms/hclaims.html

Chapter 14
The Business of Nutrition

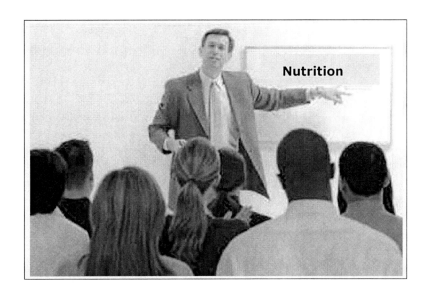

This chapter will focus on the business of nutrition - how to earn an income from incorporating nutrition services.

Objectives

After reading and studying this chapter you should:

1. Be able to define EMyth and discuss the "Business Development Model".

2. Be able to discuss the pros and cons of becoming an entrepreneur.

3. Describe the initial steps in starting a business.

4. Be able to explain how to develop a pricing scheme for the business of nutrition.

5. Be able to discuss how to attract new business.

6. Be able to discuss a successful marketing strategy.

INTRODUCTION

Whether you work for yourself or another company, implementing a nutrition component requires an understanding of entrepreneurial skills. Starting a new business - the Business of Nutrition - can be a daunting task. Every year, over a million people in this country start a business. Statistics indicate that over 40 percent of these businesses will fail by the end of the first year. Within five years that number will rise to more than 80%.

We want you to be in the 20% of businesses that succeed well beyond five years. To succeed you will need not only passion and fortitude, you will need to understand business "disciplines". You will need to become a "juggler" combining the roles of boss, employee and technician.

This chapter will focus on helping you get started. However, to be successful you will need to go beyond the information presented in this textbook. There are many great books about owning and running your own business. Beyond books, there are courses available. The federal government subsidizes many universities that offer start-up business courses. One-day courses can cost less than $100 and can provide invaluable assistance.

If you read only one book to get started, a very helpful book is *The EMyth Revisited*, by Michael Gerber.[2] This book takes the "guesswork" out of starting a business.   When it comes to running a successful business there are "rules" you can follow. Michael calls these rules "The Business Development Process. His book outlines a process that can maximize success and help avoid the common mistakes that most new business owners make. His next book - *EMyth Mastery*[1] Michael discusses the "Seven Essential Disciplines for Building a World Class Company".[3]

> "Every single, solitary person on this earth, no matter what his job might be or what his experience has been, can discover within himself the brilliance, the genius, the captivating and captivated soul of an entrepreneur, once he knows where to look."
> Michael Gerber, "E-Myth Mastery".[1]

EMYTH

What is the EMyth? The "EMyth," or Entrepreneurial Myth, is the flawed assumption that people who are expert at a certain technical skill will therefore be successful running a business of the same kind.[3]

 · "I want to be my own boss"
 · "I want to make more money"
 · "I want to have more time to enjoy my life"

In Michael Gerber's first book, The EMyth Revisited, he describes many common mistakes small business owners make. "It's a common misconception that because someone understands the nuts-and-bolts technical work, they will similarly understand how a business providing that sort of product or service should function." From the EMyth point of view, small business owners struggle to achieve success because they are working *in* their business when they need to be working *on* their business. Eventually the day comes when they realize that just as they invested time and effort learning their technical skills, they now need to acquire business development and management skills.[2]

The exciting process, developed by Michael Gerber, ensures that building a successful business does not depends on "luck" or "magic. A successful business follows the "Business Development Process." Its foundation is three distinct, yet thoroughly integrated, activities through which a business can pursue its natural evolution. They are Innovation, Quantification, and Orchestration.[2]

The difference between creativity and innovation is the difference between thinking about getting things done in the world and getting them done. Creativity <u>thinks</u> up new things, innovation <u>does</u> new things. Innovation is the signature of a bold, imaginative hand.[2]

To be effective all innovations need to be quantified. Without quantification, one would not know whether the innovation worked. Quantification is the numbers related to the impact an innovation makes. These numbers enable you to determine the precise value of your innovation. Eventually, you will think of your entire business in terms of the numbers. Without the numbers you can't possibly know where you are, let alone where you are going. With the numbers, your business will take on a new meaning. It will come alive with possibilities. Once you innovate a process and quantify its impact on your business, its time to orchestrate the whole thing.[2]

Orchestration is the elimination of discretion, or choice, at the operating level of your business. Without orchestration, nothing could be planned, and nothing anticipated. If you're doing everything differently each time you do it, if everyone in your company is doing it by their own discretion, their own choice, rather than creating order, you're creating chaos. And unless your unique way of doing business can be replicated every single time, you don't own it. You have lost it. And once you've lost it, you're out of business! Orchestration is as simple as doing what you do, saying what you say, looking like you look – being how and who you are – for as long as it works. For as long as it produces the results you want. And when it doesn't work any longer, change it![2]

In Michael Gerber's second book, The EMyth Mastery, he describes the "Seven Essential Disciplines for Building a World Class Company.[1] In great detail, Michael defines the qualities required to build a successful business.

The exciting take-home point is running a successful business requires following predetermined "rules". Success does not depend on "chance". Each one of us can be successful in business if we follow the steps. Not following the rules, however, is a "recipe" for disaster. So before you begin your journey into "entrepreneurship" take the time to understand the "process".

BEFORE GETTING STARTED

Before getting started it is critical to weigh the pros and cons of being an entrepreneur. Prepare for crazy-long hours, including weekends, and a work load that's also taxing for an entrepreneur's family. Many spouses/partners don't understand this and won't tolerate it." Aside, from these considerations, here's what the experts say is required to be a successful entrepreneur.[4]

It's Not Just the Money[4]

Two of the USA's most famous entrepreneurs — Bill Gates at Microsoft and Warren Buffett at Berkshire Hathaway — are also the two richest Americans. But they were driven to create great companies, not just huge fortunes. Indeed, Gates and Buffett are combining their riches to create a $60 billion philanthropic powerhouse in the Bill & Melinda Gates Foundation. "Entrepreneurs are much more interested in 'wealth' rather than 'riches,' "says Scott Laughlin, director of the University of Maryland's tech entrepreneurship program. Riches are piles of money, he says; wealth is broader, encompassing less-tangible rewards such as respect and independence. So, would-be entrepreneurs need to examine how they expect to be rewarded. "If the compensation is just cash," Laughlin says, "then the practice of entrepreneurship will not be very rewarding."

Passion[4]

You don't just think you've built a better mousetrap — you feel it in your gut, and know the world will be much better if only you can get your idea to market. "When something is important to you, then you know it with your heart as well as your brain," says Bob Barbato, a management and entrepreneurship professor at Rochester Institute of Technology. "You infect others with your passion, and they believe in you."

Risk-taking[4]

Business success isn't guaranteed. Would-be entrepreneurs are calculated risk-takers — like world-class mountaineers, says Vineet Buch, a principal at venture-capital firm BlueRun Ventures in Silicon Valley's Menlo Park. "They hammer in protection on the way to the top, but don't let the thought of falling slow their steps as the slope gets steeper and narrower," he says. "True entrepreneurs strive to control risk while still thriving on it."

Strong Ethics[4]

Start-ups depend heavily on good first impressions when entrepreneurs hire employees, court investors and line up customers. In a hyper-competitive economy, any whiff of dishonesty can deep-six a new enterprise. Penn State University's Anthony Warren, who advises venture capitalists, says honesty and trustworthiness are high on the list of attributes he looks for when he considers recommending a venture to potential investors. "Who wants to be in business with someone you cannot fully trust, especially in the start-up phase where the stress levels are high?" says Warren, director of the school's Farrell Center for Corporate Innovation and Entrepreneurship. The founders of Google, Sergey Brin and Larry Page, famously created a "don't be evil" mantra when they took their online search giant public.

Tech Ease[4]

Feeling comfortable with technology is crucial, because computers, software and other gadgets are key to launching a business in the fastest-growing economy, the service sector. Start-up costs have plummeted as prices fell for powerful computers and software. Those lower prices came as the internet let entrepreneurs tap global markets for engineering, accounting and other services. Setting up a small office with a laptop, fax machine, cellphone and other gizmos costs as little as $5,000. Add a professional-looking website for $500 or so, and you can compete with bigger, more established companies. But you can't take advantage of those lower costs if you aren't comfortable using popular word-processing, database, spreadsheet and presentation programs.

Tenacity[4]

Sometimes the best business ideas fail to take hold — not because there isn't demand, but because the start-up was undercapitalized, or the entrepreneur lacked management know-how or simply gave up too soon. "If you really believe in it, you keep fighting for it," says Earl "Butch" Graves, president and CEO of *Black Enterprise*, the magazine founded by his father, Earl Sr. A nobody entrepreneur who started a variety store in Arkansas in 1945 eventually lost the business when his landlord wouldn't renew his lease. But he didn't give up. "I've never been one to dwell on reverses," Sam Walton recalled in his autobiography, "and I didn't do so then." The company he fought to start, Wal-Mart, is now the USA's biggest private employer, with more than 1.3 million workers.

Pros and Cons

Benefits of having your own business are numerous. As a consultant you are your own boss. You decide how much to charge, you decide when you want to work and when you want to play. You don't have a boss telling you what to do and when to do it. You negotiate percentages when consulting with health facilities. You decide where to work, whether it's in a health setting, a corporate setting, club setting, physical therapy setting, or your own facility. Another reason to work as an independent consultant is the tax benefits. As a businessd owner, you get to deduct expenses, in some circumstances travel (when it is related to your work), home office space and much more.

Some of the problems associated with owning your own business is "you are your own boss". Now it's your job to accumulate income, pay bills, find new business, etc.

For some the benefits far outweigh any negatives. For others, the "uncertainty" and lack of "guaranteed" income are terrifying. Before you begin a journey as an entrepreneur be sure you are in the former category, not the latter.

New businesses face many challenges, from planning and licensing to opening a bank account and creating a Web site. Regardless of where you are in the process, the following preparatory steps are required for success in implementing a new business.[5]

Write a business plan and form goals and objectives for your new company. A successful start to any business requires a detailed outline of what you plan to accomplish. Whether you use your own savings or obtain loans, starting a business requires money. The loan process can take months to complete, so start early. Lenders often request a completed business plan prior to approval of funding. Forming a corporation or LLC can protect owners' personal assets from business debts. Additionally, incorporating can provide credibility and tax benefits.[5]

Will your corporation or LLC do business under a name other than its legal name filed with the Secretary of State? If so, it must file a DBA (Doing Business As) name. Businesses must maintain an address for service of process where legal documents can be received. Businesses file names on a per-state basis, so other companies may be using the same or a similar name in other states. Conducting a trademark search ensures your unique company name isn't already in use. Obtain a Federal Employer Identification Number (EIN). Incorporated businesses and companies that hire

C Corporation	S Corporation	LLC	Sole Proprietorship
Personal liability protection for owners	Personal liability protection for owners	Personal liability protection for owners	No personal liability protection for owners
Taxed at corporate and individual level	Income/loss passed directly to shareholders	Income/loss passed directly to members	Income/loss passed directly to proprietor
Formal meetings and corporate minutes	Formal meeting and corporate minutes	Option to be taxed as corporation or LLC	No annual reports
Annual state reports	Annual state reports	Annual state reports	
No membership restrictions	Membership restricted to 100 shareholders	No Membership restriction	

employees must obtain an EIN. Most state, county, and local governments require businesses to obtain licensing before they begin to operate.[5] Incorporating or forming an LLC does not provide a company with business insurance. Most companies obtain general business insurance from an insurance provider. Corporations and LLCs that hire employees also typically obtain unemployment and workers compensation insurance.[5]

Identify a location for the business and establish a business address. Establish a Web presence. Not having an effective Web site eliminates opportunities for new customers and more profit. Businesses use customized letterhead, cards, and forms with their company name and logo to establish credibility.[5]

To protect their corporate or LLC veil, businesses must maintain separate business and personal accounts and records. Establish a separate business bank account so that your personal assets are not co-mingled with business funds. Establish proper accounting procedures and follow government rules. Operating a small business means satisfying ongoing government and legal requirements to maintain the company's good standing. Identify where to get help. Smart business owners know where and when to seek advice from other sources.[5]

Visit http://www.irs.gov/businesses/small/article/0,,id=98810,00.html to obtain a checklist from the IRS "For Starting a Business".[6] Free information is also available from the Small Business Administration (http://www.sba.gov/smallbusinessplanner/index.html).[7] Free business courses are available at http://www.myownbusiness.org/.[8]

After all these steps have been taken, you're still not quite ready to get started. There are several more steps before "opening day".

Your Unique Perspective

Your business must reflect "you". What is it that makes you unique? What is it that draws you to this profession? Success rests on your ability to differentiate your services from others. Your personal reasons are what will make your business different and successful. After answering these questions you are ready to go on to the next step.

Choosing a Client Base

In Chapter 10 we discussed identifying clients that are ready to make lifestyle changes. It must be reiterated again if an individual is in the "precontemplative" stage no changes will be made. You will simply be frustrating yourself and setting your business up for failure. This type of individual will "blame" you for their lack of success. There is no quicker way to destroy a business that this type of "bad publicity.[9]

Choosing your client base means deciding on which "type" of client you would like to work with. To answer this question, begin scripting an answer to what it is you do. Have you ever met someone who asked you what you do? How did you answer? Many entrepreneurs don't know how to answer this simple questions. Often people respond with their job title or general profession. "I'm a per-sonal trainer" or "I'm a nutrition coach." For example, let's say you bumped into someone you hadn't seen in several years. You ask them, "What do you do?" They respond, "I'm a teacher." Well that's nice, but it doesn't tell you very much. Now say they responded with, "I enrich young minds and inspire children to follow their passion." This statement provides a much better understanding of "what this person does". What would be an appropriate answer for a fitness/wellness professional? How about, "I help people pursue their health and wellness goals."? Not bad, but what do **you** do? What unique group do you serve? Your response should be unique to you and your target market. Do the responses excite you? Are you comfortable using them? Get out and practice. Ask others what they do and they'll certainly ask you what you do – now's your chance, get out and practice.[9]

After answering the question "What do you do" you now have a clearer idea of the group that you want to work with. You now have an individual introduction that inspires you and gets you excited to meet new people. You can generate even more interest by leading off with a question before using the introduction you just developed. After you're asked "What do you do?" try something simple like, "You know how lots of people are trying to lose weight? Well what I do is help (your target popula-tion) to adjust their lifestyle to pursue their goals." Another example might be, "You know how there is all kinds of confusion about the healthiest way to eat? Well what I do is help (your target popula-tion) to sift through the information and develop an individual healthy eating plan." These examples are referred to as "scripting". Scripting may seem artificial at first, but as you get more comfortable with your personal script, it will come across natural. Scripting clarifies thoughts and produces confidence.[9]

Developing a Pricing Scheme

Before deciding on pricing options, it is important to research other "diet" programs in you community. When incorporating nutrition services it is important to price your program relative to other programs in your area. One mistake many fitness professionals make in pricing is to price a nutrition program relative to personal training programs. The public pays much more for nutrition/diet programs than personal training. There is also hidden preparation time that must be included in your pricing scheme.

Lifestyle Management Associates completed a pilot program in 2005. The comparison chart below shows the pricing for the Nutrition Manager program versus other popular diet programs. Neither the Atkins diet nor the Hollywood diet provides one-on-one counseling, exercise prescription, diet analysis, menu plan, or dietitian coverage. EAS provides exercise advice, but does not provide any of these other services. Jenny Craig and LA Weight Loss provide one on one counseling but do not provide exercise prescription or diet analysis. Nutrition Manager Consultant was the only program that provided all of these services AND included dietitian coverage.

The Atkins diet cost approximately $200. You need to buy their books, starter kit, supplements, and ketone strips. The Hollywood diet on line costs approximately $175 for the starter kit, energy bars, fat metabolizers and guide. EAS Body For Life requires that you purchase their Personal Fitness Guide, transformation kit, and supplements, which cost over $400. Jenny Craig, on average, costs

	Atkins	Hollywood	EAS	Jenny Craig	LA Wt Loss	Nutrition Manager
One on One Counseling	NO	NO	NO	YES	YES	YES
Exercise Prescription	NO	NO	?	NO	NO	YES
Diet Analysis	NO	NO	NO	NO	NO	YES
Menu Plan	NO	NO	YES*	YES*	YES*	YES

$199 for the membership and $96 per week for food; LA Weight Loss Center costs approximately the same as Jenny Craig. The price for Nutrition Manager was $299 for a five session program with body composition, diet analysis and menu plan. So, clearly, these consultants provided more services at a reasonable cost.

Again, taken from the pilot program, the following graph depicts how much income can be generated when consulting with health facilities. In the pilot program, completed by Lifestyle Management Associates, Nutrition Manager consultants took home 70% of the client fees and the health facility received 30%. To many facility owners this may not appear adequate; however, there are time consuming hours behind the scenes which consultants must include in the pricing scheme. Also, there are no expenses for facility owners and no liability issues.

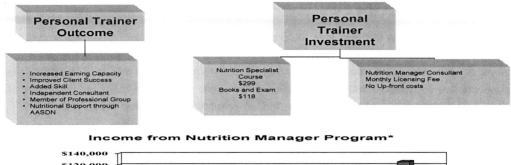

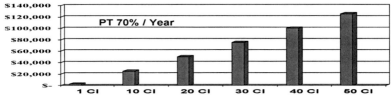

* Income based on $299 per client per month (20 clients per month provides income of over $50,000)

Nutrition Managers that saw 20 clients a month (not a week), at the $299 (low end of pricing) increased their income by $50,000. Nutrition Managers that were aggressive and saw 40 clients per month increased income by almost $100,000.

The following graph depicts income for facility owners receiving 30% of the fees charged for the Nutrition Manager program. If one facility consulted with ten trainers, who saw 10 clients each per month, the facility would increase its income by over $100,000 annually; and if 60 trainers were to work with 10 clients each per month, the facility would increase its income by over $600,000 annually. Clearly there is tremendous potential for health clubs to make large sums of money by offering this service.

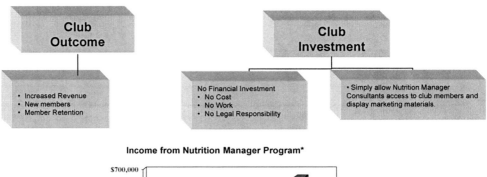

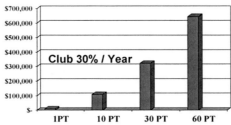

* Income based on results of pilot program with average of 10 clients/month per personal trainer and average of $299 for six to eight session program. (Inexpensive when compared to other weight loss programs such as Jenny Craig, Hollywood Diet, and other weight loss products).

A simplified calculation to detemine pricing is to multiply personal training fees by 1.5% to 1.75%.

PT/hour	3 sessions	50% uplift	75% uplift
$40	$120	$180	$210
$50	$150	$225	$263
$60	$180	$270	$315
$70	$210	$315	$368
$80	$240	$360	$420
$90	$270	$405	$473
$100	$300	$450	$525
$110	$330	$495	$578
$120	$360	$540	$630

Other components to consider when pricing a program include: Will you accept credits; will you accept PO numbers; will you accept consulting fees versus individual dollar amounts?   You also will need to define a refund policy? Check out refund policies of similar businesses before you decide on a refund policy.

ATTRACTING BUSINESS - SALES

Thoughts determine actions and actions determine your results. So the first step to attracting new business is better thinking. How do you feel when you think of selling or promoting your business? Many nutrition professionals mention all kinds of negative emotions when it comes to sales, marketing and public relations. It's important to feel comfortable with promoting your services. If you appear uncomfortable or uneasy about your services, you will attract uncomfortable and uneasy clients. Your confidence attracts confident clients. Although you may not have any formal training, it has more to do with your attitude than your aptitude on the subject. You want to display a confidence in the quality of your services, the belief that you can truly help your clients, and a passion for helping people. These may never be spoken, but will emanate a level of confidence that your clients can feel. This confidence will motivate and inspire them to work harder and believe in their abilities to succeed when working with you.[9]

Making the Sale[9]

Sales may be the most uncomfortable aspect of business for many nutrition professionals. However, sales **is** positive for everyone involved. Selling your services to a client is what's going to help that client gain the knowledge and skills needed to reach his/her goals. Free doesn't provide success. Clients need to have some financial investment to truly grasp the importance of what's being provided. There are circumstances where a complimentary session or a free lecture are excellent marketing. But producing "accountability" in clients requires a financial investment on their part.

In order to stay in business and remain competitive in the field, we **must** earn money. Money is not the only driving force behind what we do. We absolutely want to help people achieve their goals, to stretch themselves and to be better than they ever thought they could be.

The truth is selling **is** positive and in order to be successful selling your services, you need to believe it's okay, not just okay, it's great to sell! What both you and your client are really looking for is a positive relationship. Sure, a one time sale is okay but in order to build a strong nutrition business you need to attract repeat and long-term customers who will refer more business in your direction. Nutrition is an intimate business and it typically takes several sessions to get results. You'll be learning a lot about your client and you will want to develop a strong relationship **during** the promotion and sale. Knowing that you are looking for a relationship and not just a sale can help you to relax and enjoy talking to new and potential clients. Most people in health care professions enjoy people. Talking to people typically comes natural. However, if you feel like you're trying to "sell" then you may feel uncomfortable and appear less confident. You also may seem stiff and tend to lack the passion that most clients are seeking. So forget about "selling" and simply get to know the person. Ask questions, develop rapport and enjoy the process. Remember, you are providing a service that they should be desperate to receive. You have the solutions to their questions.

Although many people think "closing" a sale is complex, if you've effectively used questions to attract your client to your services, the close is relatively easy. Here are several examples of effective closing statements:

· "The nutrition coaching seems to appeal to you. When would you like to get started?"

- "It sounds like you are ready to make an investment in your health. When is a good time for your first appointment?"
- "You look eager to get started. The next step is for us to set-up an initial 1-hour appointment. Do you prefer mornings or afternoons?"
- "If I can fit you in my schedule this week, would you like to get started?"
- "If it's okay with you, I'll grab my schedule book so we can get you started right away."

In the ideal world, everyone would say "yes" and sign-up right then. However, there are two other things to consider. One is that you may feel your services don't meet the client's needs. In which case an easy way to check is, "Based on what you're telling me this may not be for you, what do you think?" This is an easy way to let the client out of an uncomfortable situation and leave the door open for future business opportunities.

The second thing that may happen is the client has some objection. You should immediately go back to asking questions. Have the client explain their objection in more detail and remember to never disagree – this is a sure way to lose a new client. Before providing an alternative solution, you need to know more about the objections. Here are some potential questions used to further discuss the objection:

- "Obviously you have a good reason for saying that. May I ask what it is?"
- "I understand how you feel. Others have felt the same way when I spoke to them. But after our initial appointment, they found this was the perfect solution for them. What do you think?" (this particular style is often referred to as a "feel, felt, found statement")
- "Let me see if I understand your concerns, (restate what they said) you're worried that you won't be able to follow the plan."

After spending so much time attracting a new client, it's important to continue the relationship even after the coaching sessions are complete. One of the best ways to gain new business is through results and referrals. If your clients get results others will see this and ask them about it. Most people are thrilled to send more business your way if you helped them achieve their goals. Referrals do not always come that easily though. Sometimes you have to ask for them. This may be as simple as asking a question at the end of a session: "Do you know anyone else who could benefit from my services?" It can also be beneficial to ask for referrals at the end of the initial sale, "Can you give me the names of three people who are in a similar situation?" I would even encourage you to ask for referrals from people who choose not to work with you. Try, "Who do you know who could benefit from the services we've just discussed?"

Other ways to obtain referrals include letters, emails and newsletters. Thank you cards, special offers, etc, all provide opportunities to gain qualified referrals.

Preparation[9]

Preparation is a key aspect of attracting new business. Whether your nutrition services include individual counseling or coaching, group sessions, or corporate workshops, you need to take the necessary time to prepare. Start the process by taking some time to write out your objectives.

Professional[9]

Another aspect of preparation is being professional. If you want people to believe in you and your services, they have to see you as a professional. There are many aspects to being professional. One of the basics is dressing professionally and appropriately for the services you're offering. If you're trying to close a sale for a nutrition presentation at a local gym, a suit may be overdressed, while shorts and a tank top are probably too casual (unless you're Richard Simmons). It's important to know your audience and dress appropriately.

Certainly your attitude and speech are critical to a professional demeanor. Carry yourself confidently and avoid sarcasm and arrogance. Be careful with the types of humor you use. There's also danger in being over confident and almost coming across as arrogant. The best way to open with a new client is to compliment them or something they own. Let's say you are meeting a potential new client in her office to discuss your nutrition services. When you enter the room, find a nice picture or piece of art, say something positive and ask a simple question. "That's a beautiful picture, where did you find it?" If the new client is coming to you, compliment him on his decision to improve his health. Make sure your compliment is sincere and something you really believe to be admirable or positive. Once again, follow with a question. For example if I walked into your office to learn more about your services, you might say, "How did you hear about me? (or) What have you heard about my services?" This will get the meeting off to a great start, as the potential client immediately feels you are interested in them.

Research[9]

The next part of preparation is research - research your competition. It's important to know what's available in your area that's competing for the same business. Some of the obvious services are Weight Watchers, fad diets, internet based programs and the latest "best selling" book. Compare what you are offering to what's available. Look at all the benefits of what you provide. Some examples might include individual attention, personal training, availability, experience, flexibility, and investment. It's important not to bad mouth your competition – the focus is what do you offer that is unique to you – not what they don't offer.

As part of your research, look into why some people are choosing other services. Are they offering something unique that you might want to add to your service or product line? Investigate the pricing structure. Typically clients are looking for the best "deal" not necessarily the lowest price. What makes your service a better deal to the client? Don't try to be all things to all people. Remember what you are offering and stay true to your vision.

It's important not to make promises you can't keep or offer services that you are not positioned to provide at a high standard of quality. This shows in your speech and in the energy you bring to the initial meeting. If you have positioned yourself to provide a service that you are not prepared to offer, it shows and the client will recognize the discomfort.

Another aspect of knowing your competition is that sometimes you are actually better off referring clients to your competition. This might sound like a poor business tactic, but it is actually a sound business tool. If a client asks about a group setting and your services are based on one-on-one nutrition coaching, then you're better off referring this client to a another program. In the long run you're both going to be more successful. The client will respect you for providing an option that is more appropriate.

MARKETING

Marketing is the wide range of activities involved in making sure that you're continuing to meet the needs of your customers and getting value in return. Marketing is usually focused on one product or service. Thus, a marketing plan for one product might be very different than for another product. Marketing activities include "inbound marketing," such as market research to find out what groups of potential customers exist, what their needs are, which of those needs you can meet, how you should meet them, etc. Inbound marketing also includes analyzing the competition, positioning your new product or service (finding your market niche), and pricing your products and services. "Outbound marketing" includes promoting a product through continued advertising, promotions, public relations and sales.[10,11]

If you are like the majority of small business owners your marketing budget is limited. The most effective way to market a small business is to create a well rounded program that combines sales activities with your marketing tactics. Your sales activities will not only decrease your out-of-pocket marketing expense but it also adds the value of interacting with your prospective customers and clients. This interaction will provide you with research that is priceless.[10]

Does having a limited marketing budget mean you can't run with the big dogs? Absolutely not. It just means you have to think a little more creatively. How about launching your marketing campaign by doing one of the following:
· Call your vendors or associates and ask them to participate with you in co-op advertising.
· Take some time to send your existing customers' referrals and buying incentives.
· Have you thought about introducing yourself to the media? Free publicity has the potential to boost your business. By doing this you position yourself as an expert in your field.
· Invite people into your place of business by piggybacking onto an event. Is there a "race" coming to town? Are you willing to help? It could mean free radio publicity.
· When you do spend money on marketing, do not forget to create a way to track those marketing efforts. You can do this by coding your ads, using multiple toll-free telephone numbers, and asking prospects where they heard about you. This enables you to notice when a marketing tactic stops working. You can then quickly replace it with a better choice or method.
· By being diligent in your marketing and creating an easy strategy, such as holding yourself accountable to contact ten customers or potential customers daily five days a week, you will see your business grow at an exceptional rate. The great thing is it will not take a large marketing budget to make it happen.

Marketing materials to consider include: Print advertising (fliers, brochures, postcards); newspaper article/ advertisements; TV and radio ads, website (own website, links to other websites); special events and trade shows; free advertising; referral relationships; and testimonials.

Print Advertising

Most small businesses budget more for print advertising than any other type. Print ads include postcards, brochures, ads in journals and magazines, and sales support materials. Print ads should always include a headline, a subhead, a visual and an action statement.

The headline is the most important aspect of any print materials.[14] Seventy to eighty percent of sales are decided on the headline alone. Your headline must attract the reader to want to continue reading. A visual is optional but pictures catch people's eye. You, of course, want to include your logo and contact information. A second crucial component (second to the headline) is an action statement. You want the reader to be moved to perform an action. The action may be to visit your website, call you or send you an email. Action statements include, but are not limited to, providing something for free. Pay attention to ads you see that attract your attention. What attracted you? Were you moved to perform an action?   A word of caution! Some ads attract a particular portion of the population and the same ad can upset another segment of the population. Which is why it is equally important to test your ad. Send it friends, family, acquaintances and ask for their opinions. You'll be amazed at how much you can learn from people's first impressions.

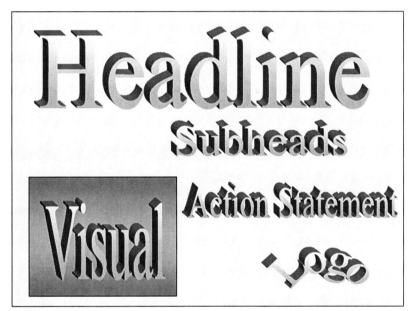

Television and Radio Advertising[14]

TV combines visual and verbal exposure in real-time. We all have our favorite TV ads. What is it that makes some ads memorable and others we "want to forget"? TV differs by combining action, audio and video. You can also demonstrate a product feature through TV advertising. The visual and verbal modes reinforce each other. TV advertising is also great for evoking emotions. A good ad generates the right emotion for the product. So when you think TV advertising, think emotion. Which TV venues work best for your ad? What programs provide the best audience for your services and/or products?

Radio is similar to television advertising. Listeners see through "imagination". Sound can be used to provoke images in the mind of the listener. A car screeching, a child crying, a phone ringing all invoke images. These images can be used in a similar manner as a television ad.

Website advertising[15]

Should you develop your own website? The answer is ABSOLUTELY! Hosting a website is inexpensive and a great way for your clients to learn about you and your services without the expense of color brochures, etc. Some internet providers offer a free site. Many of the same rules used in print advertising apply to websites. We've all been on websites that we find frustrating and websites we can navigate easily. Visit many, many websites and pattern your website after the ones you like. Just as with print ad, your website should reflect you.

Special Events and Trade Shows

Purchasing tables at special events and trade shows can become an expensive venture. Often, however, you can barter for a free table by providing a lecture or volunteering to help. Preparing for these shows is also crucial. Determine the demographics of your audience in advance. Ask for names of other presenters. If you know any presenters personally, contact them and let them know that you will be available to discuss your programs. Ask the event organizers if there are any avenues for you to advertise. Be sure to have marketing materials on hand.   Before the event let everyone you know that you will be there. Have lots of brochures and business cards on hand. It is also a great idea to have a "giveaway" for people who will provide you with contact information.

Free Advertising

Take advantage of free advertising by writing articles for you local newspapers, local clubs, local churches and other local organizations. Provide free lectures. At the end of the lecture provide details about your program and be sure to have business cards and brochures. Free lectures entice people to come listen to you discuss a "hot topic". The ad below filled an entire room and provided many great leads.

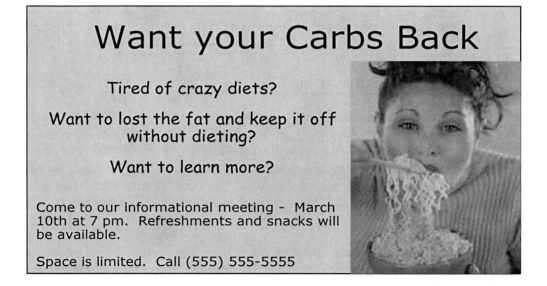

Want your Carbs Back

Tired of crazy diets?

Want to lost the fat and keep it off without dieting?

Want to learn more?

Come to our informational meeting - March 10th at 7 pm. Refreshments and snacks will be available.

Space is limited. Call (555) 555-5555

Attend meetings for local organizations and clubs. If you are a runner attend a local race. If you are interested in working with new moms, attend a local mother's group, etc. Volunteering for your favorite organization is also a great way to get people to know "what you do".

Referral relationships

Good relationships with your clients are paramount for generating positive word of mouth and referrals. For this very reason you should only accept clients that are ready to make lifestyle changes (see Stages of Readiness to Change). Provide present clients with brochures, your website, etc. Provide present client's with incentives for referrals (discount on sessions, etc.). Other trainers that are not providing nutrition services can benefit by referring clients to you for your nutrition program. You can provide incentives to the trainers for such referrals.

Ask all of your clients for permission to contact their doctors and periodically provide the physicians with the clients progress (fax a one page summary monthly). This is a great way for physicians to get use to seeing your name and will connect your name with patient improvement. Once you have one physician referring clients to you, send letters to other physicians letting them know that one of their colleagues is referring patients. Before you know it you will have other physicians referring patients.

Testimonials

Happy clients are more than willing to provide a testimonial. Testimonials are a great way for prospective clients to learn about how others have benefited from your services.

Many health facilities are shying away from incorporating nutrition services because of "litigation" worries. You can promote the benefits of consulting (remove litigation worries and increase income with absolutely no work on their part).

Many supermarkets are now getting into providing healthy choices for their customers. You can provide valuable services such as fliers, handouts, label reading, demonstrations, etc.

Physical therapists understand the need for providing nutrition counseling. They are often too busy to perform the service themselves and are "thrilled" to "outsource" and earn income.

Over age 55 communities are an untapped market. It's a great place to hold group programs as well as provide one-on-one counseling and seminars.

SUMMARY

Whether you work for yourself or another company, implementing a nutrition component requires an understanding of entrepreneurial skills. Starting a new business - the Business of Nutrition - can be a daunting task. Before getting started it is critical to weigh the pros and cons of being an entrepreneur. Prepare for crazy-long hours, including weekends.

Benefits of having your own business are numerous. As a consultant you are your own boss. You decide how much to charge, you decide when you want to work and when you want to play. You don't have a boss telling you what to do and when to do it. You negotiate percentages when consulting with health facilities. You decide where to work, whether it's in a health setting, a corporate setting, club setting, physical therapy setting, or your own facility. Another reason to work as an independent consultant is the tax benefits. As a business owner, you get to deduct expenses, in some circumstances travel (when it is related to your work), home office space and much more.

Some of the problems associated with owning your own business is "you are your own boss". Now it's your job to accumulate income, pay bills, find new business, etc.

For some the benefits far outweigh any negatives. For others, the "uncertainty" and lack of "guaranteed" income are terrifying. Before you begin a journey as an entrepreneur be sure you are in the former category, not the latter.

New businesses face many challenges, from planning and licensing to opening a bank account and creating a Web site. Regardless of where you are in the process, the following preparatory steps are required for success: create a business plan; obtain financial capital; decide on your business type; identify a location, establish a web presence; establish a business bank account; set up an accounting method and method of maintaining records; and follow government rules.

Your business must reflect "you". What is it that makes you unique? What is it that draws you to this profession? Success rests on your ability to differentiate your services from others. Your personal reasons are what will make your business different and successful.

Choosing a client base means deciding on which "type" of client you would like to work with. To answer this question, begin scripting an answer to what it is you do. After answering the question "What do you do" you will have a clearer idea of the group you want to work with.

Before deciding on pricing options, it is important to research other "diet" programs in your community. When incorporating nutrition services it is important to price your program relative to other programs in your area. One mistake many fitness professionals make is to price a nutrition program relative to personal training programs. The public pays much more for nutrition/diet programs than personal training. There is also hidden preparation time that must be included in your pricing scheme.

Other components to consider when pricing a program include: Will you accept credits cards; will you accept PO numbers; will you accept consulting fees versus individual dollar amounts? You will also need to define a refund policy. Check out refund policies of similar businesses before you decide on your policy.

Sales may be the most uncomfortable aspect of business for many professionals. However, selling **is** positive for everyone involved. Selling your services to a client is what's going to help that client gain the knowledge and skills needed to reach his/her goals. Free doesn't provide success. Clients need to have some financial investment to truly grasp the importance of what's being provided. There are circumstances where a complimentary session or a free lecture are excellent marketing. But producing "accountability" in clients requires a financial investment.

Preparation is a key aspect of attracting new business. Whether you're nutrition services include individual counseling, coaching, group sessions, or corporate workshops, you need to take the necessary time to prepare. Just like you prepare yourself before an initial personal training session or nutrition consult, preparation makes it easy to attract new business. Start the process by taking some time to write out your objectives. At the end of a day, week, year, how do you know you are successful?

The final aspect of preparation is being professional. If you want people to believe in you and your services, they have to see you as a professional. There are many aspects to being professional. One of the basics is dressing professionally and appropriately for the services you're offering. If you're trying to close a sale for a nutrition presentation at a local gym, a suit may be overdressed, while shorts and a tank top are probably too casual (unless you're Richard Simmons). It's important to know your audience and dress appropriately.

The next part of preparation is research - research your competition. It's important to know what's available in your area that's competing for the same business. Some of the obvious services are Weight Watchers, fad diets, internet based programs and the latest "best selling" book. Compare what you are offering to what's available. Look at all the benefits of what you provide. Some examples might include individual attention, personal training, availability, experience, flexibility, and investment. It's important not to bad mouth your competition – the focus is what do you offer that is unique to you – not what they don't offer.

Marketing is the wide range of activities involved in making sure that you're continuing to meet the needs of your customers and getting value in return. Marketing is usually focused on one product or service. Thus, a marketing plan for one product might be very different than for another product. Marketing activities include "inbound marketing," such as market research to find out what groups of potential customers exist, what their needs are, which of those needs you can meet, how you should meet them, etc. Inbound marketing also includes analyzing the competition, positioning your new product or service (finding your market niche), and pricing your products and services.[8,9]

If you are like the majority of small business owners your marketing budget is limited. The most effective way to market a small business is to create a well rounded program that combines sales activities with your marketing tactics.

Marketing materials to consider include: Print advertising (fliers, brochures, postcards); newspaper article/ advertisements; TV and radio ads, website (own website, links to other websites); special events and trade shows; free advertising; referral relationships; and testimonials.

CHAPTER 14 - SAMPLE TEST

1. What does EMyth refer to and provide details of the "Business Development Process".

2. List and provide details of the requirements to become a successful entrepreneur.

3. What are the pros and cons of running your own business?

4. Describe the types of businesses and the benefits of each.

5. Describe the details in choosing a client base.

6. Describe the details in developing a pricing scheme.

7. List and provide details of the steps involved in making a sale.

8. Define marketing and discuss the types of marketing materials to consider when establishing a small business.

REFERENCES

1. Gerber, M. E-Myth Mastery. Harper Collins, USA, 2005.

2. Gerber, M. EMyth Revisited, Harper Collins, USA, 2002.

3. http://www.e-myth.com/pub/htdocs/about

4. http://entrepreneurs.about.com/b/2005/09/15/the-8-toughest-questions-before-starting-a-business.htm.

5. http://www.incorporate.com/completing_startup_tasks.html?.
utm_source=google&utm_medium=ppc&iq_id =5261827&cid=5261827&utm_keyword=5261827.

6. http://www.irs.gov/businesses/small/article/0,,id=98810,00.html.

7. http://www.sba.gov/smallbusinessplanner/index.html.

8. http://www.myownbusiness.org/.

9. Salgueiro, G. *The Business of Nutrition 1 - Attracting New Business*. LMA Publishing. MA, 2006.

10. http://www.managementhelp.org/mrktng/basics/basics.htm.

11. http://www.managementhelp.org/ad_prmot/defntion.htm.

12. http://marketing.about.com/od/marketingbasics/a/smmktgbasics.htm.

13. http://www.sba.gov/smallbusinessplanner/manage/marketandprice/SERV_100MIDEAS.html.

14. Hiam, A. Marketing for Dummies. IDG Books. USA, 1997.

Appendix

A. Equations / Conversions

B. Definitions

C. Nutrient Content Sheets

D. Individual Session Handouts Outline

E. Group Program Outline

F. Youth Program Outline

G. Athletes Handouts

Equations / Conversions

Volume

1 cup = 1/2 pint = 8 fluid ounces = 237 milliliters

4 cups = 1 quart = 32 fluid ounces = 0.946 liter

4 quarts = 1 gallon = 128 fluid ounces = 3.785 liters

1 milliliter = .03 ounces

2 tablespoons = 1 fluid ounce = 30 milliliters

16 tablespoons = 1 cup = 237 milliliters

3 teaspoons = 1 tablespoon = 15 milliliters

4 cups = 1 quart

1 gallon = 3.79 liters

Weight

one ounce = 28.35 grams

3 1/2 ounces = 100 grams

1 pound = 16 ounces = 453.6 grams

1 kilogram = 1000 grams = 2.2 pounds

1 gram = 100 micrograms

Length

1 inch = 2.54 centimeters

1 foot = 30.48 centimeters

1 meter = 39.37 inches

Equations:

waist to hip ratio = waist/hip (increased risk for disease if above .8 for women and .9 for men)

Body Mass Index = $\dfrac{\text{weight} \div 2.2}{(\text{height} \times .0254)^2}$

total energy expenditure = (BMR + P.A. + TEF) x (100% - (% fat - normal)

water recommendations: 1.0 to 1.5 ml per calorie expended

Definitions

absorption: absorption is the process by which nutrients enter the intestinal cells in the small intestine and are absorbed into the body.

amenorrhea: cessation of menstruation.

anabolic: building; reactions in which small molecules are put together to build larger ones (these reactions require energy).

antibodies: large proteins in the blood and body fluids, produced by the immune system in response to the invasion of the body by foreign molecules called antigens (also proteins).

antioxidants: nutrients that are capable of neutralizing radicals and thereby protecting the cell from destruction.

bile: compound made from cholesterol which is an emulsifier, i.e. can disperse and stabilize fat droplets in a watery solution.

BMR: Basal metabolic rate is the energy expended during rest, i.e., calories consumed for metabolic processes during total rest.

bolus: the portion of food swallowed at one time.

calorie: the amount of heat needed to raise the temperature of 1 gram of water by 1 degree centigrade.

catabolic: reactions in which large molecules are broken down to smaller ones (these reactions release energy).

chylomicrons: the class of lipoproteins that transport lipids from the intestinal cells into the body.

chyme: the semiliquid mass of partly digested food expelled by the stomach into the duodenum.

complete protein: a protein containing all the amino acids essential to human nutrition and in amounts adequate for human use.

complementary proteins: two or more proteins whose amino acids complement each other in such a way that the essential amino acids missing from one are supplied by the other.

cytosol: the aqueous solution of a cell in which the contents of the cell are suspended.

digestion: is the process by which ingested foods are broken down into smaller segments in preparation for absorption.

edema: the swelling of body tissue caused by leakage of fluid from the blood vessels, seen in protein deficiency and other conditions.

emulsion: mixture of liquids that do not dissolve in each other.

enzyme: a protein that facilitates chemical reactions without itself being changed in the process (a protein catalyst).

ergogenic: tending to increase work.

essential nutrients: essential for life; the body must obtain them from foods because the body cannot make them.

element: a substance composed of atoms that are alike (calcium or iron).

enzyme: any of numerous proteins or conjugated proteins produced by living organisms and functioning as biochemical catalysts.

fiber: loose term denoting the substances in plant foods that are not attacked by human digestive enzymes.

fiber-crude: the residue of plant food remaining after extraction with harsh chemicals.

fiber-dietary: the residue of plant food resistant to hydrolysis by human digestive enzymes—so dietary fiber is the fiber that remains after digestion in the body.

gland: a group of cells that secrete materials for special purposes in the body. They may be exocrine glands (secreting their material into the digestive tract or onto the surface of the skin) or endocrine glands (secreting their materials into the blood).

gluconeogenesis: the making of glucose from noncarbohydrate sources.

glycogen: the term used when plant food carbohydrates are stored in the body.

hepatic vein: the vein that collects blood from the liver capillaries and returns it to the heart.

HDL: the type of lipoprotein that transports cholesterol back to the liver from peripheral cells (packaging system composed mostly of proteins).

hormone: a substance, usually a peptide or steroid, produced by one tissue and conveyed to another to effect physiological activity, such as growth.

hydrogenation: a chemical process by which hydrogens are added to unsaturated fats to reduce the number of double bonds, making them more saturated.

hypoglycemia: abnormally low blood sugar concentration.

iron-deficiency anemia: a blood iron deficiency that results in small pale, red blood cells.

ketones: compounds formed from the incomplete oxidation of fatty acids.

ketosis: occurs when ketone levels rise in the blood and spill into the urine.

kilocalorie: amount of heat needed to raise the temperature of 1000 grams of water by 1 degree centigrade.

LDL: The type of lipoprotein that transports triglycerides and cholesterol from the diet to peripheral cells (usually fat cells).

lecithin: one of the phospholipids with a glycerol molecule, two fatty acids, and a choline molecule; used in the food industry to combine ingredients that do not ordinarily mix, such as oil and water.

legumes: plants of the bean and pea family that have the capacity to fix nitrogen (bacteria in the root of the plants trap nitrogen from the air into the soil which then becomes part of the protein in the beans).

lipoproteins: packaging system that transports fats throughout the body, consisting of proteins, cholesterol, and phospholipids.

lymphatic system: a loosely organized system of vessels and ducts that convey the products of digestion toward the heart; provides a one way route for fluid from the tissue spaces to enter the blood.

macromolecule: a huge molecule composed of hundreds of atoms.

metabolism: a complex set of physical and chemical processes occurring within a living cell or organism that are necessary for the maintenance of life (provide energy for maintaining life).

molecule: two or more atoms of the same or different elements (O_2, H_2O).

neurotransmitter: a substance that is released at the end of one nerve cell when a nerve impulse arrives there; diffuses across the gap to the next cell, and alters the membrane of that cell in such a way that it becomes less or more likely to fire.

nutrient: substance obtained from food and used in the body to provide energy and structural materials and to regulate growth, maintenance, and repair of the body's tissues.

nutrient density: the amount of nutrients per calorie, or per gram.

photosynthesis: ability of plant cells to absorb sunlight and to convert solar energy to chemical energy.

phytic acid: a nonnutrient component of plant seeds which occurs in the husks of grains, legumes, and seeds; is capable of binding minerals such as zinc, iron, calcium, magnesium, and copper in the intestine which the body then excretes unused.

portal vein: the vein that collects blood from the GI tract and conducts it to capillaries in the liver.

protein: organic macromolecule, contains carbon, hydrogen, oxygen, and nitrogen. Usually composed of one or more chains of amino acids.

RDA: Recommended Dietary Allowances are published guidelines by the U. S. Government concerning appropriate nutrient intakes for Americans.

respiration: energy release in the aerobic oxidation of food molecules.

thermal effect of food: an estimation of the energy required to process food (digestion, absorption, transportation, metabolism, and storage of ingested foods).

tofu: a curd made from soybeans, often fortified with calcium.

vegetarian-vegan: pure vegetarian who excludes all foods except plant foods.

vegetarian-lacto-ovo: consumes milk and eggs but excludes meat, fish, and poultry from the diet.

NUTRIENT CONTENT SHEETS

WATER SOLUBLE VITAMINS

Nutrient	Richest to Poorest Sources
Thiamin	Brewer's yeast, pork chops, sunflower seeds, ham, wheat germ, green peas, black beans, watermelon, oysters, split peas, black-eyed peas, kidney beans, oatmeal, acorn squash, baked potato, winter squash, asparagus
Riboflavin	Yogurt, mushrooms, ricotta cheese, spinach, cottage cheese, beet greens, oysters milk, buttermilk, goat's milk, brewer's yeast, mushrooms, peaches
Niacin	Tuna (in water), mushroom, chicken breast, halibut, peaches, pink salmon, salmon, turkey, beef, lamb, sardines, port chops, peanuts, oysters, baked potato, brewer's yeast, shrimp, wheat bran, asparagus, sole, flounder
Biotin	Widespread in foods in small amounts and some is made by bacteria in GI tract.
Pantothenic Acid	Also widespread in foods
Vitamin B6	Baked potato, watermelon, banana, spinach, soybeans, Brewer's yeast, trout, turkey, sirloin steak, pork chop, wheat germ, cantaloupe, tuna (in water), navy beans, bok choy, avocado, sunflower seeds, chicken breast, beef, turnip greens, asparagus
Folate	Black-eyed peas, Brewer's yeast, pinto beans, spinach, navy beans, great northern beans, asparagus, turnip greens, lima beans, kidney beans, parsley, spinach, beets, bean sprouts, sunflower seeds, broccoli, wheat germ, winter squash, bok choy, cauliflower, bean sprouts, cantaloupe, green beans, peanuts, orange
Vitamin B12	Found exclusively in animal products. Fermented soy products (miso) or sea algae do not provide vitamin B12. Vegans need a reliable source such as B12 fortified soy products or supplement with Vitamin B12.
Vitamin C	Papaya, orange juice, broccoli, cantaloupe, Brussels sprouts, grapefruit juice, strawberries, orange, cauliflower, green pepper, mango, parsley, asparagus, grapefruit, watermelon, tomato juice, bok choy, turnip greens, butternut squash, tomatoes, mustard greens, honeydew melon, raspberries, cabbage, baked potato

FAT SOLUBLE VITAMINS

Nutrient	Richest to Poorest Sources
Vitamin A	Pumpkin, sweet potato, carrot, spinach, butternut squash, winter squash, cantaloupe, mango, turnip greens, papaya, bok choy, mustard greens, collard greens, parsley, apricot, oysters, broccoli, watermelon, asparagus, tomato juice, egg, cheddar cheese, green beans, tomato, milk, summer squash
Vitamin D	Fortified milk, egg yolks, liver, fatty fish, butter. A plant version of vitamin D contributes very little to needs. Without adequate sunshine, fortification, or supplementation, vitamin D needs cannot be met.
Vitamin E	Wheat germ oil, sunflower seeds, sweet potato, sunflower seed oil, almond oil, peanut butter, shrimp, corn oil, canola oil, soybean oil, peanut oil, peanuts, olive oil, brazilnuts roasted cashews, salmon, avocado
Vitamin K	Leafy green vegetables, members of the cabbage family, milk, meats, eggs, cereals, fruits

Visit www.lifestylemanagement.com to print your own copy.

MAJOR MINERALS

Nutrient   Richest to Poorest Sources

Sodium   Diets rarely lack sodium. Table salt is sodium chloride which contains about 40% sodium.

Chloride   Chloride is never naturally lacking in the diet. It abounds in foods as part of sodium chloride and other salts.

Potassium   Potassium is found in both plant and animal foods.

Calcium   Yogurt, sardines, goat's milk, milk, romano cheese, buttermilk, turnip greens, kale, salmon, soybeans, beet greens, bok choy, cottage cheese, dandelion greens, tofu, oysters, mustard greens, parsley

Phosphorus   Phosphorus is abundant in animal protein, soft drinks containing phosphorus.

Magnesium   Spinach, tofu, sesame seeds, lentils, vegetables, brewer's yeast, and fruits.

Sulfur   The body does not use sulfur as a nutrient. Sulfur occurs in essential nutrients. Two amino acids are sulfur containing amino acids—methionine and cysteine. Sulfur forms bridges in proteins and is crucial to the contour of protein molecules. There is no recommended intake for sulfur and no deficiencies are known.

TRACE MINERALS

Nutrient   Richest to Poorest Sources

Iron   Heme iron from animal products (meats, oysters, clams), and nonheme sources from plant products (soybeans, tofu, spinach, lentils, wheat germ, potatoes).

Zinc   Oysters, beef, lamb, wheat germ, poultry, lentils, spinach, milk, tofu, brewer's yeast.

Iodide   Iodized salt, seafood, bread, dairy products, plants grown in most parts of this country, and animals fed these plants.

Copper   Legumes, grains, nuts, seeds.

Manganese   Most plant foods contain significant amounts.

Fluoride   Fish, tea, and almost all foods contain small amounts. Water is the largest source.

Chromium   Unrefined foods (brewers yeast), whole grains, nuts and cheeses.

Selenium   Meats and other animal products.

Molybdenum   Legumes, breads and other grains, leafy green vegetables, milk, and liver.

Ten Session Handouts

1. Why Diets Don't Work

2. Reading Labels

3. Ten Commandments for Families

4. Stress Reduction

5. Eating Out

6. Motivation

7. Water

8. Caffeine and Alcohol

9. Fiber

10. How to Choose A Supplement

Visit www.lifestylemanagement.com for each session handout.

Group Program Outline

1. Keys to Success
2. Informational Meeting
   Questionnaire
3. First Class – Program Introduction
   Ten Commandments
   Legal Agreement
   Responsibility Clause
   Why Diets Don't Work
   Keeping a Lifestyle Journal
   Portion Sizes
   Exercise Information
   Body Composition Instructions
   Homework Assignment (journal)
   Wrap Up
4. First Individual Appointment
   Body Composition Testing
   Diet Analysis Software Training
   Goals and Objectives Discussion
5. Second Class – Exercise
   Discuss Homework
   Discuss Exercise
   Set up Weekly Exercise Program
   Homework
6. Third Class – Nutrition
   Discuss Homework
   Discuss Diet Analysis Printouts
   Set up Eating Strategy Worksheet
   Homework

7. Fourth Class – Fiber
   Discuss Homework
   Discuss Fiber Handouts
   Set up Fiber Strategy Worksheet
   Homework
8. Second Individual Appointment
   Check exercise/eating programs)
   Review Strategy Worksheets
   Listen/Listen/Listen
9. Fifth Class – Labels and Supplements
   Discuss Homework
   Discuss Reading Labels Handouts
   Discuss Supplement Handouts
   Homework
10. Sixth Class – Stress
    Discuss Homework
    Discuss Stress Handouts
    Set up Stress Worksheet
    Homework
11. Seventh Class – Defensive Eating
    Discuss Homework
    Discuss Eating Out Handouts
    Assign Recipes for last class party
12. Eighth Class – Program Wrap-up
    Party
    Completion Certificates
    Week 12 Follow up Appointments
    Exit Survey

Visit www.lifestylemanagement.com for more details.

Youth Program Outline

The Healthy Kids and Families 5 Stages of Progression and Proficiency address healthy lifestyles for youth grades K through 6th. Critical health information is imparted through five stages of progression and proficiency using exciting games, fun physical activities, and hands-on projects. Each stage has a variable number of lessons. Each lesson has a "Take Home Project" assignment that must be completed. Before proceeding to the next stage, all students must pass the proficiency testing procedure.

Informational Meeting

Before beginning the program all parents must sign a program waiver and understand details of the program. At least one parent/guardian must attend the informational meeting before a child can participate.

Program Introduction - Introductory Lesson

Learning objectives:

Children will learn the importance of working together as a family through "The Ten Commandments for Families"; your child will learn how to "log" his/her physical activity; learn details of the program including point system, reward system, and "leadership" opportunities; complete an entrance survey and fitness testing.

Lesson Plan: Each time a class gets together, the class begins with the nutrition component and ends with the "Exercise Plan" (see Exercise Plan details). In the initial class children will complete the exercise testing procedure. Children will be introduced to program details including the 5 stages of progression, take home projects, details of the "Point System. In this initial class children will complete the exercise testing procedure.

- Age, Height, Weight, and BMI measurements
  - $BMI = weight(kg)/height(m)^2$
  - 1 kg = 2.22 lbs

The Entrance Program Survey (see appendix) Entrance Survey:

- Each child will complete the program entrance survey (see appendix). Each child has a copy of the survey in their accompanying documents workbook
- Exercise Portion – President's Physical Fitness Testing
  - ¼ mile timed run
  - Push ups in 30 sec
  - Sit ups in 30 sec
  - Sit and reach

Stage 1 – My Pyramid

Learning objectives:

Identify food groups, serving sizes, and components of exercise using the new USDA Pyramid (www.mypyramid.com)

Lesson Plan: Each time a class gets together, the class begins with the nutrition component and ends with the "Exercise Plan" (see Exercise Plan and DVD for details). Several new exercises are introduced per class and formerly taught exercises are reviewed.

Stage 2 – Understanding Labels

Learning objectives:

Using the nutrition facts panel and ingredient lists on food labels, children will learn to identify and understand the following: requirements for listing of ingredients, portion size, calories, calories from fat.

Lesson Plan: Each time a class gets together, the class begins with the nutrition component and ends with the "Exercise Plan" (see Exercise Plan details). Previously taught exercises are completed and several new exercises are introduced.

Visit www.lifestylemanagement.com for more details.

Stage 3 –Nutrition

Learning objectives:

Children will learn basics of nutrition, digestion absorption, transport and metabolism through Horatio's Magical Journeys Part 1 and Horatio Flash Cards

Lesson Plan: Each time a class gets together, the class begins with the nutrition component and ends with the "Exercise Plan" (see Exercise Plan details). Previously taught exercises are completed and several new exercises are introduced.

Stage 4 –Energy

Learning objectives:

Children will learn basics of energy and energy production: energy nutrients, energy utilization, etc. through handouts, a question/answer game - "Bring Horatio Home", and through "Horatio's Magical Journeys Part 2".

Lesson Plan: Each time a class gets together, the class begins with the nutrition component and ends with the "Exercise Plan" (see Exercise Plan details). No new exercises are introduced in this stage. Children are asked to take a leadership role in which they will lead the class in the exercise portion.

Stage 5 – Program Completion - Healthy Lifestyle Changes

Learning objectives:

Taking the information presented in the previous 4 stages, children will learn how to implement healthy lifestyle changes through completing a new pyramid and comparing the initial pyramid with the final pyramid.

Lesson Plan: Each time a class gets together, the class begins with the nutrition component and ends with the "Exercise Plan" (see Exercise Plan details). No new exercises are introduced in this stage. Children are asked to continue a leadership role in which they will lead the class in the exercise portion and develop their own exercise plan. See exercise DVD for more details.

The ultimate goal of the program is for healthy changes to be made in both exercise and nutrition.

Visit www.lifestylemanagement.com for more details.

ATHLETES HANDOUTS

Water or Sports Drink

Day Long Tournament

Day Long Tournament

Liquid Meals

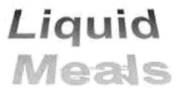

Visit www.lifestylemanagement.com for a copy of all 12 handouts.

Index

LaVergne, TN USA
29 August 2010
194676LV00004BA/2/P